T0203233

Clinics in Developmental Medicine No. 189

Fetal Behaviour: A Neurodevelopmental Approach

CHRISTA EINSPIELER
Associate Professor of Physiology, Institute of Physiology, Center for Physiological Medicine, Medical University of Graz, Austria

DANIELA PRAYER
Professor of Radiology, Division of Musculoskeletal Radiology and Neuroradiology, Medical Department of Radiology, Medical University of Vienna, Austria

HEINZ FR PRECHTL
Emeritus Professor of Developmental Neurology, University of Groningen, the Netherlands and Medical University of Graz, Austria

2012
Mac Keith Press

© 2012 Mac Keith Press
6 Market Road, London, N7 9PW

Editor: Hilary Hart
Managing Director: Ann-Marie Halligan
Production Manager: Udoka Ohuonu
Copy Editor: Penny Howes
Indexer: Laurence Errington

First published in this edition 2012

British Library Cataloguing-in-Publication data
A catalogue record for this book is available from the British Library

ISBN: 978-1-898683-87-2

Printed by Latimer Trend & Company, Plymouth, Devon, UK
Mac Keith Press is supported by Scope

CONTENTS

AUTHORS' APPOINTMENTS   vi

ACKNOWLEDGEMENTS   vii

FOREWORD   viii

INTRODUCTION   x

1. OBSERVATION OF FETAL BEHAVIOUR   1

2. SPONTANEOUS MOTOR BEHAVIOUR   17

3. PRENATAL LATERALITY   69

4. BEHAVIOURAL STATES   72

5. FETAL RESPONSIVENESS   91

6. FETAL BEHAVIOUR IN TWINS   120

7. DETERMINANTS OF FETAL BEHAVIOUR   124

8. FUNCTIONAL ASSESSMENT OF THE FETAL NERVOUS SYSTEM   158

EPILOGUE   188

LIST OF VIDEOS   190

INDEX   192

AUTHORS' APPOINTMENTS

Christa Einspieler Associate Professor of Physiology, Institute of Physiology, Center for Physiological Medicine, Medical University of Graz, Austria

Daniela Prayer Professor of Radiology, Division of Musculoskeletal Radiology and Neuroradiology, Medical Department of Radiology, University of Vienna, Austria

Heinz FR Prechtl Professor Emeritus of Developmental Neurology, University of Groningen, the Netherlands and Medical University of Graz, Austria

ACKNOWLEDGEMENTS

By the time this book was finished the almond trees had blossomed four times. Most of the writing was done in a house somewhere in Spain, with its back nestled against a mighty yellow rock and a view of a turquoise, sometimes golden, sea. In the ever coming and going waves rests the Giant of the Venetian Army, with his ebony skin covered by salt water.

I thank you with all my heart for letting me work at your house and bringing me back to the right track after you read the first draft of the manuscript.

As for you, Miha, there are no words to express my gratitude to you for standing by my side throughout these years; I greatly enjoyed playing tennis with you, although the match point was usually yours. You helped me understand that terms such as 'may' and 'might' indicate vagueness rather than determination – not only within these pages, but even more so in life. Your humour cheered me up when I struggled with a language that is not mine.

Christa Einspieler
Graz, January 2011

FOREWORD

It is a pleasure to write a Foreword for this fascinating volume. It is a remarkable account of the progressive development of knowledge in the field of fetal behaviour through the assessment of fetal movements and behavioural states. This approach is based on the premise of developmental neurology and provides important clues for the recognition of the age-specific functional repertoire of the nervous system. Some of the assessments are similar to those applied in the study of the behaviour of preterm and term born infants and this makes the book relevant to a large audience including the many paediatricians and paediatric neurologists who are familiar with such assessments.

The book is well structured, beginning with an accurate historical perspective and a description of the classic approaches to the assessment of fetal behaviour. It is good to see that the book pays due tribute to the historical methods of assessment but at the same time provides a review of other techniques that have improved our ability to assess fetal behaviour.

The book moves on to provide detailed descriptions of the pattern of movements and the mechanisms underlying them. As the authors state in the introduction, behaviour is an expression of neural activity and fetal behaviour and movements not only give an insight into the developing brain but are also necessary for the further development of the neural structure and of other organs.

The book provides a well-balanced account of the state of the art on the assessment of behavioural states, paying tribute to the seminal description of Prechtl's work on fetal behavioural states and updated with new findings based on more recent techniques.

This information provides an excellent background to the section that follows where determinants of fetal behaviour are reported, explaining the impact of different pregnancy-related and maternal factors on fetal behaviour.

Other chapters describe important aspects such as fetal responsiveness or laterality and the development of handedness. The description of different behaviour in twins is particularly interesting.

The final chapters on functional assessment of the fetal nervous system are an important contribution to the developing jigsaw of knowledge on this topic. At a time when fetal imaging has provided increasingly accurate modalities for assessing the complexity of motor patterns in fetuses, the emergence of this structured and standardised description of fetal behaviour will enable better understanding of the mechanisms underlying various aspects of behaviour in healthy fetuses and in those with brain lesions or other risk factors. Because of this, the volume will be of great relevance not only to scientists interested in this field but also to those working in neonatology, paediatrics and paediatric neurology.

Eugenio Mercuri
Department of Neurology and Psychiatry
Catholic University of Rome
Largo A Gemelli
Rome, Italy.

INTRODUCTION

Structure only fully realises itself through function.
   Gilbert Gottlieb (1971)

First and foremost, behaviour is an expression of neural activity. Embryonic or fetal behaviour, therefore, gives an insight into the developing brain: in no other stage of development is the neural structure so closely and directly related to its own function. It only takes a few neurones to generate the first movements, which in turn are necessary for the further development of the neural structure. We shall see, for instance, that spontaneous body movements, so-called general movements, are vital for the proper development of the skeletal, muscular and neural systems; sucking movements are essential for the evolution of the gastrointestinal tract; eye movements are necessary for the development of amacrine cells in the retina; and breathing movements promote lung development. In 1955, the neurobiologist Paul Weiss wrote: 'No account of neurogenesis can be complete without relating itself to the problems of behavior' (Weiss 1955, p 390). It is the utilisation of an immature structure that enables a continual, normal development of the same structure.

In spite of the immediacy in fetuses between the neural structure and its function, it is amazing just how individually distinct behaviour is from the very beginning. The first movements, which appear at 7.5–8 weeks' gestation, still lack complex patterning and sequencing, and yet they are different in every embryo. One week later, the variability in behaviour increases: the speed, amplitude and direction of the movements start to vary. At 9.5 weeks' gestation – and thus still in the embryonic stage – the sequence of movements shows a remarkable degree of variation. Even genetically identical embryos/fetuses develop their own individual ways of acting and reacting from the very beginning. More than other types of assessment, the observation of twins reveals the predominance of spontaneous, endogenously generated movements over elicited movements (although the ability of the fetus to respond to stimulation represents another landmark in the development of fetal behaviour). The auditory, olfactory and tactile senses in particular, unlike external stimuli, provide continuous stimulation of a suitable intensity. Interestingly, however, the various sensory systems respond to stimulation even before they are fully developed. Again, it turns out that activation of the sensory systems is necessary for the continuous development and maturation of sensory pathways.

Apart from the general interest in the evolution of individual human behaviour, the study of spontaneous and elicited fetal motility has also been based on clinical considerations: it seems obvious that deviations from normal behaviour indicate fetal compromise and that, vice versa, normal behaviour indicates fetal well-being. We shall see, however, that the latter is not always the case: in spite of their severity, a number of precarious neurological conditions do not hinder the fetus from reacting properly to external stimulation, whereas his or her spontaneous movements are clearly impaired. Thus, even fetuses with severe malformations show normal heart rate or movement alterations in response to acoustic or vibroacoustic stimulation; their spontaneous motility, by contrast, is abnormal long before this.

Unfortunately, in a variety of studies, isolated behavioural aspects such as the responsiveness to vibroacoustic stimulation or the number of eye- and no-eye-movement episodes were singled out – or even only the fetal heart rate was measured. Such a reductionist approach must inevitably fail to give a comprehensive insight into the nervous system, the most complex of organs. No matter how the fetus behaves (especially during the last 2 months of pregnancy), it is determined by the respective behavioural state. Since the concept of fetal behaviour refers to both motility and heart rate, not taking into account the behavioural states (which represent the linkage between motility and heart rate) will hazard inconsistencies in findings and, worse still, inappropriate patient management. Fetal heart rate accelerations, which are considered to be a sign of fetal well-being, cannot occur during quiet sleep, that is, behavioural state 1F (see Chapter 4). In other words, a so-called silent fetal heart rate pattern can, physiologically speaking, reflect behavioural state 1F, but in order for it to be a sign of fetal stress it must occur during a different behavioural state. Another example is the widely used method of vibroacoustic stimulation: applied during state 1F, it can even cause harm to the fetus. It is of utmost importance, therefore, that fetal behaviour is seen in its entirety and is strictly age and state related.

When we use the term 'behaviour', what we mean is overt behaviour, i.e. observable motility and heart rate patterns. We strongly disapprove of speculations about the fetus' subjective experiences, feelings, intentions, emotions or mood. There is no scientific evidence of the assumption, for example, that fetuses like to 'explore' the uterine wall because concepts like this clearly imply intentionality. What the fetus really 'performs' – thus coming in contact with the uterine wall – is a number of endogenously generated general movements.

The present description of fetal movements and behavioural states is based on the premises of developmental neurology, which implies the recognition of the age-specific functional repertoire of the nervous system and its ontogenetic adaptation. The advantage of this approach is that the fetus can be studied in terms that are similar to those applied in the study of the behaviour of preterm infants and term newborns. Such an approach promotes the homogeneity of terminology and provides an opportunity to compare prenatal with postnatal neural activity and, thus, to capture the transition from intrauterine to extrauterine life.

Authors' note

Throughout the book we use the term 'gestational age', which is synonymous with 'postmenstrual age' and represents the number of weeks from the first day of the mother's last menstrual period. Wherever necessary, the embryologist's dating of pregnancy (i.e. the 'developmental age' after fertilisation) has been converted into the gestational age, to avoid confusion. The gestational age is approximately 2 weeks greater than the developmental age when referring to a fetus at the same point of development.

The present work is based solely on studies on the human fetus, although animal studies have doubtlessly contributed to our understanding of human behaviour.

Unless otherwise stated, the findings described in Chapters 2 to 6 refer to low-risk fetuses, delivered as healthy full-term infants.

DVD

The DVD that accompanies this book contains 26 videos showing aspects of fetal movement and behaviour. References to each video are in Chapters 2, 6, and 8. A full list of the videos can be found at the end of the book.

REFERENCES

Gottlieb G. (1971) *Development of Species Identification in Birds: An Enquiry into the Prenatal Determinents of Perception*. Chicago: University of Chicago Press: 156.
Weiss P. (1955) Nervous system (neurogenesis). In: Willier BH, Weiss P, Hamburger V, editors. *Analysis of Development*. Philadelphia: Saunders: 346–401.

1
OBSERVATION OF FETAL BEHAVIOUR

Historical conjectures and studies

Probably the first written account of human fetal movements is to be found in the Bible, where Rebecca, Isaac's wife, describes how 'the children struggled within her' (Genesis 25:22). In fact, women have always sensed fetal movements to be a sign of life. The term 'quickening', which refers to the moment in pregnancy when the woman first feels the fetus move, has historically been attributed to the beginning of individual life and has, therefore, been regarded as a criterion to determine the point in time at which a fetus is conceded the right to life (de Bracton 1250, Blackstone 1765). Interestingly enough, Hippocrates (460–370bc) already suspected that fetal movements might in fact set in a few weeks earlier than the expectant mother feels them. More precisely, he suggested that the fetus could actually start moving as soon as 70–90 days after conception, which corresponds to a gestational age of 12–15 weeks (Needham 1959). Leonardo da Vinci, too, made a contribution to embryology: with his famous drawings of a fetus in a womb (1510–1512), he illustrated that embryos and fetuses could actually be measured and assessed, with regard not only to their dimension at a particular moment but also to their development (O'Rahilly 1988).

THE FIRST STEPS IN THE CLINICAL EVALUATION OF FETAL WELL-BEING

In the second century, the Greek physician Soranus of Ephesus, who practised in Alexandria and subsequently in Rome, was very clear about the presence of fetal movements, which, in his view, indicated that the course of pregnancy was normal. After that, however, it was not until the 16th century that this issue was brought up again. Eucharius Rösslin (1470–1526), a physician in Worms, Germany, regarded the midwives' practice as being careless and substandard. Animated by his observations, he wrote a handbook on childbirth called *Der Rosengarten* (The Rose Garden). The book was an immediate success and was translated into English by Thomas Raynalde (1545) with the title *Byrth of Mankynde*. Crucial to the work was the realisation that a decrease of fetal movements and their subsequent absence indicated intrauterine death.

In 1869, the German obstetrician Johann F Ahlfeld came to realise that maternal perception of lively fetal movements was a valuable indicator of fetal well-being (Ahlfeld 1869). At around the same time, Charles Pajot (1876) found another sign of good fetal

1

health, namely audible sounds produced by the fetus, which he believed were caused by movements of the fetal extremities. On this, Ahlfeld disagreed, for he deemed it incredible that movements of fetal extremities could possibly be perceived acoustically, even though he did agree on the presence of sounds, interpreting them as spasmodic contractions of the fetal diaphragm (Ahlfeld 1888). It was also during these years that James Whitehead (1867) observed an increase of fetal movements elicited by maternal emotional stress – an observation that would only be proven a long time later (see Chapter 7).

KNOWLEDGE OF SPONTANEOUS FETAL MOVEMENTS DATES BACK TO 1885
The English–German physiologist William T Preyer (1841–1897) placed a stethoscope on a mother's abdomen and thus 'heard' the fetal movements. He concluded that the movements were definitely present by a gestational age of 12 weeks, but most probably earlier (Preyer 1885). Furthermore, Preyer was convinced that those early movements were spontaneously generated (Preyer 1885). Strassmann (1903) and Yanase (1907) took the same line, as they speculated in their early reports that fetal movements might resemble the movements of a newborn. Ahlfeld, who recorded fetal breathing movements by means of a kymograph, also considered those movements to be spontaneously generated (Ahlfeld 1888, 1905). In spite of all the speculation, the phenomenon of spontaneous movements was not yet pursued, since, at that time, scientists were convinced that such movements had to be evoked.

THE FELS INSTITUTE CARRIES OUT THE FIRST NON-INVASIVE STUDY OF FETAL BEHAVIOUR
The Fels Research Institute was founded in 1929 with a single, albeit complex, research project known as the Fels Longitudinal Study, which was originally designed to analyse the effects of the Great Depression on child development. Arthur Morgan, then President of the Antioch College in Yellow Springs, Ohio, posed the question: 'what makes people different?'. He approached Samuel Fels, a Philadelphia businessman and philanthropist, and so the idea was born to study individuals from prenatal life to adulthood, in order to shed some light on the issue. Lester Sontag, a physician, was appointed as the first Director for the Fels Longitudinal Study in 1929 (http://www.med.wright.edu /lhrc/fels.html). The first participants were enrolled prenatally by their parents; examinations began in 1930, applying the following equipment and procedure (Sontag and Wallace 1934): the fetal heart rate was measured by means of a stethoscope and a stop watch, while fetal movements were recorded with an apparatus consisting of four rubber bags sewn into a cloth container, each connected with a tambour and a recording drum. Over this group of rubber bags, which corresponded to the four quadrants of the abdomen, the examiner placed a plaster of Paris cast, which had been made especially for the participant and was replaced with a new one each week as the fetus grew. This combination of four bags and four tambours allowed the constantly present respiratory movements of the mother to be ruled out. The recordings were made in 260 fetuses for 2

hours a week. Sontag and Wallace (1934) were thus able to differentiate between (1) slow squirming or writhing movements, which increased until about 28 weeks' gestation and then decreased; (2) sharp kicking or punching movements of the extremities, which increased with age; and (3) rare, small rhythmic movements, possibly hiccups. Even more interesting is the description of 'a great deal of variability' among fetuses as well as of the daily change in individual fetuses (Sontag 1941).

The Fels study confirmed what Whitehead (1867) had observed some 70 years before, namely that maternal emotional stress is linked to an increase in fetal movements. The study went further in claiming that those infants remained irritable and hyperactive for weeks. They cried a great deal and only slept for short periods at a stretch (Sontag 1941).

Fetal activity was also observed to increase during pre-eclampsia. And, finally, fetal movements and the fetal heart rate increased after a vibratory stimulus was applied to the maternal abdomen (Sontag and Wallace 1934). It was rightly observed that, after a sudden increase, the movements and heart rate elicited in such a way remained high for some time, before eventually returning to normal. In this context, habituation was also observed: an unstimulated fetus responded violently with movements when a vibratory stimulus was applied 15 times at 1 minute intervals, whereas a fetus that underwent daily stimulation stopped responding after five or six stimuli.

STUDIES ON EXTERIORISED FETUSES

Other systematic studies on human fetal motility were carried out in the form of examinations of embryos and fetuses after spontaneous miscarriages (Hooker 1938, 1952) or after Caesarean sections in early pregnancy (Minkowsky 1928). However, this work was done through the perspective of the reflexology doctrine, that is, the view that motility was merely a response to exogenous stimuli. On the same theme, studies were carried out that applied tactile stimulations of embryos and fetuses of amphibians (Coghill 1929), sheep (Barcroft and Barron 1939) or cats (Windle and Becker 1940). Coghill's (1929) thesis was that reflex mass movements preceded individual reflex movements, while Windle (1940) suggested that complex coordinated movements developed by the integration of local reflex circuits. This reflex-integration approach ultimately contributed to a 'reflexology' that was in line with the radical *zeitgeist* of the 1930s and 1940s.

Davenport Hooker had been carrying out studies on fetal activity in humans since 1932, mostly at the University of Pittsburgh. In his book *The Prenatal Origin of Behavior* (1952), he summarised the results of his studies as well as the animal studies of George E Coghill, who preceded and influenced his work. Hooker had examined 149 human fetuses, spontaneously delivered at 6–45 weeks' gestational age. The fetuses had been given specific tactile stimuli with von Frey hairs immediately upon delivery to obviate the effects of anoxia. The appearance of reflexes (Figure 1.1) was taken as evidence of early central nervous system function (Hooker 1938, 1952; Humphrey and Hooker 1959, 1961; Humphrey 1964).

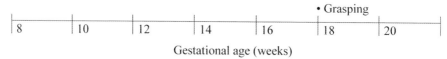

• Neck flexion (i.e. sideward bending of the head
    • Finger closure followed by wrist flexion
      • Elbow flexion
        • Plantar flexion
          • Babinski-like reaction accompanied by hip and knee flexion
            • Complete finger closure
                    • Grasping

  8   10   12   14   16   18   20

Gestational age (weeks)

Figure 1.1 First appearance of movements elicited by cutaneous stimulation of exteriorised fetuses (Hooker 1932, 1952, Humphrey 1966).

Since motility was considered to be evoked, little attention was given to spontaneous movements. In some cases, movements were indeed observed without any evidence of prior stimulation, but they were either not classified as important or described as a 'spontaneous reflex for which the stimulus was not yet known' (Hooker 1952). Furthermore, we must always bear in mind that these observations were essentially made in dying fetuses. By the time of examination, the fetal nervous system was presumably in a depressed state and spontaneous activity may already have ceased, even though responses could still be triggered by way of stimulation (de Vries et al 1982; Prechtl 1989).

THE FIRST ULTRASOUND RECORDINGS OF FETAL MOVEMENTS

The first sonar studies of fetal movements, although not yet real time, were reported by the Viennese obstetrician Emil Reinold in 1971. He described the following two types of movements: (1) a lively movement beginning with a short impulse and ending with a motionless or almost motionless phase. Here, the impression was that the body was kicked away from the wall of the amniotic cavity and then continued to swim, before eventually resettling in its original position; and (2) a slow and lazy movement, generally followed by a pause of 1–5 minutes (Reinold 1971a). In the same year, Reinold got the impression that fetal movements were actually comparable to the darting movements of fish (Reinold 1971b). He further stated that fetal movements were not forceful enough to alter the position of the fetal body before the 10th week of gestation (Reinold 1973). And, lastly, he came to the conclusion that the observed movements of the fetus were spontaneous rather than caused by external influences.

    The use of B-mode linear scanners to obtain two-dimensional images of cross-sections through the uterus soon proved a major advance in the documentation of fetal anatomy

4

(Tuck 1986). In addition, a rapid succession of linear scans on a video screen in real-time allowed comprehensive observation of fetal movements. From these earliest reports, most of which were by Jouppila and Piiroinen (1975) and Reinold (1976), a categorisation scheme of fetal motion emerged (Birnholz et al 1978). Influenced by Hooker (1952) and Humphrey (1964), Birnholz drew particular attention to the extension of the head or limbs relative to the trunk; to the rotation or displacement of the torso; and to individual phenomena related to specific limb, regional or organ activity. He thus categorised twitches; independent limb movements; combined/repetitive movements; quasi-startles; limb–joint movements; hand–face contacts; diaphragm movements; and respiratory movements (Birnholz et al 1978).

With the advent of real-time ultrasound scanners, an attempt was made to determine the age at which fetal movements first occur. Van Dongen and Goudie (1980) observed embryos with a crown–rump length of 5–12mm, and saw the heart pulsating at 6 weeks' gestation, with tiny movements occurring in one pole of the embryo at 7.5 weeks of age.

At that time, the number of images that could be recorded per second became sufficiently high to provide real-time recordings. From that point on, examinations were mainly carried out by obstetricians, some of whom evaluated the onset of motility and behaviour (Ianniruberto and Tajani 1981, de Vries et al 1982) in collaboration with the neuropaediatrician Adriano Milani Comparetti and the developmental neurologist Heinz Prechtl.

Fetal movements as reported by the mother
Expectant mothers sense the first quickening between 14 and 22 weeks' gestation, when fetal movements are forceful enough to press against the maternal abdominal wall (Tuffnell et al 1991, Hijazi and East 2009). Quickening is noticed earlier (1) by multigravidae, at an average gestational age of 17 weeks, as opposed to 19 weeks in primigravidae (O'Dowd and O'Dowd 1985); and (2) if the placental site is on the posterior instead of the anterior uterine wall (Gillieson et al 1984, Hijazi and East 2009). At first, fetal movements are infrequent, weak, and sometimes indistinguishable from other abdominal sensations, but they gradually become stronger, more frequent and easily distinguishable from other types of movement. They reach a maximum between 30 and 38 weeks and then decrease somewhat until delivery (Sadovsky and Yaffe 1973, Sadovsky and Polishuk 1977).

What mothers describe are kicks (quick jerks and thrusts of the extremities); squirms (slow stretching, pushing and turning movements); hiccups (rhythmic series of quick convulsive movements); ripples (light, rapid, constant-intensity movements consisting of a back-and-forth and up-and-down movement); and rolling or rotating movements (Walters 1964, Sadovsky et al 1979, Rayburn and Mc Kean 1980). Most fetal movements are noticed by the mother when she is lying; fewer are felt when she is sitting, and hardly any when standing (Minors and Waterhouse 1979).

Charting the mother's perception of fetal motion is the oldest and simplest method of monitoring fetal well-being during the second half of pregnancy (Figure 1.2). However, the agreement between maternally perceived and ultrasonographically recorded fetal movements is between 33% and 82% (Gettinger et al 1978, Hertogs et al 1979, Rayburn 1980, Schmidt et al 1984, Valentin and Maršál 1987, Kisilevsky et al 1991, Nishihara et al 2008). Quite often – in 30% of all cases – mothers perceive movements that cannot be sonographically confirmed (Schmidt et al 1984).

The Groningen fetal ultrasound studies
The use of real-time ultrasound has opened the door to both behavioural and neurological assessment of the human fetus. High-resolution, real-time ultrasound scanning has become an indispensable tool in the longitudinal investigation of the emergence and differentiation of an individual's prenatal movement repertoire (de Vries et al 1982, 1985, 1988, Nijhuis et al 1982, Roodenburg et al 1991). From a methodological point of view, this comes very close to the approach of developmental neurology, where the observation of movement patterns, of their quantity and, above all, their quality, serves as a basis for the investigation of neural development and for assessment of the condition of the nervous system. Aiming to acquire a sound knowledge of normal development, the first questions posed in the Groningen studies were the following:

- How should fetal movement patterns be classified?
- At what age do they appear for the first time?
- Do they change in the course of intrauterine development?
- Are there any age-related preferences with regard to the fetal position?
- Are there any specific motor patterns which are responsible for changes in the fetal position?

The attempts to answer these questions were based on many years of experience in infant observation (Prechtl and Schleidt 1950, Prechtl 1953, 1958, 1977, Prechtl et al 1979). At the beginning of the ultrasound studies, Heinz Prechtl, the founder and leading figure of the Groningen studies, was hoping that familiarity with motor patterns in preterm and term infants would help with recognition of similar patterns in the fetuses. It came as somewhat of a surprise that the repertoire of fetal movements exclusively comprised motor patterns that could also be observed postnatally (Prechtl 1984, 1985, 1989, 2001). This striking coherence greatly facilitated a consistent and comprehensive descriptive classification and terminology.

Three- and four-dimensional ultrasonography: what do they add?
Whereas three-dimensional (3D) ultrasound is a static display of the various reformatting techniques based upon the acquisition of a static volume, 4D ultrasound displays a continuously updated and newly acquired volume in any rendering modality, creating the

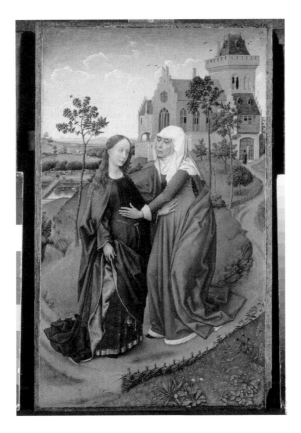

Figure 1.2 'Now at this time Mary... entered the house of Zacharias and greeted Elizabeth. And it came about that when Elizabeth heard Mary's greeting, the baby leaped in her womb; ... and she cried out with a loud voice, ... "when the sound of your greeting reached my ear, the baby leaped in my womb for joy"' (Luke 1:39–44). Painting by Rogier van der Weyden (c. 1440–1445): *Visitation of Mary*, oil on panel. Museum der Bildenden Künste, Leipzig, Germany (© bpk / Museum der bildenden Künste, Leipzig, Ursula Gerstenberger), reproduced with permission.

impression of a moving structure (Campbell 2002, Timor-Tritsch and Platt 2002). A high acquisition speed (volume per second) makes the perceivable transition between images more fluid; real-time, however, is yet to be realised. Hence, movements are of staggering appearance, and the quality of movements is especially difficult to assess from 4D ultrasound images. During the first trimester of gestation, the 4D technique may not provide a clear picture of specific movement patterns, such as hiccups, fetal breathing movements or jaw opening (Andonotopo et al 2005); but apart from the better detectability of malformations and anomalies, this technique clearly serves as a novel means for the evaluation of fetal facial expressions, especially during the last trimester (DiPietro 2005, Gonçalves et al 2005). Nevertheless, 4D is no alternative to 2D ultrasound recordings (Campbell 2002).

The effects of ultrasound examination on the parents and the fetus

Maternal–fetal attachment or bonding is literally kick-started by the onset of fetal movements. It is further intensified during the third trimester of gestation, as the mother responds to her unborn baby's distinct patterns of rest and activity. Visualisation of the fetus by the parents may arouse emotions that are capable of triggering the parental–fetal bonding much earlier, or of improving it. This, in turn, may lead to changes in behaviour and lifestyle that promote maternal and fetal health (Arabin et al 1996, Gonçalves et al 2005, Campbell 2006, Sedgmen et al 2006). Mothers who undergo 3D ultrasound show their ultrasound images to other people more often than mothers with 2D ultrasound examinations do (Ji et al 2005). The quality or intensity of the maternal–fetal attachment, however, is independent of the type of ultrasound – 2D, 3D or 4D – that the expectant mothers choose (Rustico et al 2005).

Obviously, ultrasound is a form of energy that has both thermal and mechanical effects on the tissues it runs through. Some 30 years ago, conjectures were made as to whether ultrasound could enhance fetal motion (David et al 1975), but subsequent studies did not corroborate these ideas (Powell Phillips and Towell 1979, Weinstein et al 1981, Murrils et al 1983). In a more recent study, on the other hand, fetuses moved more frequently when exposed to pulsed ultrasound in pulsed Doppler and B modes than they did in continuous wave Doppler mode (Fatemi et al 2001).

After a number of studies had shown that there was no adverse outcome associated with fetal ultrasound recording (Stark et al 1984, Reece et al 1990, Visser et al 1993), a study by Newnham and associates (1993) caused quite a stir, as it documented a higher number of intrauterine growth restrictions in an intensive ultrasound examination group than in fetuses that had only been exposed to a single sonographic examination. The same 3000 children of the study were re-examined when aged 8 years: their physical size, language, behaviour and neurological outcome bore no relationship to the number of ultrasound examinations during fetal life (Newnham et al 2004). It must, however, be stressed that there is no epidemiological study published on populations scanned after 1992, when regulations were altered and the acoustic output of ultrasound instruments was permitted to reach levels that were many times higher than previously allowed (Abramovicz et al 2008, Torloni et al 2009).

In 2006, Ang and colleagues from Pasko Rakic's well-known laboratory at Yale University published results on neuronal migration in the embryonic mouse brain and on the effects of prenatal exposure to ultrasound. The authors of the study exposed immobilised, unanaesthetised, pregnant mice to ultrasound on days 16.5–19.5 of gestation, which is the time of neuronal migration from the proliferative zone towards the brain surface. Exposure time varied from 5 to 420 minutes. Their conclusion, based on the examination of more than 335 animals, was that ultrasound exposure of 30 minutes or more caused a derangement in the migration of neurones from the deep to the more superficial layers of the brain. The authors postulated that, because of the device's low output, a non-thermal mechanism, radiation force or microstreaming was probably operating. In his comment on this study, Abramovicz (2007) questioned whether a relatively small misplacement in a relatively small number of cells could be of clinical consequence. At the same time, he supported ultrasound scanning in principle, but argued that it should be carried out for the shortest possible time and with the lowest possible output in order to achieve high diagnostic acuity.

There may be some issues if ultrasound examinations are not performed by trained experts but in commercial settings with no physicians present. In the United States (US) in particular, ultrasound scanners are operated in shopping malls and similar public places, offering non-diagnostic 'baby pictures'. Obviously, such boutique-like fetal imaging is clinically and ethically deficient, if only for the lack of counselling that some women may need (Bly and van den Hof 2005, Chervenak and McCullough 2005, Gorincour et al 2006, Abramovicz 2007, Sheiner et al 2007).

Other methods of assessing fetal behaviour
Lindsey (1942) claimed to have obtained a fetal electroencephalogram (EEG) by means of electrodes placed on the abdominal wall of a pregnant woman. Borkowski and Bernstine (1955), who applied abdominal and cervical electrodes, also produced positive EEG recordings of irregular slow-wave activity with superimposed fast waves in two fetuses. Garcia-Austt (1969) inserted hook-shaped platinum needles into the fetal vertex to study term fetuses during labour. He recorded a deceleration in all leads of the fetal EEG during a uterine contraction – apparently a consequence of the fetal head moulding.

While these EEG recordings are mainly of historical interest, various other methods have been applied to record fetal activity, employing strain gauges (Timor-Tritsch et al 1976, Wood et al 1977); electromagnetic devices, which created an electromagnetic field around the maternal abdomen and thus recorded movements inside it (Sadovsky et al 1973); impedance plethysmography (Ehrström 1979); or piezo-electric sensors, which are sensitive to rapid strained forces like fetal movements but relatively insensitive to steady or slowly changing movements such as uterine contractions or maternal respiratory movements (Sadovsky and Polishuk 1977).

A number of fetal behaviour studies by DiPietro and associates are based on the actocardiotocograph (Maeda et al 1991), which records both the fetal heart rate and body movements by means of a single wide-array Doppler transducer positioned on the maternal abdomen. It filters out the highest-frequency signal, which represents the fetal heart motion, and the lowest-frequency signals, representing maternal movements and respiration. The signals are generated by a change in the returned Doppler waveform; if there is no movement, the returned signal will retain the same frequency as the emitted signal. If the fetus moves, the echo will be returned at a different frequency, which is commensurate with the velocity with which the fetal body part moves towards or away from the transducer (Maeda et al 1991, 2009, DiPietro et al 1999, Witter et al 2007). Thus, the method is accurate in detecting periods of quiescence and activity (Maeda et al 1999); it achieves an overall kappa of 0.88 for agreement with ultrasonography (DiPietro et al 1999).

Fetal magnetoencephalography (MEG) is a new promising technique of studying the development of neuronal processing properties directly and non-invasively. It has an excellent temporal resolution but does not provide anatomical information. The current technology makes it possible to record fetal auditory and visual evoked fields, spontaneous brain activity, and, as a by-product, fetal heart rate parameters (Blum et al 1985, Wakai et al 1996, Schleussner et al 2001, Sheridan et al 2010). Most researchers have been working in the acoustic mode. The general approach is to search for an evoked component around 200ms, which is interpreted as a delayed component corresponding to the adult N100. As several factors, such as the variable position of the fetal head to the probe and differences in fetal behavioural states in different sessions of measurement, may limit detection, the detection rate is between 30% and 50% (Schleussner et al 2001, Preissl et al 2004, Eswaran et al 2007, Sheridan et al 2008).

Finally, fetal magnetocardiography (MCG) enables an accurate assessment of fetal heart rate variability. Owing to the high sensitivity of the signal to the position and orientation of the fetal heart, fetal MCG also allows an indirect assessment of fetal activity, especially of trunk movements (Wakai 2004).

Magnetic resonance imaging: spotlight on fetal behaviour

The limitations of fetal ultrasonography include the non-specific appearance of some abnormalities, and problems when there is associated maternal obesity (Pistorius et al 2008, Parkar et al 2010). Therefore, magnetic resonance imaging (MRI) has primarily been utilised as a complementary device in fetal imaging (Prayer 2006, Glenn and Coakley 2009, Limperopoulos and Clouchoux 2009, Weston 2010).

Naturally, safety is a major issue when scanning a fetus (Leithner et al 2009, Baysinger 2010, Hand et al 2010, Kikuchi et al 2010). In the UK, for instance, health authorities advise against scanning pregnant women above 3T (Gowland and Fulford 2004). The fetus can only lose heat via conduction and convection processes within the placenta and amniotic fluid; and, certainly, a greater fractional volume of the fetus is irradiated compared with the adult. A real issue of concern is that of acoustic noise. So far, there is no evidence of alterations in the short-term heart rate variability or the number of fetal movements that can be attributed to the exposure to noise (Michel et al 2003, Gowland and Fulford 2004).

Dynamic magnetic resonance imaging: a revolutionary approach

At present, dynamic MRI allows detailed behavioural studies of the fetus (Prayer 2006, Chung et al 2009). These dynamic studies are based on a so-called steady-state sequence with free precession (SSFP-sequence). A slice thickness of up to 50mm and a large field of view create a 3D-like impression of the whole fetus. Five to six images per second are sufficient to visualise fetal movements in a real-time fashion (Prayer and Brugger 2007). The images are not confined to gross body movements but also comprise swallowing, yawning, breathing excursions of the diaphragm and cardiac activity. Usually, a series of 30–60 second episodes of fetal movements is recorded during a 30–40 minute magnetic resonance (MR) examination. It is possible to make an assessment of movement patterns, but interpretation has to be made cautiously: if the fetus does not move during the MR examination, this should not be interpreted as pathological, especially if the morphological findings are normal.

FUNCTIONAL MAGNETIC RESONANCE IMAGING

Functional magnetic resonance imaging (fMRI) is a method of measuring the change in the MRI signal in response to a stimulus. Although single-trial fMRI is possible at very high field, it is usually necessary to repeat the stimulus up to 30 times, at 1 minute intervals. Blocked paradigms use extended stimuli of approximately 10 seconds, whereas event-related paradigms use short stimuli (<5 seconds). When stimulating a fetus, it is crucial to choose a stimulus that does not elicit a gross movement response (Gowland and Fulford 2004, Fulford and Gowland 2009). When averaged over the first three studies (Moore et al 2001, Fulford et al 2003, 2004), activation was found in 45% of the fetuses scanned, with 21% unsuccessful data sets because of susceptibility artefacts from the bowel or excessive fetal motion.

REFERENCES

Abramowicz JS. (2007) Prenatal exposure to ultrasound waves: is there a risk? *Ultrasound Obstet Gynecol* 29: 363–367.

Abramowicz JS, Fowlkes JB, Skelly AC, Stratmeyer ME, Ziskin MC. (2008) Conclusions regarding epidemiology for obstetric ultrasound. *J Ultrasound Med* 27: 637–644.

Ahlfeld F. (1869) [On the duration of pregnancy]. *Monatsschr Geburtsh Gynäkol* 19: 155–165. (In German)

Ahlfeld F. (1888) [Prior undescribed intrauterin movements of the child]. *Verhandl Dt Gesell Gynäkol* 2: 203–210. (In German)

Ahlfeld F. (1905) [Intrauterine movements of thoracic and diaphragmatic muscles. Intrauterine Breathing]. *Monatsschr Geburtshilfe Gynäkol* 21: 143–163. (In German)

Andonotopo W, Medic M, Salihagic-Kadic A, Milenkovic D, Maiz N, Scazzocchio E. (2005) The assessment of fetal behaviour in early pregnancy: comparison between 2D and 4D sonographic scanning. *J Perinat Med* 33: 406–414.

Ang ESBC, Glunic V, Duque A, Shafer ME, Rakic P. (2006) Prenatal exposure to ultrasound waves impacts neuronal migration in mice. *Proc Natl Acad Sci U S A* 103: 12903–12910.

Arabin B, Bos R, Rijlaarsdam R, Mohnhaupt A, van Eyck J. (1996) The onset of inter-human contacts: longitudinal ultrasound observations in early twin pregnancies. *Ultrasound Obstet Gynecol* 8: 166–173.

Barcroft J, Barron DH. (1939) [Movement in the mammalian foetus]. In: Asher L, Spiro K, editors. *Ergebnisse der Physiologie*. München: Bergman Verlag. p 107–152. (In German)

Baysinger CL. (2010) Imaging during pregnancy. *Anesth Analg* 110: 863–867.

Birnholz JC, Stephens JC, Faria M. (1978) Fetal movement patterns: a possible means of defining neurological developmental milestones in utero. *Am J Roentgenol* 130: 537–540.

Blackstone W. (1765) *Commentaries on the Laws of England. Vol 5. Amendment IX; Document 1.* Chigaco: University of Chicago Press.

Blum T, Saling E, Bauer R. (1985) First magnetoencephalographic recordings of the brain activity of the human fetus. *Br J Obstet Gynaecol* 92: 1224–1229.

Bly S, van den Hof MC. (2005) Obstetric ultrasound biological effects and safety. *J Obstet Gynaecol Can* 27: 572–580.

Borkowski WJ, Bernstine RL. (1955) Electroencephalography of fetus. *Neurology* 5: 362–365.

Campbell S. (2002) 4D, or not 4D: that is the question. *Ultrasound Obstet Gynecol* 19: 1–4.

Campbell S. (2006) 4D and prenatal bonding: still more questions than answers. *Ultrasound Obstet Gynecol* 27: 243–244.

Chervenak FA, McCullough LB. (2005) An ethical critique of boutique fetal imaging: a case for the medicalization of fetal imaging. *Am J Obstet Gynecol* 192: 31–33.

Chung R, Kasparian G, Brugger PC, Prayer D. (2009) The current state and future of fetal imaging. *Clin Perinatol* 36: 685–699.

Coghill GE. (1929) *Anatomy and the Problem of Behaviour.* Cambridge: Cambridge University Press.

David H, Weaver JB, Pearson JP. (1975) Doppler ultrasound and fetal activity. *Br Med J* 2: 62–64.

de Bracton H. (1250) The crime of homicide and the divisions into which it falls. In: Thorne SE. (1968) *Bracton on the Laws and Customs of England. Vol 2.* Cambridge MA: Belknap. p 340–344.

de Vries JIP, Visser GHA, Prechtl HFR. (1982) The emergence of fetal behaviour. I. Qualitative aspects. *Early Hum Dev* 7: 301–322.

de Vries JIP, Visser GHA, Prechtl HFR. (1985) The emergence of fetal behaviour. II: Quantitative aspects. *Early Hum Dev* 12: 99–120.

de Vries JIP, Visser GHA, Prechtl HFR. (1988) The emergence of fetal behaviour. III. Individual differences and consistencies. *Early Hum Dev* 16: 85–103.

DiPietro JA. (2005) Neurobehavioural assessment before birth. *Ment Retard Dev Disabil Res Rev* 11: 4–13.

DiPietro JA, Costigan KA, Pressman EK. (1999) Fetal movement detection: comparison of the Toitu actograph with ultrasound from 20 weeks gestation. *J Matern Fetal Med* 8: 237–242.

Ehrström C. (1979) Fetal movement monitoring in normal and high risk pregnancy. *Acta Obstet Gynecol Scand Suppl* 80: 6–32.

Eswaran H, Haddad NI, Shihabuddin BS, Preissl H, Siegel ER, Murphy P, Lowery CL. (2007) Non-invasive detection and identification of brain activity patterns in the developing fetus. *Clin Neurophysiol* 118: 1940–1946.

Fatemi M, Ogburn PL Jr, Greenleaf JF. (2001) Fetal stimulation by pulsed diagnostic ultrasound. *J Ultrasound Med* 20: 883–889.

Fulford J, Gowland PA. (2009) The emerging role of functional MRI for evaluating fetal brain activity. *Semin Perinatol* 33: 281–288.

Fulford J, Vadeyar SH, Dodampahala SH, Moore RJ, Young P, Baker PN, James DK, Gowland PA. (2003) Fetal brain activity to a visual stimulus. *Hum Brain Mapp* 20: 239–245.

Fulford J, Vadeyar S, Dodampahala SH, Ong S, Moore RJ, Baker PN, James DK, Gowland P. (2004) Fetal brain activity and hemodynamic response to a vibroacoustic stimulus. *Hum Brain Mapp* 22: 116–121.

Garcia-Austt E. (1969) *Perinatal Factors Affecting Human Development.* Washington DC: Pan American Health Organization.

Gettinger A, Roberts Ab, Campbell S. (1978) Comparison between subjective and ultrasound assessment of fetal movements. *Br Med J* 2: 88–90.

Gillieson M, Dunlap H, Nair R, Pilon M. (1984) Placental side, parity, and date of quickening. *Obstet Gynecol* 64: 44–45.

Glenn OA, Coakley FV. (2009) MRI of the fetal central nervous system and body. *Clin Perinatol* 36: 273–300.

Gonçalves LF, Lee W, Espinoza J, Romero R. (2005) Three- and 4-dimensional ultrasound in obstetric practice. Does it help? *J Ultrasound Med* 24: 1599–1624.

Gorincour G, Tassy S, LeCoz P. (2006) The moving face of the fetus – the changing face of medicine. *Ultrasound Obstet Gynecol* 28: 979–980.

Gowland P, Fulford J. (2004) Initial experiences of performing fetal fMRI. *Exp Neurol* 190: S22–S27.

Hand JW, Li Y, Hajnal JV. (2010) Numerical study of RF exposure and the resulting temperature rise in the foetus during a magnetic resonance procedure. *Phys Med Biol* 55: 913–930.

Hertogs K, Roberts A, Cooper D, Griffin D. (1979) Maternal perception of fetal motor activity. *Br Med J* 2: 1183–1185.

Hijazi ZR, East CE. (2009) Factors affecting maternal perception of fetal movement. *Obstet Gynecol Survey* 64: 489–497.

Hooker D. (1938) *Evidence of Prenatal Function of the Central Nervous System in Man*. New York: American Museum of Natural History.

Hooker D. (1952) *The Prenatal Origin of Behavior*. Lawrence: University of Kansas Press.

Humphrey T. (1964) Some correlations between the appearance of human fetal reflexes and the development of the nervous system. *Prog Brain Res* 4: 93–135.

Humphrey T, Hooker D. (1959) Double simultaneous stimulation of human fetuses and the anatomical patterns underlying the reflexes elicited. *J Comp Neurol* 112: 75–102.

Humphrey T, Hooker D. (1961) Reflexes elicited by stimulating perineal and adjacent areas of human fetuses. *Trans Am Neurol Assoc* 86: 147–152.

Ianniruberto A, Tajani E. (1981) Ultrasonographic study of fetal movements. *Semin Perinatol* 5: 175–181.

Ji EK, Pretorius DH, Newton R, Uyan K, Hull AD, Hollenbach K, Nelson TR. (2005) Effects of ultrasound on maternal–fetal bonding: a comparison of two- and three-dimensional imaging. *Ultrasound Obstet Gynecol* 25: 473–477.

Jouppila P, Piiroinen O. (1975) Ultrasonic diagnosis of fetal life in early pregnancy. *Obstet Gynecol* 46: 616–620.

Kikuchi S, Saito K, Takahashi M, Ito K. (2010) Temperature elevation in the fetus from electromagnetic exposure during magnetic resonance imaging. *Phys Med Biol* 55: 2411–2426.

Kisilevsky BS, Killen H, Muir DW, Low JA. (1991) Maternal and ultrasound measurements of elicited fetal movements: a methodological consideraton. *Obstet Gynecol* 77: 889–892.

Leithner K, Pörnbacher S, Assem-Hilger E, Krampl-Bettelheim E, Prayer D. (2009) Prenatal magnetic resonance imaging: towards optimized patient information. *Ultrasound Obstet Gynecol* 34: 182–187.

Limperopoulos C, Clouchoux C. (2009) Advancing fetal brain MRI: targets for future. *Semin Perinatol* 33: 289–298.

Lindsey DB. (1942) Head and brain potentials of human fetuses in utero. *Am J Psychol* 55: 412–416.

Maeda K, Tatsumura M, Nakajima K. (1991) Objective and quantitative evaluation of fetal movement with ultrasonic Doppler actocardiogram. *Biol Neonate* 60(Suppl): 41–51.

Maeda K, Tatsumura M, Utsu M. (1999) Analyses of fetal movements by Doppler actocardiogram and fetal B-mode imaging. *Clin Perinatol* 26: 829–851.

Maeda K, Iwabe T, Yoshida S, Ito T, Minagawa Y, Morokuma S, Pooh RK, Fuchiwaki T. (2009) Detailed multigrade evaluation of fetal disorders with the quantified actocardiogram. *J Perinat Med* 37: 392–396.

Michel SC, Rake A, Keller TM, Huch R, König V, Seifert B, Marincek B, Kubik-Huch RA. (2003) Fetal cardiographic monitoring during 1.5-T MR imaging. *Am J Roentgenol* 180: 1159–1164.

Minkowsky M. (1928) *[Neurobiological studies on the human fetus]*. *Handbuch Biol Arbeitsmeth Abt V Teil* 5B: 511–618. (In German)

Minors D, Waterhouse J. (1979) The effect of maternal posture, meals, and time of day on fetal movements. *Br J Obstet Gynaecol* 86: 717–723.

Moore JR, Vadeyar S, Fulford J, Tyler DJ, Gribben C, Baker PN, James D, Gowland PA. (2001) Antenatal determination of fetal brain activity in response to acoustic stimulus using functional magnetic resonance imaging. *Hum Brain Mapping* 12: 94–99.

Murrils AJ, Barrington P, Harris PD, Wheeler T. (1983) The influence of Doppler ultrasound on fetal activity. *Br Med J* 286: 1009–1012.

Needham J. (1959) *A History of Embryology*. Cambridge: Cambridge University Press.

Newnham JP, Evans SF, Michael CA, Stanley FJ, Landau LI. (1993) Effects of frequent ultrasound during pregnancy: a randomised controlled trial. *Lancet* 342: 887–891.

Newnham JP, Doherty DA, Kendall GE, Zubrick SR, Landau LI, Stanley FJ. (2004) Effects of repeated prenatal ultrasound examinations on childhood outcome up to 8 years: follow-up of a randomised controlled trial. *Lancet* 364: 2038–2044.

13

Nijhuis JG, Prechtl HFR, Martin CB, Bots RSGM. (1982) Are there behavioural states in the human fetus? *Early Hum Dev* 6: 177–195.

Nishihara K, Horiuchi S, Eto H, Honda M. (2008) A long-term monitoring of fetal movement at home using a newly developed sensor: an introduction of maternal micro-arousals evoked by fetal movement during maternal sleep. *Early Hum Dev* 84: 595–603.

O'Dowd MJ, O'Dowd TM. (1985) Quickening – a re-evaluation. *Br J Obstet Gynaecol* 92: 1037–1039.

O'Rahilly R. (1988) One hundred years of human embryology. In: Kalter H, editor. *Issues and Reviews in Teratology. Vol 4*. New York: Plenum Publishing Corporation. p 81–128.

Pajot C. (1876) A treatise on gynaecology, clinical and operative. *Ann Gynecol* 6: 241–351.

Parkar AP, Olsen ØE, Gjelland K, Kiserud T, Rosendahl K. (2010) Common fetal measurements: a comparison between ultrasound and magnetic resonance imaging. *Acta Radiol* 51: 85–91.

Pistorius LR, Hellmann PM, Visser GH, Malinger G, Prayer D. (2008) Fetal neuroimaging: ultrasound, MRI, or both? *Obstet Gynecol Surv* 63: 733–745.

Powell Phillips WD, Towell ME. (1979) Doppler ultrasound and subjective assessment of fetal action. *Br Med J* 2: 101–102.

Prayer D. (2006) Fetal MR. *Eur J Radiol* 57: 171.

Prayer D, Brugger PC. (2007) Investigation of normal organ development with fetal MRI. *Eur Radiol* 17: 2458–2471.

Prechtl HFR. (1953) [Coupling of suction and the grasp reflex in infants]. *Naturwissensch* 12: 347–348. (In German)

Prechtl HFR. (1958) The directed head turning response and allied movements of the human body. *Behaviour* 8: 212–242.

Prechtl HFR. (1977) *The Neurological Examination of the Fullterm Newborn Infant. Second Revised and Enlarged Edition. Clinics in Developmental Medicine No. 63*. London: Heinemann.

Prechtl HFR. (1984) Continuity and change in early neural development. In: Prechtl HFR, editor. *Continuity of Neural Functions From Prenatal to Postnatal Life. Clinics in Developmental Medicine No. 94*. Oxford: Blackwell. p 1–15.

Prechtl HFR. (1985) Ultrasound studies of human fetal behaviour. *Early Hum Dev* 12: 91–98.

Prechtl HFR. (1989) Fetal behavior. In Hill A, Volpe JJ, editors. *Fetal Neurology*. New York: Raven Press. p 1–16.

Prechtl HFR. (2001) Prenatal and postnatal development of human motor behaviour. In: Kalverboer AF, Gramsbergen A, editors. *Handbook of Brain and Behaviour in Human Development*. Dordrecht, Boston, London: Kluwer Academic Publ. p 415–428.

Prechtl HFR, Schleidt WM. (1950) [Inititating and controlling mechanisms of the act of sucking] I. *Ztschr Vergl Physiol* 32: 257–262. (In German)

Prechtl HFR, Fargel JW, Weinmann HM, Bakker HH. (1979) Postures, motility and respiration of low-risk preterm infants. *Dev Med Child Neurol* 21: 3–27.

Preissl H, Lowery CL, Eswaran H. (2004) Fetal magnetoencephalography: current progress and trends. *Exp Neurol* 190: S28–S36.

Preyer W. (1985) *[Special Physiology of the Embryo]*. Leipzig: Grieben. (In German)

Rayburn WF. (1980) Clinical significance of perceptible fetal motion. *Am J Obstet Gynecol* 138: 210–212.

Rayburn WF, Mc Kean HE. (1980) Maternal perception of fetal movement and perinatal outcome. *Obstet Gynecol* 56: 161–164.

Reece EA, Assimakopoulos E, Zheng XZ, Hagay Z, Hobbins JC. (1990) The safety of obstetric ultrasonography: concern for the fetus. *Obstet Gynecol* 76: 139–146.

Reinold E. (1971a) [Fetal movements in early pregnancy] *Z Geburtsh Gynäkol* 174: 220–225. (In German)

Reinold E. (1971b) [Observation of fetal movement in the first half of pregnancy with ultrasound]. *Pädiat Pädol* 6: 274–279. (In German)

Reinold E. (1973) Clinical value of fetal spontaneous movements in early pregnancy. *J Perinat Med* 1: 65–69.

Reinold E. (1976) *Ultrasonics in Early Pregnancy. Diagnostic Scanning and Fetal Motor Activity*. Basel: Karger.

Roodenburg PJ, Wladimiroff JW, van Es A, Prechtl HFR. (1991) Classification and quantitative aspects of fetal movements during the second half of normal pregnancy. *Early Hum Dev* 25: 19–35.

Rustico MA, Mastromatteo C, Grigio M, Maggioni C, Gregori D, Nicolini U. (2005) Two-dimensional vs. two- plus four-dimensional ultrasound in pregnancy and the effect on maternal emotional status: a randomised study. *Ultrasound Obstet Gynecol* 25: 468–472.

Sadovsky E, Polishuk WZ. (1977) Fetal movements in utero. Nature, assessment, prognostic value, timing of delivery. *Obstet Gynecol* 50: 49–55.

Sadovsky E, Yaffe H. (1973) Daily fetal movement recording and fetal prognosis. *Obstet Gynecol* 41:845–850.

Sadovsky E, Mahler Y, Polishuk WZ, Molkin A. (1973) Correlation between electromagnetic recording and maternal assessment of fetal movements. *Lancet* 1(7813): 1141–1143.

Sadovsky E, Laufer N, Allen JW. (1979) The incidence of different types of fetal movements during pregnancy. *Br J Obstet Gynaecol* 86: 10–14.

Schleussner E, Schneider U, Kausch S, Kähler C, Haueisen J, Seewald HJ. (2001) Fetal magnetoencephalography: a non-invasive method for the assessment of fetal neuronal maturation. *Br J Obstet Gynaecol* 108: 1291–1294.

Schmidt W, Cseh I, Hara K, Kubli F. (1984) Maternal perception of fetal movements and real-time ultrasound findings. *J Perinat Med* 12: 313–318.

Sedgmen B, McMahon C, Cairns D, Benzie RJ, Woodfield RL. (2006) The impact of two-dimensional versus three-dimensional ultrasound exposure on maternal-fetal attachment and maternal health behaviour in pregnancy. *Ultrasound Obstet Gynecol* 27: 245–251.

Sheiner E, Shoham-Vardi I, Hussey MJ, Pombar X, Strassner HT, Freeman J, Abramovicz JS. (2007) First-trimester sonography: is the fetus exposed to high levels of acoustic energy? *J Clin Ultrasound* 35: 245–249.

Sheridan CJ, Preissl H, Siegel ER, Murphy P, Ware M, Lowery CL, Eswaran H. (2008) Neonatal and fetal response decrement of evoked responses: a MEG study. *Clin Neurophysiol* 119: 796–804.

Sheridan CJ, Matuz T, Draganova R, Eswaran H, Preissl H. (2010) Fetal magnetoencephalography – achievements and challenges in the study of prenatal and early postnatal brain responses: a review. *Infant Child Dev* 19: 80–93.

Sontag LW. (1941) The significance of fetal environmental differences. *Am J Obstet Gynecol* 42: 86–103.

Sontag LW, Wallace RF. (1934) Preliminary report of the Fels Fund study of fetal activity. *Am J Dis Child* 48: 1050–1057.

Stark CR, Orleans M, Haverkamp AD, Murphy J. (1984) Short- and long-term risks after exposure to diagnostic ultrasound in utero. *Obstet Gynaecol* 63: 194–200.

Strassmann P. (1903) *[Life Before Birth. Collection of Clinical Presentations. No. 353]*. Leipzig: Breitkopf und Härtel. (In German)

Timor-Tritsch I, Platt L. (2002) Three-dimensional ultrasound experience in obstetrics. Curr Opin Obstet Gynecol 14: 569–575.

Timor-Tritsch I, Zador I, Hertz RH, Rosen MG. (1976) Classification of human fetal movement. *Am J Obstet Gynecol* 126: 70–77.

Torloni MR, Vedmedovska N, Merialdi M, Betrán AP, Allen T, Gonzáles R. Platt LD, ISUOG-WHO Fetal Growth Study Group. (2009) Safety of ultrasonography in pregnancy: WHO systematic review of the literature and meta-analysis. *Ultrasound Obstet Gynecol* 33: 599–608.

Tuck SM. (1986) Ultrasound monitoring of fetal behaviour. *Ultrasound Med Biol* 12: 307–317.

Tuffnell DJ, Cartmill RSV, Lilford RJ. (1991) Fetal movements – factors affecting their perception. *Eur J Obstet Gynecol Reprod Biol* 39: 165–167.

Valentin L, Maršál K. (1987) Recording of fetal movements. A comparison of three methods. *Eur J Obstet Gynecol Reprod Biol* 24: 23–32.

van Dongen LGR, Goudie EG. (1980) Fetal movement patterns in the first trimester of pregnancy. *Br J Obstet Gynaecol* 87: 191–193.

Visser GHA, de Vries JIP, Mulder EJH, Ververs IA, van Geijn HP. (1993) Effects of frequent ultrasound during pregnancy. *Lancet* 342: 1359–1360.

Wakai RT. (2004) Assessment of fetal neurodevelopment via fetal magnetocardiography. *Exp Neurol* 190 (Suppl 1): S65–S71.

Wakai RT, Leuthold MS, Martin MD. (1996) Fetal auditory evoked responses detected by magnetoencephalography. *Am J Obstet Gynecol* 174: 1484–1486.

Walters CE. (1964) Reliability and comparison of four types of foetal activity and of total activity. *Child Dev* 35: 1249–1256.

Weinstein D, Navot D, Sadovsky E. (1981) Antepartum ultrasound fetal heart rate monitoring and fetal movements. *J Obstet Gynaecol* 2: 85–87.

Weston MJ. (2010) Magnetic resonance imaging in fetal medicine: a pictorial review of current and developing indications. *Postgrad Med J* 86: 42–51.

Whitehead J. (1867) Convulsions in utero. *Br Med J* 2: 59–61.

Windle WF. (1940) *Physiology of the Fetus. Origin and Extent of Function in Fetal Life.* Philadelphia: WB Saunders.

Windle WF, Becker RF. (1940) Relation of anoxemia to early activity in the fetal nervous system. *Arch Neurol Psychiatr* 43: 90–101

Witter F, DiPietro J, Costigan K, Nelson P. (2007) The relationship between hiccups and heart rate in the fetus. *J Matern Fetal Neonatal Med* 20: 289–292.

Wood C, Walter WAW, Trigg P. (1977) Methods of recording fetal movements. *Br J Obstet Gynaecol* 84: 561–567.

Yanase J. (1907) [Observations in human fetuses]. *Pflügers Arch* 119: 451–464. (In German)

2
SPONTANEOUS MOTOR BEHAVIOUR

Right from the beginning of pregnancy, early spontaneously generated motility shows a rich repertoire of coordinated and identifiable patterns (Figure 2.1). Once a movement pattern is stabilised, it remains present at least until term, but usually for longer, sometimes even for life.

The evidence of endogenously generated motility

Preyer (1885) was the first to draw attention to embryonic motility originating in endogenous processes. He realised that the chick embryo exhibited overt motor activity several days before sensory stimulation effectively evoked reflexes, which implied that the efferent motor system began to function before the sensory system. It turns out that, once the motor neurones have innervated the muscles, the sensory reflex arc is not completed (Windle and Orr 1934, Oppenheim 1982). In other words, there is a motor output to the muscles that can occur in the absence of an input from the sensory receptors.

Similar results have been found in amphibian larvae, which exhibit complex and often highly coordinated spontaneous locomotor activity in spite of being surgically deafferented at the embryonic stage (Weiss 1941). Bullfrog embryos and larvae exhibit endogenously generated, patterned, motoneuronal discharges that are the specific neural correlate of swimming (Stehouwer and Farel 1980); both the motoneuronal discharges and the swimming pattern persist after sensory deafferentation. Similarly, newborn monkeys, whose limbs are deafferented in utero display a remarkable repertoire of spontaneous motor activity (Taub 1976), although definite abnormalities in voluntary fine motor movements also exist.

The most convincing evidence that embryonic motility is not dependent on sensory input but is centrally generated comes from the work of Viktor Hamburger and his associates. They extirpated several segments of the thoracic neural tube (immature spinal cord) of a 2-day-old chick embryo. The lumbosacral cord was thus isolated from input from the brain and the rostral cord regions. In a second operation, the dorsal half of the neural tube caudal to the thoracic spinal gap and the associated neural crest areas – i.e. the precursors of the dorsal root sensory ganglia – were removed; thereby the sensory input to the residual, postgap cord was eliminated. The ventral root efferents remained intact. Thus, the leg movements of the operated embryo were the product of neuronal discharges

17

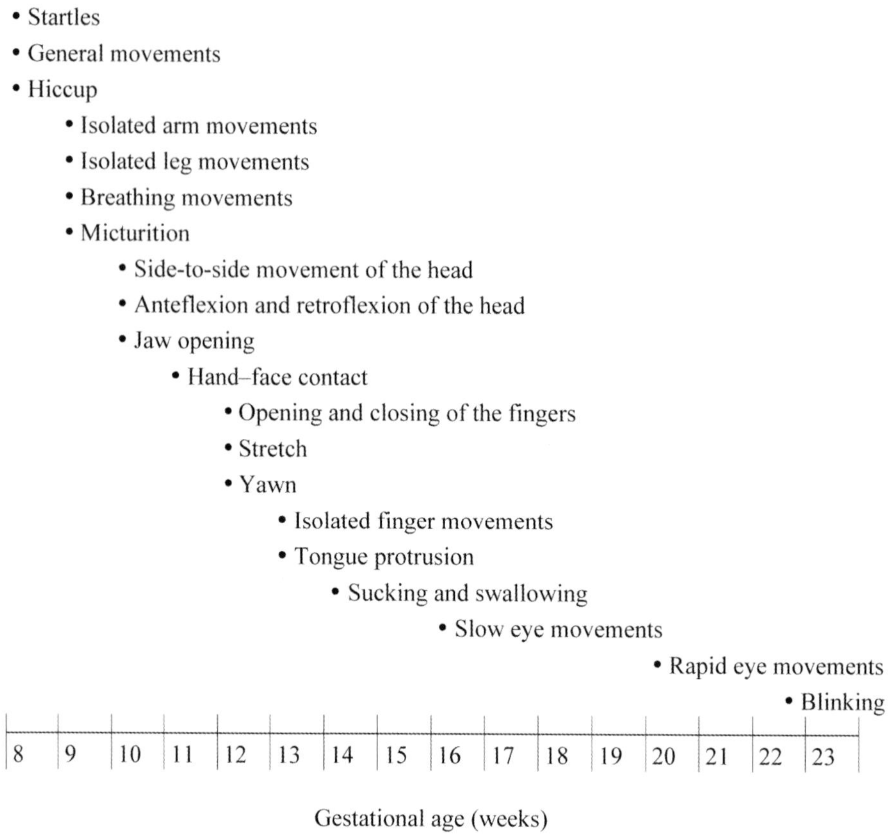

- Startles
- General movements
- Hiccup
    - Isolated arm movements
    - Isolated leg movements
    - Breathing movements
    - Micturition
        - Side-to-side movement of the head
        - Anteflexion and retroflexion of the head
        - Jaw opening
            - Hand–face contact
                - Opening and closing of the fingers
                - Stretch
                - Yawn
                    - Isolated finger movements
                    - Tongue protrusion
                        - Sucking and swallowing
                            - Slow eye movements
                                - Rapid eye movements
                                    - Blinking

| 8 | 9 | 10 | 11 | 12 | 13 | 14 | 15 | 16 | 17 | 18 | 19 | 20 | 21 | 22 | 23 |

Gestational age (weeks)

Figure 2.1 The first occurrence of specific spontaneous embryonic and fetal movement patterns (Ianniruberto and Tajani 1981, Birnholz 1981, Bots et al 1981, de Vries et al 1982, de Elejalde and Elejalde 1985, Campbell 2002, Pooh and Ogura 2004, Hata et al 2005, Lüchinger et al 2008).

within the surgical isolated lumbosacral spinal cord segment that innervated them. The legs of the operated embryo were highly motile during most of the embryonic period, which indicated that the embryonic motility was both spontaneous and patterned by neural circuitry within the residual spinal cord (Hamburger et al 1966).

Modern neurobiology has provided extensive experimental evidence for the existence of endogenously generated activity and its underlying neural network, the so-called central pattern generators (Grillner 1999). Well-known examples of central pattern generators are the central mechanisms for breathing, sucking and chewing, as well as those for locomotion, such as swimming, crawling and walking (Onimaru 1995, Roberts and Perrins 1995, Prechtl 1997, Forssberg 1999, Tabak et al 2000, Prechtl 2001a, Cheng et al 2002, Staras et al 2003, Einspieler et al 2004, Guertin 2009).

18

Ultimately, we need to acknowledge that centrally generated and reflexive behaviours are not mutually exclusive (Hamburger 1963). In fact, certain reflex and central mechanisms work together to produce adaptive coordinated behaviours (Pearson 2000).

Why does the fetus move in the first place?
Traditionally, three different explanations have been given as to the function of embryonic and fetal movements.

1. The *epiphenomenal concept* proceeds on the assumption that fetal behaviour has no adaptive significance whatsoever. In this view, the fetus's movement simply represents an incidental epiphenomenon of structural development. Support for this view was particularly strong during the days of fetal reflexology, between the 1920s and the 1940s, when fetal motility was widely used as an index of neuromuscular development (Windle 1940).

2. According to the *preparatory hypothesis*, fetal movements represent incipient stages that foreshadow the development of postnatal patterns of adaptive behaviour. Fetal movements may provide practice, or experience, which is crucial for the development of motor coordination and its expression in organised postnatal behaviour (Bekoff et al 1980). Further, prenatal activity and behavioural development may be influenced by information obtained in utero.

3. Complementary to the preparatory hypothesis, the *functional hypothesis* suggests that fetal behaviour is functional and adaptive during the prenatal period (Oppenheim 1981a). Amniote embryos (reptiles, birds, mammals) develop in environments that are totally different from the external world of their postnatal life, which indicates that anatomical and behavioural features could be functional during prenatal development to promote the survival and well-being of the embryo and fetus.

Today, there is increasing evidence that embryonic and fetal movements are necessary for the proper development of the skeletal, muscular and neural systems, or vice versa, that normal fetal development requires adequate fetal activity (see also Chapter 8, p 173). Function is an integral part of normal development, and the prenatal use of a structure (albeit immature) is necessary for the continuing and normal development of that structure.

If the neuromuscular activity underlying the movement is silenced pharmacologically or by disease, the population of the spinal motor neurones, the distribution of neurotransmitter receptors on the muscle fibres, and the pattern of neuromuscular synaptic contacts develop abnormally (Pena and Shokeir 1974, Gottlieb 1976, Purves and Lichtman 1980, Harris 1981, Oppenheim 1981b, Moessinger 1983).

The number of motor neurones undergoing genetically determined cell death (apoptosis) is closely related to muscle activity. Chick embryos immobilised by means of neuromuscular blocking agents show an increase of motor neurones in the brachial and lumbar lateral motor columns that would otherwise degenerate. When administration of the immobilising agents is stopped, allowing the embryo's motility to return to control level, the excess neurones undergo a delayed cell death and the total cell number falls below the control level (Pittman and Oppenheim 1979, Usiak and Landmesser 1999, Oppenheim et al 2003). On the other hand, there is a delay in the disappearance of early multiple motor endplates when muscle activity is reduced by means of tenotomy in young rats (Benoit and Changeux 1975). Conversely, this disappearance is accelerated when muscle activity is increased by way of electrical stimulation of the corresponding nerve (O'Brien et al 1978). In this case, the increased release of proteolytic enzymes from an active muscle seems to be responsible for the removal of superfluous endplates and innervations.

Prolonged experimental blocking of the neuromuscular junction of the chick embryo leads to malformation of the joints (Oppenheim et al 1978). Initial buds can differentiate, but adequate development of joint cavities and even proper shaping of synovial plates require motion of the limb (Sissons 1956). Reserpine-induced changes in chick embryo motility entail modifications in the development of the joint cavities, which become larger than normal when the movements are enhanced, whereas they are replaced by undifferentiated mesenchyme after drug-induced restricted motility (Ruano-Gil et al 1978). In the context of the human fetal akinesia deformation sequence (Chapter 8, p 174), it has been reported that, in the same fetus, a partial absence of movements results in contractures or hypoplasia in the respective regions (e.g. upper limbs, part of the face, thorax), while the active regions (e.g. lower limbs) develop normally (Tongsong et al 2000).

In addition to common genetic regulatory programmes required for organogenesis, mechanical forces generated in the embryo or fetus also have an influence on how the differentiating tissues respond to gene instructions. Lack or impairment of such physical forces changes the state of the organs (Inanlou et al 2005).

Fetal movements continuously change the position of the fetus (p 51) – when, for example, the trunk follows a rotation of the head, or when the fetus somersaults backwards with the help of alternating leg movements. These active – and frequent – changes of the intrauterine position prevent adhesions and local stasis of the blood, especially in the early fetus, whose skin is very fragile (Visser and Prechtl 1988).

The first movements

BEATING OF THE HEART

The Swiss surgeon Mayor (1818) is credited with being the first to report fetal heart tones. Independently, their presence was discovered and extensively publicised by the French nobleman Jean Alexandre Le Jumeau, Viscount de Kergaradec, in 1822. Legend would have us believe that Mayor discovered the fetal heart rate as he applied his ear to the abdomen of a pregnant woman to hear the fetus move, while Le Jumeau attempted to hear, with a stethoscope, a fetus splash in its amniotic fluid (Goodlin 1979). In 1906, the first fetal electrocardiogram was successfully performed (Cremer 1906).

Heart motion sets in at 5–6 weeks of gestation. It is the first motor activity that can be observed in an embryo (Jouppila and Piiroinen 1975, van Dongen and Goudie 1980, Nijhuis 2003). The initial rate of 100–120 beats per minute increases to 160–175 beats at 9–10 weeks, followed by a gradual decrease to 155 beats at 12–16 weeks' gestation (Robinson and Shaw-Dunn 1973, van Heeswijk et al 1990). As gestation advances, the mean heart rate drops by approximately 1 beat per minute per week and eventually settles at a value of 130 beats per minutes (range: 110–150 beats per minute) at term (James et al 1995).

THE FIRST BODY MOVEMENTS

Reinold (1971) was the first to use ultrasound to document fetal movements, which he found set in at around 9 weeks' gestational age (Figure 2.2). These first movements are variously described as 'twitches' (Birnholz et al 1978); 'vermicular movements' (Ianniruberto and Tajani 1981); 'just discernible movements' (de Vries et al 1982); 'rippling' (van Doungen and Goudie 1980, Goto and Kato 1983); or 'sideways bending of the head' (Prechtl 1985). The small size of the embryo (about 2cm) and the limited resolution of ultrasound in those days impeded a more detailed analysis of the first movements, but what all studies had in common was a description of small displacements occurring between 7 and 10 weeks (Figure 2.2) and disappearing thereafter.

We know from recent transvaginal ultrasound recordings following in vitro fertilisation that the earliest body movements occur at 7 weeks and 2 days (Lüchinger et al 2008). They consist of slow, small, non-complex sideward bending of the head (Video 1) or the rump or both, sometimes accompanied by a little activity in the arms or legs a few days later (Figure 2.3). By 10 weeks' gestation, the duration of this sideward bending increases to 5 seconds, while at the same time its frequency decreases. By 8.5 weeks, the speed and amplitude of the movements start to vary to some degree, although no variation in sequence or direction can be seen as yet.

Coinciding with the appearance of the first movements, axodendritic synapses are rapidly formed in the cervical spinal cord – initially between interneurones and motor neurones, then between afferent fibres and interneurones. In the lateral motor column, axodendritic synapses increase from one synapse per $200m^2$ at 8 weeks to ten synapses at 9 weeks (Okado et al 1979, Okado 1981).

Along with the spontaneous movements, responsive flexion of the neck elicited by tactile stimulation of the perioral region (Chapter 5, p 100) occurs at 7–8 weeks' gestation (Hooker 1952, Humphrey 1964). This significant co-existence provides evidence against the hypothesis that reflexes emerge earlier than spontaneous movements. On the other hand, there is no evidence that the spontaneous movement patterns precede the corresponding reflex patterns (Prechtl 1985).

Interestingly, the sideward bending of the head and/or the rump can be found in all mammals as a highly reproducible spatiotemporal early movement pattern (Suzue and

- Single cross episodes of jerky trunk flexion and head extension without separate or associated limb movements (Birnholz et al 1978)
- Smooth vermicular movements of the embryonic body due to the pulsating cardio-circulatory system (Ianniruberto and Tajani 1981)
- A slow and small shifting of the fetal contour, lasting 0.5–2 seconds, usually occurs as a single event (de Vries et al 1982)
    - Very small movements occurring in one pole of the embryo (van Dongen and Goudie 1980)
        - First movements (Jouppila and Piiroinen 1975, Higginbottom et al 1976)
        - First body movements (Schillinger et al 1976)
        - Trunk movements (Shawker et al 1980)
        - Rippling movements (van Dongen and Goudie 1980)
        - Rapid, irregular and vermicular movements of the whole body. Quick flexion and extension movements of trunk sometimes with slight movements of the limbs but without altering the position of the embryo (Ianniruberto and Tajani 1981)
            - Brisk and uniform rhythm of changing the position and the posture (Reinold 1971)

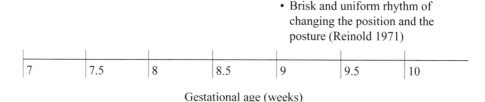

| 7 | 7.5 | 8 | 8.5 | 9 | 9.5 | 10 |

Gestational age (weeks)

Figure 2.2 The emergence and description of the first human embryonic movements documented by abdominal ultrasound, including A- and B-scan.

Shinoda 1999), and is probably induced via circuits of neural activity at the spinal level (Prechtl 1997, Bradley 2001, de Vries and Fong 2006).

Generalised movements
By 8–10 weeks' gestation, so-called generalised movements emerge in the entire body (de Vries et al 1982). They can be either quick, i.e. in the form of startles, or slower and more complex. The latter are referred to as general movements (Prechtl et al 1979), which comprise rotation and displacement of the thorax, partial rotation of the head and displacement of the limbs. Startles, on the other hand, cause a pronounced upward lift of the fetal body, followed by a subsequent fall. As startles promote a displacement of the thorax, they often induce a general movement (Piontelli 2006, Lüchinger et al 2008). It

22

- Small sideways bending of head or rump or both
- Slow, small stereotyped movements of the trunk in which one or two arms or legs also participate
- Single, slow, sideways bending of the head (about 1 second), no variation
- Single slow lateral movement of the head and rump towards each other (up to 5 seconds; exceptionally more than 20 seconds), no variation
  - Single slow sideways bending of the rump (up to 3 seconds), no variation
  - Single slow lateral bending of the head and/or rump together with an active leg movement (a few seconds), no variation in direction, but a little variation in speed and amplitude
  - Single slow lateral bending of the head and/or rump together with an active arm movement (up to 30 seconds), no variation in direction, but a little variation in speed, amplitude and participating body parts
    - Single slow lateral bending of the head and/or rump together with an active arm and leg movement (30 seconds), no variation in direction, but a little variation in speed, amplitude and participating body parts
    - Slow or abrupt extension of the spine
      - Variation in speed and amplitude emerge
        - Twitching activity in the spinal region
        - Movements become variable (i.e. general movements)

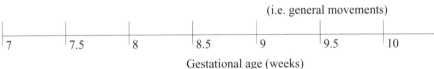

| | | | | | | |
|7|7.5|8|8.5|9|9.5|10|

Gestational age (weeks)

Figure 2.3 The earliest spontaneous motility due to transvaginal ultrasound recordings in 18 embryos after in-vitro fertilisation. Created using data from Lüchinger 2008.

would seem plausible, therefore, that the simultaneous ontogenetic onset of these two movement patterns (Figure 2.1) has an adaptive function.

STARTLE

This quick generalised movement is initiated in the limbs and spreads to the neck and trunk (Videos 2 and 3). Depending on whether the initial limb posture is extended or flexed, the limbs either flex or extend, respectively. With progressing gestational age, startles increasingly set out from flexed extremities, resulting in an extension of the limbs. A startle is a forceful movement, lasting for about 1 second (de Vries et al 1982, Roodenburg et al 1991, Prechtl 2001b). It basically occurs as an isolated event but

23

sometimes recurs in rapid succession, at an interval of a few seconds. Startles are frequent until mid-gestation (Ianniruberto and Tajani 1981, de Vries et al 1985, Piontelli 2006); thereafter their frequency decreases significantly (Figure 2.4; Birnholz et al 1978, Roodenburg et al 1991) and eventually reaches a rate that is even lower than in preterm infants of comparable age (Cioni and Prechtl 1990).

FETAL GENERAL MOVEMENTS

Several research groups discovered complex generalised movements and referred to them as 'squirming and writhing slow movements' (Sontag and Wallace 1934); 'twisting or creeping' (Reinold 1971); 'simultaneous or serial movements of the head, trunk and limbs with a smooth quality' (Birnholz et al 1978); 'moving and exercising all body parts including rolling from side to side, extension and then flexion of the back and neck, turning of the head, waving of the arms and kicking of the legs' (van Dongen and Goudie 1980); 'harmonious complex movements with wider limb movements' (Shawker et al 1980, Ianniruberto and Tajani 1981, Boué et al 1982, Kuno et al 2001); 'rolling and stretching' (Shawker et al 1980, Rayburn 1982, Kozuma et al 1997); and 'upper, lower and whole trunk activity including stepping and writhing' (Kozuma et al 1997).

In an observational study on spontaneous motility in low-risk preterm infants (Prechtl et al 1979), Prechtl coined the term 'general movements'. General movements involve the entire body and manifest themselves in a variable sequence of arm, leg, neck and trunk movements. They appear and cease gradually and vary in intensity and speed (Prechtl 1990, Prechtl 2001a, 2001b, Einspieler et al 2004). Rotations and frequent slight variations of the direction of motion make them look complex but smooth (Video 4). General movements occur until the fifth month of life but have a long prenatal history (Videos 5–7).

At 8 weeks' gestation, the whole body moves slowly and with limited range (de Vries et al 1982), but no distinctive patterning or sequencing of the body parts can yet be recognised (Lüchinger et al 2008). Just a week later, the speed, amplitude and direction start to vary a little. Thereafter, i.e. from 9 weeks' and 3 days' gestation onwards, the majority of general movements show a substantial degree of variation not only in speed, amplitude and direction but also in the sequence of the participating body parts. At this early stage, the sideward bending of the head and rump still co-exists with general movements (Lüchinger et al 2008). At 10–12 weeks' gestational age, the general movements become more forceful, albeit smooth in appearance (Video 5). They frequently cause a shift in the fetal position. After 12 weeks they come and go, but vary more in speed and amplitude (Video 6), lasting from 1 to 5 minutes. However variable these movements may be, they are always graceful and fluent in character. During the second half of pregnancy, even incidental crossing of arms over the midline of the fetal trunk can be seen as part of a general movement (Roodenburg et al 1991).

The incidence of general movements increases between 8 and 10 weeks' gestational age (Lüchinger et al 2008), when these movements appear scattered irregularly over the

Number of startles

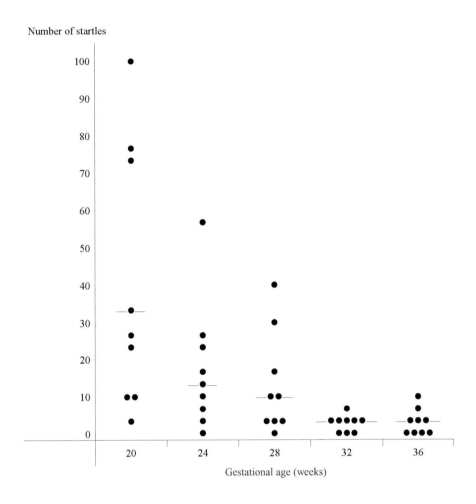

Figure 2.4 Incidence of startles (–, median; *n* = 9) per hour at 20, 24, 28, 32, and 36 weeks' gestation; the median incidence decreases from 28 per hour at 20 weeks to 1 per hour at 36 weeks. Adapted from Roodenburg PJ, Wladimiroff JW, van Es A, Prechtl HFR. (1991) Classification and quantitative aspects of fetal movements during the second half of normal pregnancy. *Early Hum Dev* 25: 19–35, with permission.

recording. In the course of the following weeks, they occur grouped in bursts of several minutes (Figure 2.5; de Vries et al 1982). After 14 weeks, the occurrence of such bursts becomes obscured and is replaced by longer periods of fluctuating activity (see Chapter 4). While the frequency of occurrence of general movements is 16% at mid-gestation, it is only 8–10% around term (Patrick et al 1982, Visser and Prechtl 1988, Roodenburg et al 1991, ten Hof et al 1999). Although the space within the uterus becomes increasingly limited during the third trimester, it seems more likely that the decrease of general movements is a result of the central nervous system development. Interestingly enough, the incidence of general movements also decreases in low-risk preterm infants until term age, even though there is no space limitation (Prechtl et al 1979).

The variability and complexity of general movements is an indicator for the integrity of the young nervous system (Prechtl and Einspieler 1997), but we shall come back to that in Chapter 8.

EXTENSION OF THE SPINE

Between 8 and 13 weeks of gestation, two types of extension movements of the spine are observed: isolated, slow extension of the spine, and twitching activity in the spinal region. They can both be followed by movements of other body parts (Lüchinger et al 2008). Extension of the spine can be distinguished from hiccup by the absence of displacement of the diaphragm, chest or abdomen.

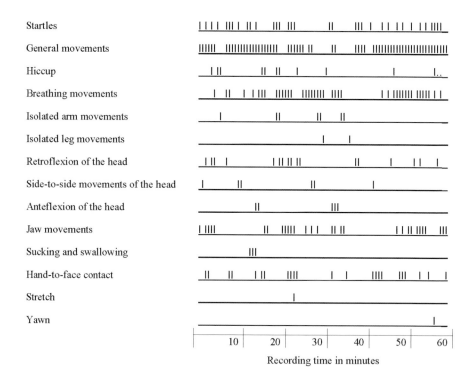

Figure 2.5 This actogram, recorded by means of an event recorder during videotape replays, indicates the incidence and temporal organisation of specific movement patterns during a 1 hour observation of a 14-week-old fetus. Adapted from de Vries JIP, Visser GHA, Prechtl HFR. (1982) The emergence of fetal behaviour. I. Qualitative aspects. *Early Hum Dev* 7: 301–322, with permission.

26

A complete change in position around the transverse axis, usually with a backwards somersault, is achieved by a complex general movement including alternating leg movements. Rotation around the longitudinal axis can either result from leg movements with hip rotation or be caused by a rotation of the head, followed by trunk rotation. A total change of the fetal position can be performed in a mere 2 seconds, but may also take longer (de Vries et al 1982).

MINIMAL NEURAL STRUCTURES ARE CAPABLE OF GENERATING WELL-ORGANISED MOVEMENTS

The synaptic innervation of cervical motor neurones only sets in at 8–9 weeks' gestation (Okado and Kojima 1984, Konstantinidou et al 1995), when a variety of fetal movements (Figure 2.1) are already present. By the end of week 10, the number of axodendritic synapses on the motor neurones has increased about eightfold, while axosomatic synapses only increase at 14–15 weeks (Okado and Kojima 1984). The majority of the synaptic boutons barely contain 20 synaptic vesicles (Okado 1980). The first appearance of definite myelinated fibres is in the lateral portion of the ventral marginal layer at 12 weeks' gestation (Okado 1982). The differentiation of skeletal muscles is also still at an early phase, as it is even several weeks after the onset of fetal movements (Fidziańska and Goebel 1991).

Transient structures and functions – whatever their specific significance – make the nervous system unique at each stage of development (Prechtl and Connolly 1981). One such transient structure is the subplate (Molliver et al 1973), which functions as a temporary goal for afferent fibres from several areas (the thalamus, basal forebrain, brainstem nuclei, contralateral and ipsilateral hemispheres) heading for cortical connections. Interestingly, the general movements become variable and complex when the subplate is formed (Lüchinger et al 2008). From this it follows that general movements are probably modulated supraspinally (Prechtl 1997). It is also remarkable that they co-occur with monotonous sideward bending and extension of the spine, which may be an expression of the local spinal circuit (Lüchinger et al 2008).

None of the fetal movements (Figure 2.1) are under corticospinal control. The corticospinal tract is the last of the major descending fibre systems to enter the spinal cord. Corticospinal axons reach the lower cervical spinal cord by 24 weeks' gestation, and functional monosynaptic corticomotoneuronal projections are likely to be present from as early as 26 weeks' gestation, while direct corticospinal projections to group Ia inhibitory interneurones only appear at term (Eyre et al 2000).

Observations on anencephalic fetuses have demonstrated that minimal neural structures are sufficient to generate fetal movements (Chapter 8, p 162). Isolated arm movements, breathing movements and hiccups can be seen, although only fetal meninges, glial tissue, ectopic motor neurones and dorsal ganglia are present at the level of the spinal cord (Visser et al 1985). However, the quality of the movements is abnormal. It is clear, therefore, that a normal fetal nervous system, albeit age-specifically still poorly developed, is needed in order for movements to be executed normally.

Specific motor patterns of the limbs

It might be assumed that, at this early stage, isolated movements should be more difficult for the nervous system to produce than global motor activity; however, isolated movements of particular limbs emerge only a few days after the generalised movements (Shawker et al 1980, de Vries et al 1982, Prechtl 1985). And there is yet another unexpected finding: it has traditionally been taken for granted that the early ontogenetic process goes from cranial to caudal (Saint-Anne Dargassies 1979). Although this assumption is primarily based on stimulation experiments (Hooker 1952, Jacobs 1967), the motor system does not follow that rule: isolated arm and isolated leg movements emerge at the same time, at 9–10 weeks (Figure 2.1). It is a fact, however, that isolated arm movements occur more frequently than isolated leg movements (Figure. 2.5), which certainly biases the results of short recordings (Prechtl 2001b).

ISOLATED ARM MOVEMENTS

Isolated arm movements, rapid or slow, may involve extension, flexion, external or internal rotation, abduction or adduction of an arm without movement in other body parts (Video 8). The amplitude varies from small to large. The extension of an arm is frequently accompanied by an extension of the fingers, at least from 12 weeks onwards. Fast, jerky arm movements can appear as either single events (twitches) or rhythmical movements at a rate of 3–4 per second (clonus). Cloni only appear after 14 weeks, but are rare even then (de Vries et al 1982). Arm twitches and cloni occur not only as isolated phenomena but may also be superimposed on general movements or, in fact, precede them. Isolated arm movements peak at 15 weeks' gestation and then decline with increasing gestational age (de Vries et al 1982, 1985).

HAND AND FINGER MOVEMENTS

Fetuses start to clench and unclench their fists at 12–13 weeks' gestation (Ianniruberto and Tajani 1981, Pooh and Ogura 2004). Isolated movements of one or more fingers appear from 13–14 weeks onwards (Pooh and Ogura 2004, Katz et al 2007). Some hand postures resemble postnatal hand gestures (Figure 2.6; Video 9).

HAND-TO-FACE CONTACT

From 11–13 weeks' gestation onwards, the hand regularly touches the head, face and mouth (Ianniruberto and Tajani 1981). These contacts are most frequent between 14 and 20 weeks, before decreasing again (van Tol-Geerdink et al 1995). The hand slowly

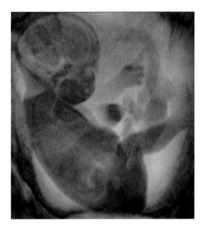

Figure 2.6 MRI print of a 27-week-old fetus with pointing index finger.

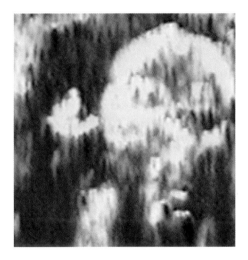

Figure 2.7 Ultrasound video print of a 14-week-old fetus whose thumb approaches the mouth.

touches the face, with the fingers extending and flexing (de Vries et al 1982). Insertion of finger(s) into the mouth, occasionally even thumb-sucking, is observable (Figure 2.7; Video 10). Hand-to-face contacts usually last for a few seconds, sometimes longer (Bowie and Clair 1982, Roodenburg et al 1991); they are either isolated events or part of a general movement.

GRASPING THE UMBILICAL CORD

There are several case reports of third-trimester fetuses who grasp (Figure 2.8), manipulate and even squeeze the umbilical cord (Sherer et al 1990, Brotanek and Lopez 1991, Petrikovsky and Kaplan 1993, Collins 1994, Heyl and Rath 1996, Habek et al 2003, 2006). Partial or intermittent complete cord occlusion alters the blood flow in the umbilical cord, increases the afterload and decreases the fetal oxygen content (Hill et al 1983, Ball and Parer 1992), which results in increased vagal activity causing variable fetal heart rate decelerations by up to 15–60 beats per minute (Petrikovsky and Kaplan 1993, Collins 1994, Habek et al 2006). Such a significant heart rate deceleration may result in diminished fetal cardiac output due to a poorly developed Frank–Starling mechanism at low fetal heart rates. Any hypoperfusion thus engendered is likely to be transient, however, because the brainstem-mediated grasp reflex would soon be abolished due to sustained hypoperfusion of the fetal central nervous system. Still, it sometimes takes a motor provocation test (vibroacoustic stimulation) for the fetus to release the umbilical cord. On release, heart rate decelerations disappear immediately (Heyl and Rath 1996) – although fetal hiccups may now set in and last for several minutes (Collins 1994).

ISOLATED LEG MOVEMENTS

Isolated leg movements (Video 11), rapid or slow, may involve extension, flexion, external or internal rotation, abduction or adduction of a leg without movements in other body parts (de Vries et al 1982, Katz et al 1999). The amplitude varies from small to large. A sporadic kick can be of sufficient strength to displace the fetus from its resting position (van Dongen and Goudie 1980). Slow leg movements are rare. Fast and jerky leg movements occur either as a single event (twitch) or as rhythmical movements at a rate of 3–4 per second (clonus). The latter only appear after 14 weeks, but are rare even then (Video 11). Leg twitches and cloni occur not only as isolated phenomena but may also be superimposed on general movements or, in fact, precede them.

ALTERNATING LEG MOVEMENTS

The so-called stepping movements, as observed after birth (Video 12) are probably a remnant of a specific fetal function, namely alternating leg movements (Figure 2.9), which enable the fetus to change position (Prechtl 2001b). Two months after birth, the stepping movements disappear (Peiper 1949).

Diaphragmatic movements

Formation of the diaphragm sets in at 8 weeks' gestation and is completed by 10 weeks (Wells 1954), providing the anatomical substrate for the onset of hiccups and breathing movements. While motor neurones need a critical number of functional synapses in order to discharge spontaneously, phrenic motor neurones in the cervical region seem to possess

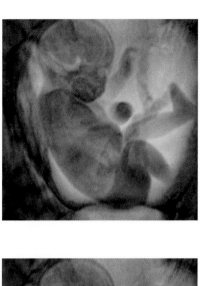

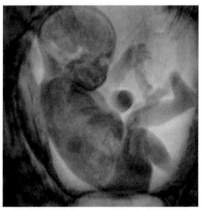

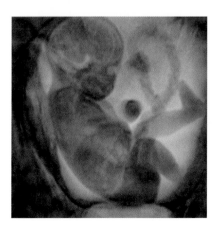

Figure 2.8 MRI prints of a 27-week-old fetus grasping the umbilical cord.

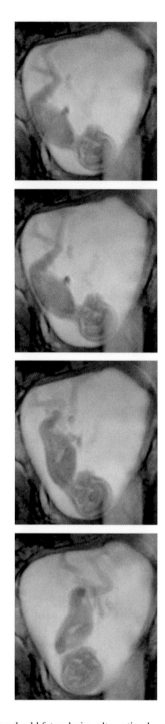

Figure 2.9 MRI prints of a 19-week-old fetus during alternating leg movements.

sufficient synapse contacts to produce hiccup by as early as 8 weeks (de Vries et al 1982). Fetal breathing movements typically follow 2–4 weeks later (de Vries et al 1982), although they can sometimes even be observed as early as 8–9 weeks (Lüchinger et al 2008).

The developmental trends of both motor patterns are quite different, with fetal hiccups being the predominant type of diaphragmatic movements until 26–30 weeks, and fetal breathing movements predominating thereafter (Pillai and James 1990a, Tatsumura 1991). The observation that hiccups decrease with advancing gestational age suggests that brain development may have an inhibitory effect on the hiccup. This assumption is corroborated by the finding that growth-retarded or otherwise compromised fetuses hiccup more often than normally growing fetuses (Bots et al 1978, James et al 1995).

HICCUPS

Pregnant women do usually notice fetal hiccups, which are forceful and jerky diaphragmatic contractions characterised by a sudden and abrupt displacement of the thorax and abdomen (Video 13; de Vries et al 1982, Zheng et al 1998). The accompanying closure of the vocal cords (Harris et al 1977) is difficult to see by means of ultrasound, especially if the amniotic fluid is reduced (Roberts and Mitchell 1995). Hiccups are often followed by passive limb or head movements, sometimes by both (de Vries et al 1982). Typically, hiccups occur episodically, in regular succession, at an interval of 2–3 seconds. Such hiccup spells can last up to 10 minutes (van Woerden et al 1989).

At an early stage of gestation, hiccups are very frequent (de Vries et al 1982, 1985). With advancing gestational age their frequency decreases, especially during the last 10 weeks (Pillai and James 1990b, Roodenburg et al 1991, Tatsumura 1991). By then, the rate is a mere 2–4 hiccup spells in 24 hours, although they sometimes last for several minutes (Patrick et al 1982). Only in compromised term fetuses is there still a high frequency of hiccup occurrence, after all other movements – including breathing movements – have ceased (James et al 1995).

By and large, the physiological significance of hiccups is still unclear. It has been suggested that fetal hiccups could be the manifestation of a programmed isometric inspiratory muscle exercise, which is supposed to smoothen the subsequent diaphragmatic motion necessary for breathing (Kahrilas and Shi 1997, Piontelli 2006). Harris and colleagues (1977) reported on a personal communication with Lendon, who suggested that hiccupping might actually stimulate blood circulation in the placenta.

Data on the baboon fetus indicate that hiccups show a diurnal variation, occurring more frequently at night (Stark et al 1994). This has not yet been confirmed for the human fetus. It is also unclear whether hiccups are related to behavioural states. Some take the view that they are more common in active states (Pillai and James 1990b), while others consider that there is no specific relation (van Woerden et al 1989), although hiccups may modulate the fetal heart rate, albeit not before 30 weeks' gestation (Levi et al 2000, Witter et al 2007). The cardiac interbeat interval that follows immediately upon a hiccup spell is longer than the interval that immediately precedes or occurs during the hiccup spell (Popescu et al 2007). A potential mechanism implies an increase in the afferent vagal activity triggered by hiccups, which induces a subsequent increase in the tonic efferent vagal activity. In addition, fetal hiccups are associated with decreased umbilical arterial and venous flow (Zheng et al 1998, Levi et al 2000). Such a transient reduced or even reversed umbilical artery flow is not associated with an adverse fetal outcome and may be a normal finding during fetal hiccups (Mueller and Sipes 1993).

BREATHING MOVEMENTS

Fetal breathing movements are paradoxical in nature: inspiratory movements consist of fluent movements of the diaphragm in a caudal direction, making the anterior chest move inwards and the abdominal wall move outwards (Video 14; de Vries et al 1982, Maršál et al 1984). The displacement of the diaphragm in the caudal direction varies in amplitude and lasts no longer than 1 second. In normal fetuses, chest wall movements are generally 2–5mm in amplitude, while abdominal wall movements are 3–8mm (Patrick et al 1978a).

Breathing movements emerge at 8–12 weeks (de Vries et al 1982, Lüchinger et al 2008), but nasal fluid flow velocity waveforms are only present from 22 weeks onwards, increasing progressively until term (Cosmi et al 2003). An absence of nasal flow at 22 weeks and thereafter is predictive for an adverse outcome such as pulmonary hypoplasia (Fox et al 1993). The intra-tracheal flow volume that is moved during inspiratory and expiratory movements increases until 36 weeks' gestation, after which the flow rate flattens. The median difference between the inspiratory volume and the expiratory volume is positive from 20 to 35 weeks and negative afterwards, which indicates that in term fetuses the effect of fetal breathing movements no longer results in an influx (Kalache et al 2002).

Breathing movements usually occur episodically; they have either a regular or an irregular pattern (Videos 7 and 15). The most common interval at early gestation is 2–3 seconds; from mid-gestation onwards it is less than 1 second (Trudinger and Knight 1980, de Vries et al 1985). From the beginning of the third trimester onwards, short episodes of breathing movements (<10 seconds) decrease, while longer episodes increase (Higuchi et al 1991). They last some 15 minutes during the preterm period (Natale et al 1988) and may increase to 2 hours at term (Patrick et al 1980).

Breathing movements vary from superficial and rapid to deep and slow (Roodenburg et al 1991). Rapid and irregular movements (both in rate and amplitude) account for more than 90% of all breathing movements (Cosmi et al 2001), while slow, deep inspiratory movements like sighs or gasps, or respiratory efforts that resemble grunting, coughing or panting, are less frequent (Cosmi et al 2001). Yet another type is shallow fetal breathing movements (Piontelli 2006), a form of superficial and regular breathing movements characterised by low synergistic outward excursions of the thorax and the abdomen. Shallow fetal breathing movements are noticed from 12 weeks onwards; they increase until 16 weeks and then level off. Because of their sporadic nature, shallow fetal breathing movements are unlikely to play a critical role in lung development.

Historical studies on fetal breathing movements

The first description of fetal breathing movements goes back to Ahlfeld (1888), who observed rhythmic excursions of the fetal thorax through the maternal abdominal wall – an observation that was confirmed by Reifferscheid (1911) and Barcroft (1946). Snyder (1949) suggested that, on occasion – and only without anoxia – the fetal chest moved rhythmically, at a rate that was comparable to respiration. Morison (1952), however, doubted whether there was any tidal movement of fluid that resembled in any way the tidal movement of air in postnatal respiration. The presence of vernix squames in the large bronchi showed that fluid penetrated into the upper respiratory passages of the fetus (Blair 1965). Windle (1971) found regular thoracic and abdominal wall movements in exteriorised human fetuses at a mere 11 weeks' gestation and described them as complex movements characterised by rhythmical episodes, by deep and shallow excursions, by opening and closing of the mouth, and sometimes by an extension of the head and cervical spine. Quite often, these features are accompanied by whole-body movements. As respiration is the most basic of all mechanisms essential for survival, Windle (1971) suggested that the component movements necessary for breathing had to develop very early in fetal life. He also noted that after placental separation, gasping is the last reflex to disappear. Following their visual representation by means of ultrasound (Dawes 1973), the existence of fetal breathing movements has been generally accepted.

Lung development depends on fetal breathing movements

Four parameters are responsible for normal fetal lung development through pulmonary distension: adequate intrathoracic space; adequate amount of amniotic fluid; normal fetal breathing movements; and normal balance of fluid volumes and pressures in prospective pulmonary conductive and respiratory systems (Wigglesworth 1988, Inanlou et al 2005, Joshi and Kotecha 2007, Hasan et al 2008). Fetal lamb preparations show that continuous drainage of the chloride-rich fluid that fills the airspaces and airways in utero results in lung hypoplasia. In addition, surgical procedures that prevent fetal breathing movements – or their associated transpulmonary pressure changes – cause severe lung hypoplasia (Wigglesworth and Desai 1982). The lack of fetal breathing movements contributes to disturbed cell-cycle kinetics. Insufficiency or absence of fetal breathing movements is associated with decreased proliferation and increased apoptosis of pulmonary cells, possibly by establishing the gradient of the thyroid transcription factor-1 expression and by regulating the expression of platelet-derived growth factors and insulin-like growth factors at the last stage of lung organogenesis (late mediators). It has also been suggested that fetal breathing movements may influence the expression of early mediators that are responsible for changes in cell-cycle kinetics at earlier stages of lung development (Inanlou et al 2005).

Aside from lung growth, fetal breathing movements are also required for lung maturation. If they are abnormal, surfactant-active material is only partially released into the alveolar or amniotic fluid (Dornan et al 1984a; see also Chapter 8, Table 8.3). Moreover, fetal breathing movements appear to be required for the accomplishment of the morphological differentiation of type I and type II pneumocytes (Inanlou et al 2005).

Fetal breathing movements change with gestational age
Apart from the fact that the amount of fetal breathing movements varies considerably from hour to hour (Roberts et al 1979), the percentage of observation time in which breathing movements are present is related to the gestational age. Starting from 3–6% at mid-gestation (de Vries et al 1985, Roodenburg et al 1991, James et al 1995), it increases to 14% at around 25 weeks (Natale et al 1988) and advances to 40% at around 30 weeks' gestation (Roodenburg et al 1991), after which is declines to 30% during the last weeks of pregnancy (Patrick et al 1980). At 40 weeks, fetal breathing movements only occur during 6–9% of the observation time (Bots et al 1978), and they decrease even further in prolonged pregnancies (Zimmer et al 1985).

Breathing movements are absent during labour
Labour inhibits fetal breathing movements (Nijhuis and Visser 2003). As early as the last 3 days before spontaneous parturition at term, fetal breathing movements decrease (Carmichael et al 1984), and they disappear entirely several hours before labour (Patrick and Challis 1980, Castle and Turnbull 1983, Carmichael et al 1984, Boylan et al 1985, Agustsson and Patel 1987, Kim et al 2003). In the case of elective labour induction, the induction period is shorter and the oxytocin requirement is lower when fetal breathing movements are already absent (Schreyer et al 1991). It has therefore been speculated that a decrease or absence of breathing movements may be predictive for preterm labour. A systematic examination of this assumption did not, however, provide clarity on the matter (Honest et al 2004).

Physiological conditions that affect breathing movements
As mentioned above, labour inhibits fetal breathing movements. During the last 10 days of pregnancy, fetal breathing movements decrease over the day and reach their lowest value between 19:00 and 24:00 hours (Patrick et al 1980). They also decrease during the ascending part of Braxton Hicks contractions, but increase when the uterus relaxes again (Wilkinson and Robinson 1982, Mulder and Visser 1987, Mulder et al 1995).

Fasting for more than 12 hours (Dornan et al 1984b, Mirghani et al 2003, Abd El Aal et al 2009), smoking (Manning et al 1975, Ritchie 1980) or methadone (Wouldes et al

2004) or alcohol ingestion (Maršál 1983, McLeod et al 1983, Pillai and James 1990a) considerably reduce the rate of fetal breathing movements (Table 2.1).

An increase of fetal breathing movements is caused by maternal meals. From 20–22 weeks onwards, a postprandial increase occurs especially during the second hour (Patrick et al 1980, Nijhuis et al 1986, de Vries et al 1987); then the incidence falls again (Patrick et al 1978a, Bocking et al 1982, Adamson et al 1983). Such an increase appears to be related to maternal plasma glucose concentrations, since glucose administered to the expectant mother causes an increase of fetal breathing movements (Adamson et al 1983, Maršál 1983, Harper et al 1987). Even around term, when fetal breathing movements are usually almost absent, they can increase by 25% after intravenous administration of glucose to the mother (Divon et al 1985). However, fetal breathing movements also increase during the night – especially between 01:00 and 07:00 hours (Patrick et al 1978b, Natale et al 1988), even though there is no obvious relation with maternal glucose concentration (Patrick et al 1980). Fetal breathing movements in mothers with diabetes are dealt with in Chapter 7 (p 140).

Whether these behavioural shifts are to be interpreted as an attempt to compensate for the effects of changes in the internal and/or external fetal environment and enable normal development of the fetal lung, or whether they mirror changes in brain development is yet to be determined (Kisilevsky et al 1999).

Maternal oxygen and carbon dioxide levels influence fetal breathing movements
Fetal breathing movements decrease with hypocapnia caused by maternal hyperventilation (Connors et al 1989), but they increase after administration of 2–4% carbon dioxide (Ritchie 1980, Connors et al 1989).

TABLE 2.1
Physiological reasons and pathophysiological conditions that result in an increase or decrease of fetal breathing movements

	Increase	Decrease
Physiological reasons	Glucose intake	Labour
	Diurnal variation: early morning	Diurnal variation: late evening
		Maternal fasting
Pathological conditions	Maternal diabetes	Smoking
	Maternal hypercapnia	Alcohol
		Methadone
		Maternal hyperventilation
		Severe fetal hypoxia
		Preterm rupture of the membranes

Maternal hyperoxia following inhalation of 50% atmospheric oxygen does not have an effect on the frequency of fetal breathing movements in either uncomplicated pregnancies (Devoe et al 1984) or insulin-dependent mothers (Ritchie and Lakhani 1980a). The fetal breathing movements do, however, increase substantially in response to maternal hyperoxia in cases in which hypoxia had obviously existed, such as in fetuses with intrauterine growth retardation or fetuses of mothers with severe pre-eclampsia (Ritchie and Lakhani 1980b, Dornan and Ritchie 1983).

The effect of hypoxia upon the fetus depends not only on the degree of hypoxia induced, but probably also on the gestational age and the initial level of fetal oxygenation. Mild hypoxia causes fetal tachycardia, while a more severe insult causes bradycardia and a decrease in fetal breathing movements. Smoking has the same effect, with an onset no later than 30 minutes after smoking and recovery by 90 minutes (Ritchie 1980).

Pathological suppression of fetal breathing movements
Acute hypoxia secondary to maternal hypoxia, anaemia, reduced uterine blood flow or umbilical cord occlusion causes a decrease of fetal breathing movements. This is believed to be due to an increase of the neuromodulator adenosine in the brainstem areas regulating fetal breathing movements (Bocking 2003).

Suppression of fetal breathing movements may follow a preterm rupture of the membranes (Kivikovski et al 1988, Roberts et al 1991) and is considered to be a predictor of fetal infection (Vintzileos et al 1985) and of pulmonary hypoplasia (Blott et al 1990, Mulder et al 2001). The presence of fetal breathing movements despite oligohydramnios, on the other hand, is regarded as a predictor of a favourable neonatal outcome (Blott and Greenough 1988).

Qualitatively abnormal fetal breathing movements
Vigorous, jerky breathing movements of large amplitude, ranging from minimum to maximum thoracic capacity in spite of a normal quantity regarding the percentage of time and frequency, were described in a 31-week-old fetus whose post-mortem diagnosis revealed tracheal atresia in combination with other congenital abnormalities, which suggested VATER (vertebrae, anal, tracheal, (o)esophageal and renal abnormalities) association (Baarsma et al 1993).

Specific motor patterns of the head
SIDE-TO-SIDE MOVEMENTS OF THE HEAD
Side-to-side movements of the head were first noticed in Hooker's stimulation experiments at 10–11 weeks' gestation (Hooker 1952), which is actually the age at which they emerge spontaneously (Figure 2.1; de Vries et al 1982). They are usually characterised by slow speed and may cover a range of approximately 160 degrees (Video

38

16). The incidence increases steadily during the first 20 weeks (de Vries et al 1985), but decreases from 65 movements per hour at 20 weeks to half that value at 28 weeks, only to increase again thereafter (Roodenburg et al 1991). At times, such head movements come in association with hand-to-face contact. Quite often, side-to-side movements succeed each other, incidentally reaching a rhythmical pattern over a longer period. Prechtl regards these rhythmical side-to-side movements, which are slightly irregular in nature, as the basis of rooting (Prechtl 1989, 2001b). In the newborn, rooting gradually comes under tactile control (Video 17) and develops into an oriented turning response of the head and mouth towards the eliciting stimulus (Prechtl 1958, Einspieler et al 2008).

RETROFLEXION OF THE HEAD

Retroflexion of the head (Figure 2.10) is usually carried out at a slow pace, but can sometimes also be quick and jerky, resembling a twitch. The displacement of the head varies in amplitude; wide displacement may cause over-extension of the fetal spine. The head may remain retroflexed for a time, from a few seconds to more than a minute. Although mostly categorised as a single, isolated event, such jerky retroflexions of the head can also occur in succession (de Vries et al 1985). Sometimes retroflexion of the head is part of a stretch or yawn (de Vries et al 1982). It emerges at 10–11 weeks (Figure 2.1) and can occur up to 12 times per hour, especially during the second half of pregnancy (de Vries et al 1982, Roodenburg et al 1991).

ANTEFLEXION OF THE HEAD

Anteflexion of the head (Figure 2.11) is carried out at a slow pace (Video 18). It sometimes occurs along with hand-to-mouth contact (de Vries et al 1982). After birth at term, it takes 4–5 months for the anteflexion of the head to reoccur, so the movement in

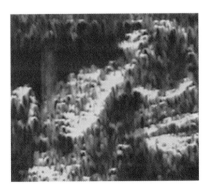

Figure 2.10 Ultrasound video print of a 14-week-old fetus during retroflexion of the head.

utero appears to be due to the buoyancy effect in the amniotic fluid (Prechtl 2001b, Velazquez and Rayburn 2002, Einspieler et al 2008).

JAW MOVEMENTS

Isolated jaw movements (Figure 2.12) may be slow or quick, with the jaw opening varying in both degree and duration (1–5 seconds). They come as a single event or in a sequence (de Vries et al 1982). At 9.5 weeks' gestation, the jaw already starts to open after perioral stimulation (Hooker 1938), with spontaneous jaw movements emerging a few days later (Figure 2.1; van Dongen and Goudie 1980, de Vries et al 1982). Elicited jaw opening is usually part of a retroflexion of the head and/or an extension of the trunk, whereas spontaneous jaw opening normally occurs unaccompanied by other movements. At this age the masseter muscle is still mainly composed of irregularly arranged myotubes, and the motor endplate is as yet simple and undeveloped (Ezure 1996). Until up to 15 weeks' gestation, single wide opening of the jaw is more common than later (de Vries et al 1982). At around 15 weeks, jaw opening may occur more quickly than jaw closing (Ianniruberto and Tajani 1981). Later on, jaw movements tend to reoccur irregularly (de Vries et al 1982).

Rhythmical mouthing

Rhythmical mouthing shows a developmental trend that is diametrically opposed to that of general movements. Its incidence increases progressively during the last 10 weeks of gestation (D'Elia et al 2001). By now the myotubes in the masseter muscle have disappeared and the muscle is composed solely of muscle fibres (Ezure 1996).

Once behavioural states are established (see Chapter 4), clusters of regular mouthing occur – in the absence of other motor activities – during behavioural state 1F (van Woerden et al 1988a, Horimoto et al 1989, D'Elia et al 2001). Accordingly, newborn infants only show regular mouthing movements during behavioural state 1, that is, quiet sleep (Prechtl 1974, Wolff 1986). Rhythmical mouthing movements like sucking can entrain a sinusoidal-like fetal heart-rate pattern that coincides with the oscillation frequency of the mouthing cluster (Nijhuis et al 1984, van Woerden et al 1988b, Nijhuis 2003). This might deceive the clinician, since a sinusoidal fetal heart rate can also reflect an underlying pathology like fetal anaemia or acute blood loss (James et al 1995, Nijhuis 2003).

TONGUE MOVEMENTS

At 13–14 weeks' gestation, mouth opening with tongue protrusion may occur (Ianniruberto and Tajani 1981). It is known from experiments on mice that tongue movements are required for normal palate development (Walker and Quarles 1962). In the human fetus, tongue expulsion, tongue thrust or tongue click can occasionally be observed

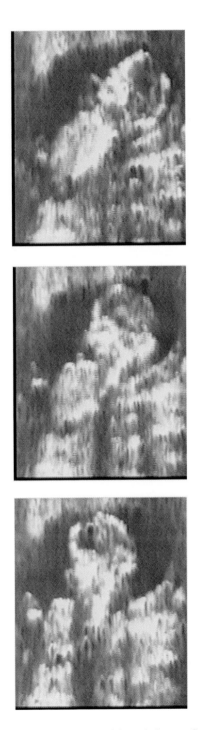

Figure 2.11 Ultrasound video prints of a 13-week-old fetus during anteflexion of the head.

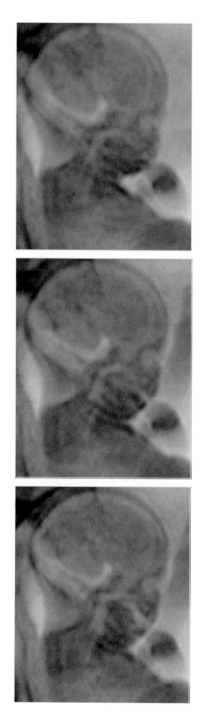

Figure 2.12 MRI prints of a 27-week-old fetus during opening of the jaw.

during the second half of pregnancy (Bowie and Clair 1982, Roodenburg et al 1991, Hata et al 2005, Yigiter and Kavak 2006), especially near term (de Vries and Fong 2006). Most of the tongue protrusions can be observed during behavioural state 2F (van Woerden et al 1988a).

Protrusion of the tongue can also co-occur with a wide opening of the mouth and extension of the neck, which looks as though the fetus were regurgitating or vomiting. This has been described in fetuses with oesophageal atresia or tracheo-oesophageal fistula (Dunne and Johnson 1979, Bowie and Clair 1982).

FACIAL EXPRESSIONS

By means of three-dimensional (3D) ultrasonography, various facial expressions can be distinguished. Smiling movements (Campbell 2002, Yigiter and Kavak 2006), like yawning (see p 47), elicit emotional reactions in the observer. Moreover, full extension of the lips in a pout and scowling can be observed (Kurjak et al 2003, Yan et al 2006). Usually 3D recordings are carried out during the last trimester, which is why the early ontogeny of these facial expressions is not yet known.

EYE MOVEMENTS

In the first study on human fetal eye movements – carried out by Hooker on exteriorised human fetuses – contraction of the orbicularis oculi muscle was observed following stimulation of the upper eyelid at 10.5 weeks' gestational age (Hooker 1952).

By means of transabdominal ultrasound scanning, the fetal lens can be seen at 14 weeks' gestation (de Elejalde and Elejalde 1985). There are two ways of making fetal eye movements visible: (1) the plane of a linear-array real-time scanner can be placed sagitally over one orbita, or horizontally over both orbitae. Since the eyeball acts as an acoustic lens, the area behind the eyeball shows a high echodensity. If the eyeball moves, a flicker can easily be observed in this area; (2) the plane of the ultrasound transducer can be placed coronally over the anterior part of the orbita, visualising the lenses as sharp contours. Displacement of the lenses indicates slow or rapid eye movements (Prechtl and Nijhuis 1983). It is important to bear in mind, however, that it is extremely difficult – and sometimes impossible – to assess eye movements while the fetus is performing general movements or head rotations.

The first report on sonographically scanned fetal eye movements is by Bots and associates (1981). At almost the same time, Birnholz (1981) came up with a description of the developmental course of four types of fetal eye movements (Figure 2.13). According to Birnholz, type I eye movements can only be observed between 16 and 25 weeks' gestation, although in preterm infants they are present until 33 weeks (Bridgeman 1983). Type III eye movements are dominant from 30 to 37 weeks' gestation, while type IV eye movements are predominant at term (Birnholz 1981).

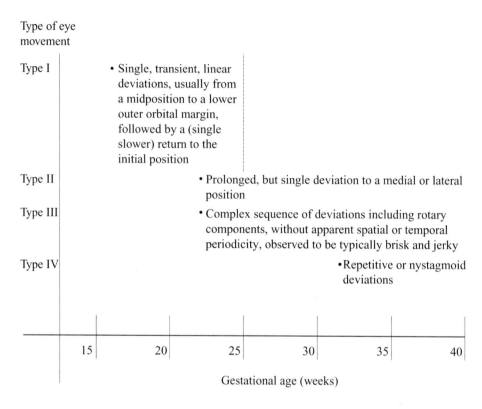

Type of eye
movement

Type I   • Single, transient, linear
            deviations, usually from
            a midposition to a lower
            outer orbital margin,
            followed by a (single
            slower) return to the
            initial position

Type II   • Prolonged, but single deviation to a medial or lateral
                    position

Type III   • Complex sequence of deviations including rotary
                    components, without apparent spatial or temporal
                    periodicity, observed to be typically brisk and jerky

Type IV   • Repetitive or nystagmoid
                                       deviations

        15   20   25   30   35   40

                    Gestational age (weeks)

Figure 2.13 Description, onset and developmental course of type I–IV eye movements. Created using data from Birnholz 1981.

Another classification distinguishes between (1) slow, rolling eye movements; (2) rapid, more regular eye movements with a duration of less than 0.6 seconds; and (3) occasional nystagmoid eye movements (Bots et al 1981, Horimoto et al 1990). Considering all eye movements together, their incidence increases from 25 per hour at 20 weeks to 100 per hour at 36 weeks (Roodenburg et al 1991). With this increase, eye movements begin to consolidate at about 24 weeks – a tendency that becomes more distinct from then onwards, as the consolidation grows into a long-term cluster of rapid eye movements from around 30 weeks onwards (Bots et al 1981, Inoue et al 1986, Koyanagi et al 1993). Isolated, slow eye movements, which are less frequent, occur only irregularly. During periods with a high frequency of eye movements, it is difficult, if not impossible, to differentiate between rapid and slow eye movements; sometimes rapid eye movements are even superimposed on slow ones. As in the neonate (Lynch and Aserinsky 1986), most eye movements in the fetus are horizontal (Figure 2.14) and conjugate (Video 19). In fact, disjunctive eye movements also exist, but they only appear sporadically and account for a mere 5% of all eye movements (Takashima et al 1991).

Episodes with no eye movements

During the third trimester of pregnancy, eye movements begin to cluster into bursts and pauses. During the last 10 weeks of pregnancy, the percentage of time in which eye movements are absent increases (Figure 2.15). Between 36 and 38 weeks, the duration of episodes with no eye movements nearly doubles, lasting for about as long as episodes with eye movements (Prechtl and Nijhuis 1983, Koyanagi et al 1993). In this respect there is no difference between fetuses in breech and fetuses in cephalic presentation, which implies that the neural system that controls the generation of eye movements, stretching from the dorsal tegmental field in the pons to the medullary ventral tegmentum, is of equal maturation in either presentation (Takashima et al 1995).

Fetal blinking

From 23–26 weeks onwards, opening and closing of the eyelids can be observed (Figure 2.16; Video 20; de Elejalde and Elejalde 1985, Campbell 2002, Hata et al 2005). Repeated blinking is associated with the central dopaminergic system (Karson 1982). It occurs during the last weeks of pregnancy (Hata et al 2005, Yigiter and Kavak 2006) at a frequency of 6.2 blinks per hour (Petrikovsky et al 2003). Blinking can also be elicited by means of light (Birnholz 1985) or vibroacoustic stimulation (Birnholz and Benacerraf 1983, Petrikovsky et al 2003), but habituates rather quickly (Bellieni et al 2005).

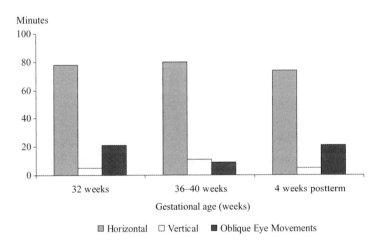

Figure 2.14 The proportion of horizontal (grey), vertical (white) and oblique (black) eye movements in the fetus at 32 weeks (Hepper and Shahidulla 1992) and at 36–40 weeks (Takashima et al 1995) as well as in the neonate at 4 weeks of age (Lynch and Aserinsky 1986).

45

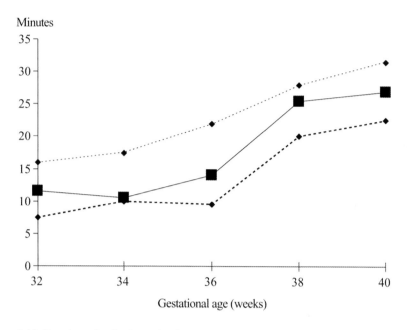

Minutes

Figure 2.15 Duration of episodes (min) in which eye movements are absent (■, median; ♦, interquartiles). Adapted from Prechtl HFR, Nijhuis JG. (1983) Eye movements in the human fetus and newborn. *Behav Brain Res* 10: 119–124, with permission.

Stretches and yawns: lifelong motor patterns

One striking phenomenon in fetal motor development is the early emergence of stretches and yawns. They can both be observed from 12 weeks onwards (de Vries et al 1982), but it is interesting to note that they continue to exist throughout life with virtually no change in form or pattern.

FETAL STRETCHING

A stretch (Video 21) is a complex motor pattern that is always carried out at a slow pace. It consists of the following components: marked extension of the trunk, retroflexion of the head and elevation of the arms in outward rotation. The pattern lasts for several seconds and only occurs in the form of isolated events (de Vries et al 1982). At mid-gestation, there are about six stretches per hour; this incidence decreases to one stretch per hour by term (Roodenburg et al 1991). Sometimes a stretch is accompanied by a short-lasting heart-rate deceleration.

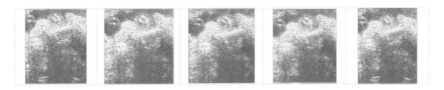

Figure 2.16 Ultrasound video prints of a 36-week-old fetus during opening and closing of the eyelid(s).

FETAL YAWNING

Yawning is a phylogenetically old, stereotyped event that occurs either alone or associated with stretching and/or penile erection in both humans and animals, that is, in fish, amphibians, reptiles, birds and mammals (Darwin 1872, Provine 1986, Argiolas and Melis 1998, Walusinski 2010). It is considered to be indicative of fatigue, drowsiness or boredom. Yawning in the presence of others is a clear but – from the point of view of social convention – inappropriate manifestation of the above-mentioned conditions (Provine 1986), although research has found no support for the popular hypotheses that it reflects boredom or fatigue (Provine et al 1987a). In fact, neither elevated carbon dioxide nor a depressed oxygen level in the blood increases yawning; and, conversely, breathing pure oxygen does not decrease yawning either (Provine et al 1987b). As for the fetus, yawning is not associated with fetal hypoxia (Sepulveda and Mangiamarchi 1995). The most curious, if least understood, aspect of human yawning is its contagiousness: people who witness or even just think about yawning cannot help but yawn themselves, which is not so much a case of imitation – since the mirror-neurone system is not involved – as an automatically released behavioural act (Schürmann et al 2005).

A fetal yawn (Video 22) starts with a slow, usually wide and prolonged opening of the jaw and a simultaneous downward movement of the tongue, as well as a retroflexion of the head, sometimes accompanied by limb stretching; this lasts for 9–13 seconds and occupies 50–75% of the yawn cycle. After reaching its maximum opening, the mouth remains open for 2–8 seconds (20–45% of the yawning cycle). The third part of the complex yawning movement consists in shutting the mouth quickly and returning to the initial position (1–2 seconds, 5–10% of the yawning cycle; de Vries et al 1982, Petrikovsky et al 1999). Once a yawn is under way, there seems to be no way back (Provine 1986). Fetal yawning is accompanied by a flow of fluid between the amniotic cavity and the fetal airway (Masuzaki et al 1996).

In most cases, a fetal yawn is an isolated event (Petrikovsky et al 1999), but repetitive yawning lasting for several minutes may also occur, especially during the second half of pregnancy (Sepulveda and Mangiamarchi 1995). An unusual amount of bursts of yawning has been observed in anaemic fetuses, where it could be a compensatory mechanism, as it changes the intrathoracic pressure and thereby increases the venous flow to the heart (Petrikovsky et al 1999).

The physiological function of yawning is still a subject of speculation. Some consider it to be a protective mechanism that prevents alveolar collapse (Twiest 1974, Sepulveda and Mangiamarchi 1995). Others regard it as a spreading activation of facial motor patterning (Giganti et al 2002). The powerful muscular contraction caused by yawning could also release arousal by activation of the locus coeruleus, to which the cranial nerves send retro-projections (Saper et al 2001). Still others consider yawning to be a mechanism for thermoregulation, providing compensatory cooling when other provisions fail to operate favourably (Gallup and Gallup 2008).

Since anencephalic neonates only yawn if they have an intact medulla oblongata (Heusner 1946), the neural circuits for this complex motor pattern are probably located in the brainstem near the respiratory and vasomotor centres. Yawning is controlled by several neurotransmitters and neuropeptides, above all by dopamine. Dopamine activates the production of oxytocin in the paraventricular nucleus of the hypothalamus. The oxytocin activates the cholinergic neurotransmission in the hippocampus and the reticular formation of the brainstem. Acetylcholine induces yawning via the muscarinic receptors of the effectors. Other neurotransmitters like serotonin, neuropeptides, hypocretin or sexual hormones can influence its occurrence (Argiolas and Melis 1998).

Sucking and swallowing
After Hooker (1952) had described sucking movements in a 14-week-old exteriorised fetus, Mori (1956), who applied hysteroscopy, found a drinking-like movement of the fetus in utero at no more than 12 weeks' gestation. We know from ultrasound recordings that from 14 weeks onwards (Figure 2.1), rhythmical bursts of regular jaw opening and closing at a rate of about 1–2 per second can be followed by swallowing movements, which indicates that the fetus is drinking amniotic fluid (Videos 7 and 23; Ianniruberto and Tajani 1981, de Vries et al 1982). Sucking and swallowing increase as pregnancy progresses (Roodenburg et al 1991). By 34 weeks, most healthy fetuses can suck and swallow well enough to sustain nutritional needs via the oral route, if born at this early age (Arvedson and Brodsky 1993, da Costa et al 2008, Delaney and Arvedson 2008). During the final weeks of fetal life, sucking increases, as does the amount of amniotic fluid swallowed: starting from 2–7ml per day, the fetus swallows 450–500ml per day by the end of pregnancy (Bosma 1986).

SUCKING
The sucking mechanism is only active when rhythmical mandibular and/or labial movements are followed by evidence of flow signals in the oronasal cavities (Grassi et al 2005). Sucking movements are controlled not only by central pattern generators but also by sensory feedback. The central pattern generator for sucking seems to consist of two

distinct parts: the brainstem (nucleus tractus solitarius and the dorsal medullar reticular formation) for motor control, and parts of the surrounding reticular formation for sensory control (da Costa et al 2008).

During the third trimester, the fetus may occasionally suck on the umbilical cord, possibly even for several minutes (Sherer et al 1991). This does not cause a cord occlusion, however, and is therefore not associated with fetal bradycardia.

FETAL SWALLOWING

During prenatal life, swallowing is both preparatory and functional. It is preparatory in the sense that the neonate must be capable of ingesting food actively; and it is functional in that fetal swallowing – along with urine flow and intramembraneous resorption of fluids – is one of the main regulators of the amniotic fluid volume. Moreover, swallowing is considered to enhance the growth and development of the mandibula (Sherer et al 1995) as well as the gastrointestinal tract (Pritchard 1966, Grassi et al 2005).

With advancing gestation, lingual movements increase in complexity – from simple forward thrusting and cupping to anterior–posterior motions; laryngeal movements change from shallow flutter-like movements along the lumen to more complex and complete adduction–abduction patterns (Miller et al 2003). At term, the fetus initiates swallowing with two to six sucking movements, before opening the mouth wide. Next, low-frequency tongue movements propel the fluid bolus into the hypopharynx (Petrikovsky et al 1995). In some fetuses, as a normal variant of fetal swallowing, the entry of the fluid bolus into the hypopharynx is followed by a prolonged pharyngeal dilatation, which is maintained for up to 40 minutes despite changes in the position of the neck (Petrikovsky et al 1996).

Liley (1972) speculated whether hunger could be the stimulus for fetal swallowing. Actually the amount of amniotic fluid that is normally swallowed contributes little to the caloric requirement of the fetus. The concentration of glucose in the amniotic fluid is somewhat less than that in blood, so the total amount of glucose normally ingested is less than 1g per day, even in late pregnancy. The amount of vernix caseosa ingested is unknown but must be rather small. Although the protein concentration in the amniotic fluid is typically less than 1g per 100ml, the ingestion of, say, 500ml of amniotic fluid per day might deliver enough protein to the gastrointestinal tract to contribute slightly to the requirements of fetal growth (Pritchard 1966, Pitkin and Reynolds 1975).

Regulation of the amniotic fluid volume

The volume of the amniotic fluid is kept in balance by constant fetal fluid production (lung liquid and urine) and resorption (swallowing and intramembranous flow). The regulatory mechanisms act on three levels: (1) placental control of water and solute transfer; (2) regulation of inflows and outflows from the fetus; and (3) a maternal effect on fetal fluid balance (Ross and Nijland 1997, Bacchi Modena and Fieni 2004). Amniotic fluid consists of water for the most part (98%). The chemical composition of its substances varies with gestational age. When fetal urine begins to enter the amniotic sac at 8–11 weeks' gestation, amniotic osmolarity decreases slightly compared with fetal blood. After keratinisation of the fetal skin at 22–25 weeks, amniotic fluid osmolarity decreases further with advancing gestational age (Gilbert and Brace 1989).

During the 40-week period of human gestation, about 4 litres of water accumulate within intrauterine compartments, with 2800ml in the fetus, 400ml in the placenta and 800ml in the amniotic fluid. At the beginning of pregnancy, the amniotic fluid exceeds the fetal volume many times over. At this point, fetal swallowing still has little effect on the amniotic fluid; in fact the volume swallowed is quite small compared with the total amniotic fluid (Pritchard 1966). Soon after mid-gestation, however, the amniotic fluid volume and the fetal volume harmonise; by 30 weeks, the amniotic fluid volume is only about half the fetal volume and at term it is no more than about a quarter (Bacchi Modena and Fieni 2004). It is estimated that the volume of amniotic fluid swallowed in late gestation averages 700ml per day (Pritchard 1966) and that swallowing occurs primarily during episodes of fetal breathing movements. Swallowing also serves to filter out some of the insoluble debris that is normally shed into the amniotic sac and sometimes excreted into it abnormally. Undigested portions remain in the intestine and can be identified in the meconium.

Increased fetal swallowing is sometimes found with polyhydramnios but it is still an intermittent activity.

Urogenital functions

MICTURITION

Leonardo da Vinci rightly suspected that the fetus micturated (Hill et al 1983). Today we know that fetal urine is a major source of amniotic fluid in the second half of pregnancy. Urine first enters the amniotic space at 8–11 weeks' gestation, after which the rate of urine production shows a steady increase (Abramovich and Page 1972). By the end of pregnancy, the urine production is approximately 50ml per hour (Rabinowitz et al 1989). It increases after furosemide has been administered to the mother intravenously (Wladimiroff 1975), which is clear evidence of fetal tubular function (i.e. reabsorption of water and electrolytes) during the latter period of gestation. At term, the fetal urine flow rate averages 700–900ml per day. It is modulated by arginine, vasopressin, aldosterone, angiotensin II and atrial natriuretic peptide in much the same way as in adults (Bacchi Modena and Fieni 2004). Voiding is a gradual process that can span over as long as 30 minutes – or be finished within a few seconds. External abdominal pressure directly on the fetal bladder (for example by means of a scanner) can stimulate voiding. Also, vibroacoustic stimulation may induce voiding (Zimmer et al 1993). The stream of urine can be strong enough to move the umbilical cord about within the amniotic cavity (Hill et al 1983).

By 16 weeks' gestation, the elongation of the genital tubercle is complete. Fetal penile erections can be observed (Jakobovits 2001, Odeh et al 2009), which implies that specific vasocongestion and myogenic irritability are present in the male external genitalia (Hitchcock et al 1980). As soon as the behavioural states are developed, fetal tumescence occurs more often and for longer periods during state 2F than during state 1F (Shirozu et al 1995).

The position and posture of the fetus

The general idea of a typical fetal posture is still one of all joints in flexion. The fetus's joints are, indeed, usually flexed, but sometimes the neck, trunk or limbs are extended. In fact, both the posture and the position of the fetus are variable, changing frequently, especially during the first half of pregnancy.

POSITIONAL CHANGES

In relation to the field of gravity, the fetal position alternates between cephalic, breech and transverse orientation (Reinold 1971, de Vries et al 1982, Ververs et al 1994). Positional changes are usually achieved by rotational movements along the longitudinal axis of the fetus, alternating leg movements, and even by somersaults. Such displacements increase from 10 weeks onwards and reach a maximum frequency at 13–15 weeks (de Vries et al 1982). Later on, positional changes decrease due to spatial constriction. At mid-gestation, the cephalic lie becomes slightly predominant and then increases dramatically week by week (Ververs et al 1994). In late pregnancy, the fetal position is influenced by the position of the placenta – which deforms the circular cross-section of the uterus to an oval – the shape of the maternal lumbar lordosis, and the inclination of the pelvic brim. The extent to which breech position influences fetal behaviour will be discussed in Chapter 7, p 125.

THERE IS NO PREFERRED POSTURE IN THE FETUS

In relation to the surface that the fetus is resting on, the posture can be supine, prone, lateral, sitting or standing upright or on the head. From 11 to 15 weeks' gestation, the supine posture predominates over all other postures; at 16–17 weeks the supine posture is as frequent as the lateral posture, but it decreases significantly at 18–19 weeks. The opposite is true of the frequency curve of the lateral posture (de Vries et al 1982). Especially during the first half of pregnancy, some fetuses raise their hands and place them behind the head; with semiflexed legs, they lie as though relaxing in a hammock. Some sit with crossed legs and an extended trunk, which resembles a yoga posture (Ianniruberto and Tajani 1981).

No fetal posture is predominant over a longer period (de Vries et al 1982). Similarly, the posture of low-risk preterm infants is intra-individually consistent, with virtually no age-specific inter-individual preference (Prechtl et al 1979, Vles et al 1989).

Fetuses may have postural deformities: asymmetrical deformities are usually caused by extrinsic factors such as uterine malformation, whereas symmetrical deformities may be caused by intrinsic factors like impairments of the central or peripheral nervous system, the muscles, the connective tissue or the skeleton (de Vries and Fong 2007).

THE FETAL ARM POSTURE IS AGE SPECIFIC

An arm posture during rest is defined by the flexion/extension of the elbow as well as the wrist and fingers. It can be observed from 12 weeks onwards (Ververs et al 1998). In contrast to the fetal body posture, the arm posture is clearly age related. It develops from a high incidence of (1) elbow flexion, wrist extension and finger extension at 12 weeks' gestation, to (2) elbow flexion, wrist extension and finger flexion from 16 to 28 weeks, and thereafter to (3) flexion of all three joints (Ververs et al 1998).

At least until mid-gestation, the fetus has plenty of space to move, which allows for large-amplitude limb movements and full extension of both arms. Hence, the early preference for elbow flexion is due to neuromaturation rather than being an expression of environmental restrictions. In fact, the ventromedial brainstem pathway that controls the proximal muscles of the upper limbs develops earlier than the lateral brainstem pathway controlling the distal muscles of the arm (Kuypers 1973).

As development advances, environmental restriction can, in fact, play a crucial role, as is shown by comparison between fetuses in a breech or cephalic position. Fetuses tend to keep their hands close to their head, which is in the upper part of the uterus when in breech position, and in the lower, narrower, part of the uterus when in cephalic position. Near term, fetuses in a breech position show less wrist flexion than cephalic fetuses, even though both groups follow the same developmental course of arm postures before that age (Fong et al 2005).

Quantitative aspects of fetal motility

There are tremendous differences in the activity levels of fetuses, even though they tend to stick to a particular scheme of motility throughout pregnancy, moving either a lot or little (Bekedam et al 1985, de Vries et al 1988, DiPietro et al 1996, ten Hof et al 2002). This intra-fetal consistency – and inter-fetal variability – is well-known to expectant mothers. Statements like 'she hardly kicked at all; this one is kicking all the time' are not without reason (Sadovsky et al 1979, Valentin et al 1984, Visser and Prechtl 1988). Furthermore, the frequency of each movement pattern varies greatly, because of the different movement generators (Figure 2.5). Some motor patterns such as isolated leg movements, yawning or stretches can be rare in a fetus that is otherwise very active (Figure 2.5); other patterns may occur relatively frequently in rather inactive fetuses (de Vries et al 1988). Finally, we must not forget that in the normal course of pregnancy several quantitative changes occur.

The movement patterns vary in their developmental courses: general movements increase during the first weeks of pregnancy; then they reach a plateau and remain at this level for the first two trimesters, only to decrease again. By contrast, isolated limb movements, breathing movements, side-to-side movements of the head, or sucking, all gradually increase in incidence. Yet another possible variant is the development of startles or hiccups, which increase rapidly during the first few weeks, followed by a gradual decline (Prechtl 1989, Roodenburg et al 1991).

Fetal motility clusters in rest/activity cycles until behavioural states set in (see Chapter 4). If all movement patterns are taken together, fetal activity decreases from 13–17% at the beginning of the third trimester to an average of 7% near term (Nasello-Paterson et al 1988, D'Elia et al 2001, ten Hof et al 2002). This decline in the amount of fetal movements at the end of pregnancy is not related to a restriction of the intrauterine space available to the growing fetus, but appears to be due to the maturation of inhibition (Prechtl 1989), since the low-risk preterm infant shows the same decline (Prechtl et al 1979).

DIURNAL VARIATIONS OF FETAL ACTIVITIES

As early as by 20–22 weeks' gestation (de Vries et al 1987), fetal activity shows a diurnal variation, with peaks of activity in the late evening (Sadovsky and Polishuk 1977, Patrick et al 1982, Visser et al 1982, Nasello-Paterson et al 1988, de Vries and Fong 2006), which corroborates mothers' reports (Goodlin and Lowe 1974, Ehrström 1984, Pillai and James 1990a). Above all, the increase in breathing movements during the afternoon (Figure 2.17) accounts for this diurnal variation (Roberts et al 1979, de Vries et al 1987). Head retroflexion and jaw opening also occur more often in the afternoon and evening than in the morning (Table 2.2). Since the percentage of general movements per hour basically remains constant throughout the day (Figure 2.18), general movements account for 50% of the total activity during the morning hours, but for only 30% during the evening hours.

At mid-gestation, diurnal variation of the basal fetal heart rate, which is closely related to the maternal heart rate variation (Lunshof et al 1998, Mirmiram et al 2003), also sets in (de Vries et al 1987). The underlying mechanism of this biological clock is poorly understood and caution is required in determining causal links. The suprachiasmatic nuclei in the anterior hypothalamus also seem to play an essential role in generating diurnal rhythms in early development (Reppert and Schwartz 1984, Lunshof et al 1997). Furthermore, maternal factors – especially maternal glucocorticoid levels – may play an important role, since heart rates of anencephalic fetuses with an aplasia that is rostral of the medulla oblongata show diurnal oscillations (Muro et al 1998).

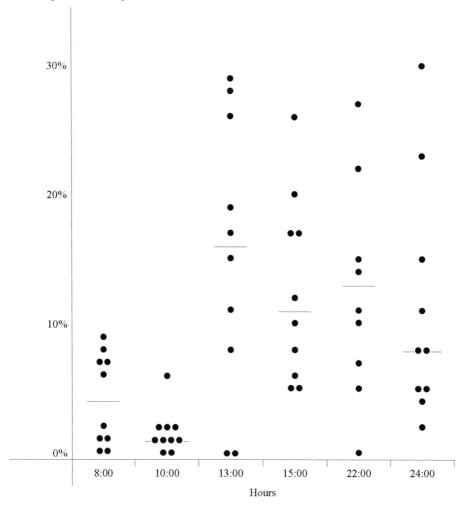

Breathing movements in per cent of time

Figure 2.17 Percentage of breathing movements per hour (median, –) observed at six different times of the day in 10 fetuses; age: 20–22 weeks' gestation. Adapted from de Vries JIP, Visser GHA, Mulder EJH, Prechtl HFR. (1987) Diurnal and other variations in fetal movements and other heart rate patterns. Early Hum Dev 15: 99–114, with permission.

Continuity of motor patterns from prenatal to postnatal life

While birth is an environmental discontinuity *par excellence*, the motor repertoire displays an impressive continuity from intrauterine to extrauterine life (Prechtl 1984a). The comparison of a third-trimester fetus (Video 7) with a preterm infant of almost the same age (Video 4) reveals that their movements are pretty much the same in spite of the fact that the respective environmental influences are quite different in terms of gravity, spatial

General movements in per cent of time

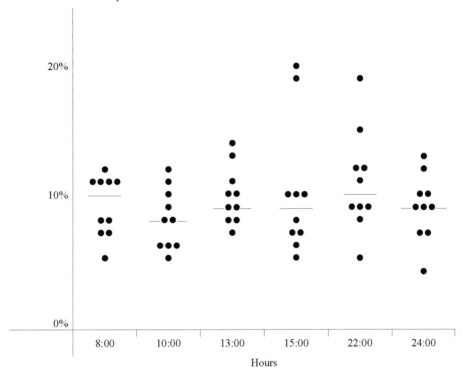

Hours

Figure 2.18 Percentage of general movements per hour (median, –) observed at six different times of the day in 10 fetuses; age: 20–22 weeks' gestation. Adapted from de Vries JIP, Visser GHA, Mulder EJH, Prechtl HFR. (1987) Diurnal and other variations in fetal movements and other heart rate patterns. *Early Hum Dev* 15: 99–114, with permission.

constriction and perceptual information. Neither preterm infants nor preterm fetuses change their motor repertoire in a way that would indicate functional reorganisation around term age (Prechtl 1986). This phenomenon was anticipated by Preyer, who wrote: 'the sometimes quick, sometimes slow, mostly uncoordinated, but sometimes coordinated extension and flexion of arms and legs of the newly born are nothing else than a continuation of the intrauterine movements' (Preyer 1890, p 161).

Some movements like stretches or yawns maintain their pattern throughout life, whereas other patterns such as general movements or sucking change at the end of the second month post-term (Hopkins and Prechtl 1984, Prechtl 1986, Iwayama and Eishima 1997, Einspieler et al 2008).

Anteflexion of the head and upward extension of the legs disappear temporarily after birth, only to reappear 15–18 weeks later (Hopkins and Prechtl 1984). It is questionable whether this striking paucity of antigravity mechanisms during the first postnatal months

TABLE 2.2
Incidence of the various movement patterns at 20-22 weeks' gestation (median [range]) in decreasing order at the morning hours, measured at three different times of the day

	8:00 to 10:00	**13:00 to 15:00**	**22:00 to 24:00**
Jaw movements	51 (11–205)	97 (19–280)[a]	85 (13–180)
Hiccup	28 (2–335)	12 (0–324)	13 (0–554)
Isolated arm movements	25 (3–70)	28 (11–62)	29 (7–84)
Side-to-side movements of the head	14 (1–63)	18 (0–43)	17 (1–45)
Retroflexion of the head	13 (2–34)	26 (8–45)[a]	28 (3–47)[a]
Sucking and swallowing	3 (0–42)	7 (0–50)	0 (0–49)
Hand-to-face contact	3 (0–35)	6 (1–39)	5 (0–32)
Startles	3 (0–15)	4 (0–22)	4 (0–21)
Anteflexion of the head	1 (0–24)	0 (0–43)	1 (0–20)
Isolated leg movements	0 (0–28)	2 (0–45)	0 (0–8)
Yawning	0 (0–0)	0 (0–2)	0 (0–1)

Breathing movements and general movements are given in separate figures (Figs 2.16 and 2.17).
[a]Significantly higher than in the morning, $p<0.01$. Adapted from de Vries JIP, Visser GHA, Mulder EJH, Prechtl HFR. (1987) Diurnal and other variations in fetal movements and other heart rate patterns. *Early Hum Dev* 15: 99–114, with permission.

is due to limited muscle power or to the slow development of adequate central neural mechanisms. The sudden onset of distinct antigravity movements at 3–4 months seems to indicate that the latter is the case.

A set of endogenously generated motor patterns gradually comes under afferent control after birth (Prechtl 1984b, 2001b). Rooting is an outstanding example: a rhythmical side-to-side head movement in the fetus (Video 16), it aligns with the stimulated perioral area in the young infant (Video 17). While in the fetus sucking movements are endogenously generated (Video 23), they need to be triggered after birth in the actual feeding situation (Video 24). Hence, it is a matter of vital biological adaptation that rooting and sucking are elicited in the proper feeding situation, which is now initiated by the caregiver. Other examples of endogenously generated motor patterns that need to come under sensory control are breathing movements and smiling movements. Endogenous smiling – often one-sided in the fetus, the preterm and term infant – is superseded by elicited social smiling at 6–8 weeks after birth or at a corresponding conceptional age for preterm infants (van Wulfften Palthe and Hopkins 1984).

REFERENCES

Abd-El-Aal DE, Shahin AY, Hamed HO. (2009) Effect of short-term maternal fasting in the third trimester on uterine, umbilical, and fetal middle cerebral artery Doppler indices. *Int J Gynaecol Obstet* 107: 23–25.

Abramovich DR, Page KR. (1972) Pathways of water exchange in the fetoplacental unit at mid-pregnancy. *J Obstet Gynaecol Br Commonw* 79: 1099–1102.

Adamson SL, Bocking A, Cousin AJ, Rapoport I, Patrick JE. (1983) Ultrasonic measurement of rate and depth of human fetal breathing: effect of glucose. *Am J Obstet Gynecol* 147: 288–295.

Agustsson P, Patel NB. (1987) The predictive value of fetal breathing movements in the diagnosis of preterm labour. *Br J Obstet Gynaecol* 94: 860–863.

Ahlfeld F. (1888) [Previously undescribed intrauterin movements of the child]. *Verhandl Dt Gesell Gynäkol* 2: 203–210. (In German)

Argiolas A, Melis MR. (1998) The neuropharmacology of yawning. *Eur J Pharmacol* 343: 1–16.

Arvedson JC, Brodsky L. (1993) *Pediatric Swallowing and Feeding. Assessment and Management.* San Diego: Singular Publishing Group.

Baarsma R, Bekedam DJ, Visser GHA. (1993) Qualitative abnormal fetal breathing movements, associated with tracheal atresia. *Early Hum Dev* 32: 63–69.

Bacchi Modena A, Fieni S. (2004) Amniotic fluid dynamics. *Acta Bio Med Ateneo Parmense* 75(Suppl): 11–13.

Ball RH, Parer JT. (1992) The physiological mechanisms of variable decelerations. *Am J Obstet Gynecol* 166: 1683–1689.

Barcroft J. (1946) *Researches on Pre-Natal Life.* Oxford: Blackwell.

Bekedam DJ, Visser GHA, de Vries JIP, Prechtl HFR. (1985) Motor behaviour of the growth retarded fetus. *Early Hum Dev* 12: 155–165.

Bekoff M, Byers JA, Bekoff A. (1980) Prenatal motility and postnatal play: functional continuity? *Dev Psychobiol* 13: 225–228.

Bellieni CV, Severi F, Bocchi C, Caparelli N, Bagnoli F, Buonocore G, Petraglia F. (2005) Blink-startle reflex habituation in 30–34-week low-risk fetuses. *J Perinat Med* 33: 33–37.

Benoit P, Changeux JP. (1975) Consequences of tenotomy on the evolution of multi-innervation in developing rat soleus muscle. *Brain Res* 99: 354–358.

Birnholz JC. (1981) The development of human fetal eye movement patterns. *Science* 213: 679–681.

Birnholz JC. (1985) Ultrasonic fetal ophthalmology. *Early Hum Dev* 12: 199–209.

Birnholz JC, Benacerraf BR. (1983) The development of human fetal hearing. *Science* 222: 516–518.

Birnholz JC, Stephens JC, Faria M. (1978) Fetal movement patterns: a possible means of defining neurological developmental milestones in utero. *Am J Roentgenol* 130: 537–540.

Blair RG. (1965) Vagitus uterinus. Crying in utero. *Lancet* 2(7423): 1164–1165.

Blott M, Greenough A. (1988) Oligohydramnios in the second trimester of pregnancy, fetal breathing and normal lung growth. *Early Hum Dev* 17: 37–40.

Blott M, Greenough A, Nicolaides KH, Campbell S. (1990) The ultrasonographic assessment of the fetal thorax and fetal breathing movements in the prediction of pulmonary hypoplasia. *Early Hum Dev* 21: 143–151.

Bocking AD. (2003) Assessment of fetal heart rate and fetal movements in detecting oxygen deprivation in-utero. *Eur J Obstet Gynecol Reprod Biol* 110: S108–S112.

Bocking AD, Adamson SL, Cousin A, Campbell K, Carmichael L, Natale R, Patrick J. (1982) Effects of intravenous glucose injections on human fetal breathing movements and gross fetal body movements at 38 to 40 weeks gestational age. *Am J Obstet Gynecol* 142: 606–611.

Bosma JF. (1986) Development of feeding. *Clin Nutr* 5: 210–218.

Bots RSGM, Broeders GHB, Farman DJ, Haverkorn MJ, Stolte LAM. (1978) Fetal breathing movements in the growth retarded human fetus: a multiscan M-mode echofetographic study. *Eur J Obstet Gynecol Reprod Biol* 8: 21–29.

Bots RSGM, Nijhuis JG, Martin CB, Prechtl HFR. (1981) Human fetal eye movements: detection in utero by means of ultrasonography. *Early Hum Dev* 5: 87–94.

Boué J, Vignal P, Aubry JP, Aubry MC, Mac Aleese J. (1982) Ultrasound movement patterns of fetuses with chromosome anomalies. *Prenat Diagn* 2: 61–65.

Bowie JD, Clair MR. (1982) Fetal swallowing and regurgitation: observation of normal and abnormal activity. *Radiol* 144: 877–878.

Boylan P, O'Donovan P, Owens OJ. (1985) Fetal breathing movements and the diagnosis of labor: a prospective analysis of 100 cases. *Obstet Gynecol* 66: 517–520.

Bradley NS. (2001) Age-related changes and condition-dependent modifications in distribution of limb movements during embryonic motility. *J Neurophysiol* 86: 1511–1522.

Bridgeman B. (1983) Phasic eye movement control appears before tonic control in human fetal development. *Invest Ophtalmol Vis Sci* 24: 658–659.

Brotanek V, Lopez JS. (1991) An unusual cause and treatment of decelerations in fetal heart rate. *Int J Gynecol Obstet* 34: 271–275.

Campbell S. (2002) 4D, or not 4D: that is the question. *Ultrasound Obstet Gynecol* 19: 1–4.

Carmichael L, Campbell K, Patrick J. (1984) Fetal breathing, gross fetal body movements, and maternal and fetal heart rates before spontaneous labor at term. *Am J Obstet Gynecol* 148: 675–679.

Castle BM, Turnbull AC. (1983) The presence or absence of fetal breathing movements predicts the outcome of preterm labour. *Lancet* 2(8348): 471–473.

Cheng J, Jovanovic K, Aoyagi Y, Bennett DJ, Han Y, Stein RB. (2002) Differential distribution of interneurons in the neural networks that control walking in the mudpuppy (*Necturus maculatus*) spinal cord. *Exp Brain Res* 145: 190–198.

Cioni G, Prechtl HFR. (1990) Preterm and early postterm motor behaviour in low-risk premature infants. *Early Hum Dev* 23: 159–191.

Collins JH. (1994) Fetal grasping of the umbilical cord with simultaneous fetal heart rate monitoring. *Am J Obstet Gynecol* 170: 1836.

Connors G, Hunse C, Carmichael L, Natale R, Richardson B. (1989) Control of fetal breathing in the human fetus between 24 and 34 weeks' gestation. *Am J Obstet Gynecol* 160: 932–938.

Cosmi EV, Cosmi E, La Torre R. (2001) The effects of fetal breathing movements on the utero-fetal-placental circulation. *Early Pregnancy* 5: 51–52.

Cosmi EV, Anceschi MM, Cosmi E, Piazze JJ, La Torre R. (2003) Ultrasonographic patterns of fetal breathing movements in normal pregnancy. *Int J Gynaecol Obstet* 80: 285–290.eosophagus on electrocardiogram of the fetus

Cremer M. (1906) [On direct recordings of action potentials of the human heart above the eosophagus on electrocardiogram of the fetus] *Münch Med Wochenschr* 53: 811–821. (In German)

da Costa SP, van den Engel-Hoek L, Bos AF. (2008) Sucking and swallowing in infants and diagnostic tools. *J Perinatol* 28: 247–257.

Darwin C. (1872/1920) *The Expressions of the Emotions in Man and Animals.* New York: Appleton.

Dawes GS. (1973) Revolutions and cyclical rhythms in prenatal life: fetal respiratory movements rediscovered. *Pediatr* 51: 965–971.

de Elejalde MM, Elejalde BR. (1985) Ultrasonographic visualization of the fetal eye. *J Craniofac Genet Dev Biol* 5: 319–326.

Delaney AL, Arvedson JC. (2008) Development of swallowing and feeding: prenatal through first year of life. *Dev Dis Res Rev* 14: 105–117.

D'Elia A, Pighetti M, Moccia G, Santangelo N. (2001) Spontaneous motor activity in normal fetuses. *Early Hum Dev* 65: 139–147.

Devoe LD, Abduljabbar H, Carmichael L, Probert C, Patrick J. (1984) The effects of maternal hyperoxia on fetal breathing movements in third-trimester pregnancies. *Am J Obstet Gynecol* 148: 790–794.

de Vries JIP, Fong BF. (2006) Normal fetal motility: an overview. *Ultrasound Obstet Gynecol* 27: 701–711.

de Vries JIP, Fong BF. (2007) Changes in fetal motility as a result of congenital disorders: an overview. *Ultrasound Obstet Gynecol* 29: 590–599.

de Vries JIP, Visser GHA, Prechtl HFR. (1982) The emergence of fetal behaviour. I. Qualitative aspects. *Early Hum Dev* 7: 301–322.

de Vries JIP, Visser GHA, Prechtl HFR. (1985) The emergence of fetal behaviour. II: Quantitative aspects. *Early Hum Dev* 12: 99–120.

de Vries JIP, Visser GHA, Mulder EJH, Prechtl HFR. (1987) Diurnal and other variations in fetal movements and other heart rate patterns. *Early Hum Dev* 15: 99–114.

de Vries JIP, Visser GHA, Prechtl HFR. (1988) The emergence of fetal behaviour. III. Individual differences and consistencies. *Early Hum Dev* 16: 85–103.

DiPietro JA, Hodgson DM, Costigan KA, Hilton SC, Johnson TR. (1996) Fetal neurobehavioural development. *Child Dev* 67: 2553–2567.

Divon MY, Zimmer EZ, Yeh SY, Vilenski A, Sarna Z, Paldi E, Platt LD. (1985) Effect of maternal intravenous glucose administration on fetal heart rate patterns and fetal breathing. *Am J Perinatol* 2: 292–294.

Dornan JC, Ritchie JW. (1983) Fetal breathing movements and maternal hyperoxia in the growth retarded fetus. *Br J Obstet Gynaecol* 90: 210–213.

Dornan JC, Ritchie JWK, Meban C. (1984a) Fetal breathing movements and lung maturation in the congenitally abnormal human fetus. *J Dev Physiol* 6: 367–374.

Dornan JC, Ritchie JW, Ruff SS. (1984b) The rate and regularity of breathing movements in the normal and growth-retarded fetus. *Br J Obstet Gynaecol* 91: 31–36.

Dunne ME, Johnson ML. (1979) The ultrasonic demonstration of fetal abnormalities in utero. *J Reprod Med* 23: 195–206.

Ehrström C. (1984) Circadian rhythm of fetal movements. *Acta Obstet Gynecol Scand* 63: 539–541.

Einspieler C, Prechtl HFR, Bos AF, Ferrari F, Cioni G. (2004) *Prechtl's Method on the Qualitative Assessment of General Movements in Preterm, Term and Young Infants. Clinics in Developmental Medicine No. 167*. London: Mac Keith Press.

Einspieler C, Marschik PB. Prechtl HFR. (2008) Human motor behaviour. Prenatal origin and early postnatal development. *J Psychol* 216: 147–153

Eyre JA, Miller S, Clowry GJ, Conway EA, Watts C. (2000) Functional corticospinal projections are established prenatally in the human foetus permitting involvement in the development of spinal motor centres. *Brain* 123: 51–64.

Ezure H. (1996) Development of the motor endplates in the masseter muscle in the human fetus. *Ann Anat* 178: 15–23.

Fidziańska A, Goebel HH. (1991) Human ontogenesis. 3. Cell death in fetal muscle. *Acta Neuropathol* 81: 572–577.

Fong B, Savelsbergh GJP, van Geijn HP, de Vries JIP. (2005) Does intra-uterine environment influence fetal head-position preference? A comparison between breech and cephalic presentation. *Early Hum Dev* 81: 507–517.

Forssberg H. (1999) Neural control of human motor development. *Curr Opin Neurobiol* 9: 676–682.

Fox HE, Badalian SS, Timor-Tritsch IE, Marks F, Stolar CJ. (1993) Fetal upper respiratory tract function in cases of antenatally diagnosed congenital diaphragmatic hernia: preliminary observation. *Ultrasound Obstet Gynecol* 3: 164–167.

Gallup AC, Gallup GG Jr. (2008) Yawning and thermoregulation. *Physiol Behav* 95: 10–16.

Giganti F, Hayes MJ, Akilesh MR, Salzarulo P. (2002) Yawning and behavioural states in premature infants. *Dev Psychobiol* 41: 289–293.

Gilbert WM, Brace RA. (1989) The missing link in amniotic fluid volume regulation: Intramembraneous absorption. *Obstet Gynecol* 74: 748–754.

Goodlin RC. (1979) History of fetal monitoring. *Am J Obstet Gynecol* 133: 323–352.

Goodlin RC, Lowe EW. (1974) Multiphasic fetal monitoring. *Am J Obstet Gynecol* 119: 341–357.

Goto S, Kato TK. (1983) Early movements are useful for estimating the gestational weeks in the first trimester of pregnancy. *Ultrasound Pregn Biol Suppl* 2: 577–582.

Gottlieb G. (1976) Conceptions of prenatal development: behavioural embryology. *Psychol Rev* 83: 215–234.

Grassi R, Farina R, Floriani I, Amodio F, Romano S. (2005) Assessment of fetal swallowing with gray-scale and color Doppler sonography. *Am J Radiol* 185: 1322–1327.

Grillner S. (1999) Bridging the gap – from ion channels to networks and behaviour. *Curr Opin Neurobiol* 9: 663–669.

Guertin PA. (2009) The mammalian central pattern generator for locomotion. *Brain Res Rev* 62: 45–56.

Habek D, Habek JC, Barbir A, Barbir M, Granić P. (2003) Fetal grasping of the umbilical cord and perinatal outcome. *Arch Gynecol Obstet* 268: 274–277.

Habek D, Kulaš, Selthofer R, Rosso M, Popović Z, Petrović D, Ugljarević M. (2006) 3D-ultrasound detection of fetal grasping of the umbilical cord and fetal outcome. *Fetal Diagn Ther* 21: 332–333.

Hamburger V. (1963) Some aspects of the embryology of behavior. *Q Rev Biol* 38: 342–365.

Hamburger V, Wenger E, Oppenheim R. (1966) Motility in the absence of sensory input. *J Exp Zool* 162: 133–160.

Harper MA, Meis PJ, Rose JC, Swain M, Burns J, Kardon B. (1987) Human fetal breathing response to intravenous glucose is directly related to gestational age. *Am J Obstet Gynceol* 157: 1403–1405.

Harris PF, Bagnali KM, Mahon M, Scott EM. (1977) Fetal hiccups and fetal movements. *Lancet* 310: 560–561.

Harris WA. (1981) Neural activity and development. *Annu Rev Physiol* 43: 689–710.

Hasan SU, Bharadwaj B, Remmers JE, Patel A, Rigaux A, Schneider J. (2008) Pulmonary feedback and gestational age-dependent regulation of fetal breathing movements. *Can J Physiol Pharmacol* 86: 691–699.

Hata T, Kanenishi K, Akiyama M, Tanaka H, Kimura K. (2005) Real-time 3-D sonographic observation of fetal facial expression. *J Obstet Gynaecol Res* 31: 337–340.

Hepper PG, Shahidullah S. (1992) Trisomy 18: Behavioural and structural abnormalities. An ultrasonographic case study. *Ultrasound Obstet Gynecol* 2: 48–50.

Heusner AP. (1946) Yawning and associated phenomena. *Physiol Rev* 25: 156–168.

Heyl W, Rath W. (1996) Intrapartum therapy-resistant fetal bradycardia-color Doppler sonographic diagnosis of umbilical cord compression due to fetal grasping. *Z Geburtshilfe Neonatol* 200: 30–32.

Higginbottom J, Bagnall KM, Harris PF, Slater JH, Porter GA. (1976) Ultrasound monitoring of fetal movements – a method for assessing fetal development? *Lancet* 1(7962): 719–723.

Higuchi M, Hirano H, Gotoh K, Otomo K, Maki M. (1991) Relationship between the duration of fetal breathing movements and gestational age and the development of the central nervous system at 25–32 weeks of gestation in normal pregnancy. *Gynecol Obstet Invest* 31: 136–140.

Hill LM, Breckle R, Wolfgram KR. (1983) An ultrasonic view of the developing fetus. *Obstet Gynecol Surv* 38: 375–398.

Hitchcock DA, Sutphen JH, Scholly TA. (1980) Demonstration of fetal penile erection in utero. *Perinatol Neonatal* 4: 59–60.

Honest H, Bachmann LM, Sengupta R, Gupta JK, Kleijnen J, Khan KS. (2004) Accuracy of absence of fetal breathing movements in predicting preterm birth: a systematic review. *Ultrasound Obstet Gynecol* 24: 94–100.

Hooker D. (1938) *Evidence of Prenatal Function of the Central Nervous System in Man*. New York: American Museum of Natural History.

Hooker D. (1952) *The Prenatal Origin of Behavior*. Lawrence: University of Kansa Press.

Hopkins B, Prechtl HFR. (1984) A qualitative approach to the development of movements during early infancy. In: Prechtl HFR, editor. *Continuity of Neural Functions From Prenatal to Postnatal Life. Clinics in Developmental Medicine No. 94.* Oxford: Blackwell. p 179–197.

Horimoto N, Koyanagi T, Nagata S, Nakahara H, Nakano H. (1989) Concurrence of mouthing movements and rapid eye movement/non rapid eye movement phases with advance in gestation of the human fetus. *Am J Obstet Gynecol* 161: 344–351.

Horimoto N, Koyanagi T, Satoh S, Yoshizato T, Nakano H. (1990) Fetal eye movement assessed with real-time ultrasonography: are there rapid and slow eye movements? *Am J Obstet Gynecol* 163: 1480–1484.

Humphrey T. (1964) Some correlations between the appearance of human fetal reflexes and the development of the nervous system. *Prog Brain Res* 4: 93–135.

Ianniruberto A, Tajani E. (1981) Ultrasonographic study of fetal movements. *Semin Perinatol* 5: 175–181.

Inanlou MR, Baguma-Nibasheka M, Kablar B. (2005) The role of fetal breathing-like movements in lung organogenesis. *Histol Histopathol* 20: 1261–1266.

Inoue M, Koyanagi T, Nakahara H, Hara K, Hori E, Nakano H. (1986) Functional development of human eye movement in utero assessed quantitatively with real-time ultrasound. *Am J Obstet Gynecol* 155: 170–174.

Iwayama K, Eishima M. (1997) Neonatal sucking behaviour and its development until 14 months. *Early Hum Dev* 47: 1–9.

Jacobs MJ. (1967) Development of normal motor behaviour. *Am J Phys Med* 46: 41–51.

Jakobovits AA. (2001) Fetal penile erection. *Ultrasound Obstet Gynecol* 18: 405.

James DJ, Pillai M, Smoleniec J. (1995) Neurobehavioural development in the human fetus. In: Lecanuet JP, Fifer WP, Krasnegor NA, Smotherman WP, editors. *Fetal Development. A Psychobiological Perspective*. Hillsdale, Hove: Lawrence Erlbaum Associates. p 101–128.

Joshi S, Kotecha S. (2007) Lung growth and development. *Early Hum Dev* 83: 789–794.

Jouppila P, Piiroinen O. (1975) Ultrasonic diagnosis of fetal life in early pregnancy. *Obstet Gynecol* 46: 616–620.

Kahrilas PJ, Shi G. (1997) Why do we hiccup? *Gut* 41: 712–713.

Kalache KD, Chaoui R, Narks B, Wauer R, Bollmann R. (2002) Does fetal tracheal fluid flow during fetal breathing movements change before the onset of labor? *Br J Obstet Gynaecol* 109: 514–519.

Karson CN. (1982) Spontaneous eye blink rates and dopaminergic system. *Brain* 106: 643–653.

Katz K, Mashiach R, Bar On A, Merlob P, Soudry M, Meizner I. (1999) Normal range of fetal knee movements. *J Pediatr Orthop* 19: 739–741.

Katz K, Mashiach R, Meizner I. (2007) Normal range of fetal finger movements. *J Pediatr Orthop B* 16: 252–255.

Kim SY, Khandelwal M, Gaughan JP, Agar MH, Reece EA. (2003) Is the intrapartum biophysical profile useful? *Obstet Gynecol* 102: 471–476.

Kisilevsky BS, Hains SMJ, Low JA. (1999) Maturation of body and breathing movements in 24–33 week-old fetuses threatening to deliver prematurely. *Early Hum Dev* 55: 25–38.

Kivikovski A, Amon E, Vaalamo PO, Pirhonen J, Kopta MM. (1988) Effect of third-trimester premature rupture of membranes on fetal breathing movements: a prospective case-control study. *Am J Obstet Gynecol* 159: 1474–1477.

Konstantinidou AD, Silos-Santiago I, Flaris N, Snider WD. (1995) Development of the primary afferent projection in human spinal cord. *J Comp Neurol* 354: 11–12.

Kozuma S, Okai T, Nemoto A, Kagawa H, Sakai M, Nishina H, Taketani Y. (1997) Developmental sequence of human fetal body movements in the second half of pregnancy. *Am J Perinatol* 14: 165–169.

Koyanagi T, Horimoto N, Takashima T, Satoh S, Maeda H, Nakano H. (1993) Ontogenesis of ultradian rhythm in the human fetus, observed through the alternation of eye movement and no eye movement periods. *J Reprod Infant Psychol* 11: 129–134.

Kuno A, Akiyama M, Yamashiro C, Tanaka H, Yanagihara T, Hata T. (2001) Three-dimensional sonographic assessment of fetal behavior in the early second trimester of pregnancy. *J Ultrasound Med* 20: 1271–1275.

Kurjak A, Azumedi G, Vecek N, Kupesic S, Solak M, Varga D, Chervenak F. (2003) Fetal hand movements and facial expression in normal pregnancy studied by four-dimensional sonography. *J Perinat Med* 31: 496–508.

Kuypers HGJM. (1973) The anatomical organization of the descending pathways and their contribution to motor control, especially in primates. In: Desmedt JE, editor. *New Developments in Electromyography and Clinical Neurophysiology. Vol 3*. Basel: Karger. p 38–68.

Levi A, Benvenisti O, David D. (2000) Significant beat-to-beat hemodynamic changes in fetal circulation: A consequence of abrupt intrathoracic pressure variation induced by hiccup. *J Am Soc Echocardiogr* 13: 295–299.

Liley AW. (1972) The fetus as a personality. *Austral New Zealand J Psychiatr* 6: 99–105.

Lüchinger AB, Hadders-Algra M, van Kan CM, de Vries JIP. (2008) Fetal onset of general movements. *Pediatr Res* 63: 191–195.

Lunshof S, Boer K, van Hoffen G, Wolf H, Mirmiran M. (1997) The diurnal rhythm in fetal heart rate in a twin pregnancy with discordant anencephaly: comparison with three normal twin pregnancies. *Early Hum Dev* 48: 47–57.

Lunshof S, Boer K, Wolf H, van Hoffen G, Bayram N, Mirmiram M. (1998) Fetal and maternal diurnal rhythms during the third trimester of normal pregnancy: outcomes of computerized analysis of continuous twenty-four-hour fetal heart rate recordings. *Am J Obstet Gynecol* 178: 247–254.

Lynch JA, Aserinsky E. (1986) Developmental changes of oculomotor characteristics in infants when awake and in the 'active state of sleep'. *Behav Brain Res* 20: 175–183.

Manning FA, Wyn Pugh E, Boddy K. (1975) Effect of cigarette smoking on fetal breathing movements in normal pregnancies. *Br Med J* 8: 552–553.

Maršál K. (1983) Ultrasonic assessment of fetal activity. *Clin Obstet Gynaecol* 10: 541–563.

Maršál K, Lindblad A, Lingman G, Eik-Nes SH. (1984) Blood flow in the fetal descending aorta; intrinsic factors affecting fetal blood flow, i.e. fetal breathing movements and cardiac arrhythmia. *Ultrasound Biol* 10: 339–348.

Masuzaki H, Masuzaki M, Ishimaru T. (1996) Color Doppler imaging of fetal yawning. *Ultrasound Obstet Gynecol* 8: 355–360.

McLeod W, Brien J, Loomis C, Carmichael L, Probert C, Patrick J. (1983) Effect of maternal ethanol ingestion on fetal breathing movements, gross body movements and heart rate at 37 to 40 weeks' gestational age. *Am J Obstet Gynecol* 145: 251–257.

Miller JL, Sonies BC, Macedonia C. (2003) Emergence of oropharyngeal, laryngeal and swallowing activity in the developing fetal upper aerodigestive tract: an ultrasound evaluation. *Early Hum Dev* 71: 61–87.

Mirghani HM, Weerasinghe DS, Ezimokhai M, Smith JR. (2003) The effect of maternal fasting on the biophysical profile. *Int J Gynaecol Obstet* 81: 17–21.

Mirmiran M, Maas YGH, Ariagno RL. (2003) Development of fetal and neonatal sleep and circadian rhythms. *Sleep Med Rev* 7: 321–334.

Moessinger AC. (1983) Fetal akinesia deformation sequence: an animal model. *Pediatr* 72: 857–863.

Molliver ME, Kostovic I, van der Loos H. (1973) The development of synapses in the cerebral cortex of the human fetus. *Brain Res* 50: 403–407.

Mori C. (1956) A study on the intrauterine self-movement of early human fetus by hysteroscopy and its recording on the film. *J Jpn Obstet Gynecol Soc* 3: 374–388.

Morison JE. (1952) *Fetal and Neonatal Pathology.* London: Butterworth.

Mueller GM, Sipes SL. (1993) Isolated reversed umbilical arterial blood flow on Doppler ultrasonography and fetal hiccups. *J Ultrasound Med* 12: 541–643.

Mulder EJH, Visser GHA. (1987) Braxton Hicks' contractions and motor behaviour in the near-term human fetus. *Am J Obstet Gynecol* 156: 543–549.

Mulder EJH, Leiblum DM, Visser GHA. (1995) Fetal breathing movements in late diabetic pregnancy: relationship to fetal heart rate patterns and Braxton Hicks' contractions. *Early Hum Dev* 43: 225–232.

Mulder EJ, Beemer FA, Stoutenbeek P. (2001) Restrictive dermopathy and fetal behaviour. *Prenatal Diagn* 21: 581–585.

Muro M, Shono H, Ito Y, Sugimori H. (1998) Diurnal variation in baseline heart rate of anencephalic fetuses. *Psychiatry Clin Neurosci* 52: 173–174.

Nasello-Paterson, C, Natale R, Connors G. (1988) Ultrasonic evaluation of fetal body movements over twenty-four hours in the human fetus at twenty-four to twenty-eight weeks gestation. *Am J Obstet Gynecol* 158: 312–316.

Natale R, Nasello-Paterson C, Connors G. (1988) Patterns of fetal breathing activity in the human fetus at 24 to 28 weeks of gestation. *Am J Obstet Gynecol* 158: 317–321.

Nijhuis JG. (2003) Fetal behaviour. *Neurobiol Aging* 24: S41–S46.

Nijhuis JG, Visser GHA. (2003) Discussion to 'Fetal behaviour' by Jan G. Nijhuis and 'Fetal behaviour: a commentary' by Gerard H.A. Visser *Neurobiol Aging* 24: S51–S52.

Nijhuis JG, Staisch KJ, Martin CB Jr, Prechtl HFR. (1984) A sinusoidal-like fetal heart-rate pattern in association with fetal sucking – report on two cases. *Eur J Obstet Gynecol Reprod Biol* 16: 353–358.

Nijhuis JG, Jongsma HW, Crijns IJMJ, de Valk IMGM, van der Velden JWHJ. (1986) Effects of maternal glucose ingestion on human fetal breathing movements at weeks 24 and 28 of gestation. *Early Hum Dev* 13: 183–188.

O'Brien RAD, Östberg AJC, Vrbová G. (1978) Observations on the elimination of polyneural innervation in developing mammalian skeletal muscle. *J Physiol* 282: 571–582.

Odeh M, Granin V, Kais M, Ophir E, Bornstein J. (2009) Sonographic fetal sex determination. *Obstet Gynecol Surv* 64: 50–57.

Okado N. (1980) Development of the human cervical spinal cord with reference to synapse formation in the motor nucleus. *J Comp Neurol* 191: 495–513.

Okado N. (1981) Onset of synapse formation in the human spinal cord. *J Comp Neurol* 201: 211–219.

Okado N. (1982) Early myelin formation and glia cell development in the human spinal cord. *Anat Rec* 202: 483–490.

Okado N, Kojima T. (1984) Ontogeny of the central nervous system: neurogenesis, fibre connection, synaptogenesis and myelination in the spinal cord. In: Prechtl HFR, editor. *Continuity of Neural Functions From Prenatal to Postnatal Life. Clinics in Developmental Medicine No. 94.* London: Spastics International Medical Publications. p 31–45.

Okado N, Kakimi S, Kojima T. (1979) Synaptogenesis in the cervical cord of the human embryo. Sequence of synapse formation in a spinal reflex pathway. *J Comp Neurol* 184: 491–518.

Onimaru H. (1995) Studies of the respiratory center using isolated brainstem-spinal cord preparations. *Neurosci Res* 21: 183–190.

Oppenheim RW. (1981a) Neuronal cell death and some related regressive phenomena during neurogenesis: a selective historical review and progress report. In: Cowan WM, editor. *Studies in Developmental Neurobiology: Essays in Honor of Viktor Hamburger.* New York: Oxford University Press. p 74–133.

Oppenheim RW. (1981b) Ontogenetic adaptations and retrogressive processes in the development of the nervous system and behaviour: A neuroembryological perspective. In: Connolly KJ, Prechtl HFR, editors. *Maturation and Development: Biological and Psychological Perspectives. Clinics in Developmental Medicine No. 77/78.* London: Spastics International Medical Publications. p 73–109.

Oppenheim RW. (1982) The neuroembryological study of behaviour: progress, problems, perspectives. In: Hunt RK, editor. *Neural Development. Part III. Curr Top Dev Biol 17.* New York: Academic Press. p 257–309.

Oppenheim RW, Pittman R, Gray M, Maderdrut JL. (1978) Embryonic behaviour, hatching and neuromuscular development in the chick following a transient reduction of spontaneous motility and sensory input by neuromuscular blocking agents. *J Comp Neurol* 179: 619–640.

Oppenheim RW, Calderó J, Cuitat D, Esquerda J, Ayala V, Prevette D, Wang S. (2003) Rescue of developing spinal motorneurons from programmes cell death by the GABAA agonist muscimol acts by blockade of neuromuscular activity and increased intramuscular nerve branching. *Mol Cell Neurosci* 22: 331–343.

Patrick C, Challis J. (1980) Measurement of human fetal breathing movements in healthy pregnancies using a real-time scanner. *Semin Perinatol* 4: 275–286.

Patrick J, Fetherston W, Vick H, Voegelin R. (1978a) Human fetal breathing movements and gross fetal body movements at weeks 34 to 35 gestation. *Am J Obstet Gynecol* 130: 693–699.

Patrick J, Natale R, Richardson B. (1978b) Patterns of human fetal breathing activity at 34 to 35 weeks gestational age. *Am J Obstet Gynecol* 132: 507–513.

Patrick J, Campbell K, Carmichael L, Natale R, Richardson B. (1980) Patterns of human fetal breathing during the last 10 days of pregnancy. *Obstet Gynecol* 56: 24–30.

Patrick J, Campbell K, Carmichael L, Natale R, Richardson B. (1982) Patterns of gross fetal body movements over 24-hour observation intervals during the last 10 weeks of pregnancy. *Am J Obstet Gynecol* 146: 363–371.

Pearson KG. (2000) Neural adaption in the generation of rhythmic behaviour. *Annu Rev Physiol* 62: 723–753.

Peiper A. (1949) [The Singularity of Childlike Brain Activity]. Leipzig: Thieme. (In German)

Pena SDJ, Shokeir MHK. (1974) Syndrome of camptodactyly, multiple ankyloses, facial anomalies and pulmonary hypoplasia: a lethal condition. *J Pediatr* 85: 373–375.

Petrikovsky BM, Kaplan GP. (1993) Fetal grasping of the umbilical cord causing variable fetal heart rate decelerations. *J Clin Ultrasound* 21: 642–644.

Petrikovsky BM, Kaplan GP, Pestrak H. (1995) The application of color Doppler technology to the study of fetal swallowing. *Obstet Gynecol* 86: 605–608.

Petrikovsky BM, Gross B, Kaplan GP. (1996) Fetal pharyngeal distention – is it a normal component of fetal swallowing? *Early Hum Dev* 46: 77–81.

Petrikovsky BM, Kaplan G, Holsten N. (1999) Fetal yawning activity in normal and high-risk fetuses: a preliminary observation. *Ultrasound Obstet Gynecol* 13: 127–130.

Petrikovsky BM, Kaplan GP, Holsten N. (2003) Eyelid movements in normal human fetuses. *J Clin Ultrasound* 31: 299–301.

Pillai M, James D. (1990a) Development of human fetal behaviour: a review. *Fetal Diagn Ther* 5: 15–32.

Pillai M, James D. (1990b) Hiccups and breathing in the human fetus. *Arch Dis Child* 65: 1072–1075.

Piontelli A. (2006) On the onset of human fetal behaviour. In: Manca M, editor. *Psychoanalysis and Neuroscience*. Mailand: Springer. p 391–418.

Pitkin RM, Reynolds WA. (1975) Fetal ingestion and metabolism of amniotic fluid protein. *Am J Obstet Gynecol* 123: 356–363.

Pittman R, Oppenheim RW. (1979) Cell death motoneurons in the chick embryo spinal cord. IV. Evidence that a functional neuromuscular interaction is involved in the regulation of naturally occurring cell death and the stabilization of synapses. *J Comp Neurol* 187: 425–446.

Pooh RK, Ogura T. (2004) Normal and abnormal fetal hand positioning and movement in early pregnancy detected by three- and four-dimensional ultrasound. *Ultrasound Rev Obstet Gynecol* 4: 46–51.

Popescu EA, Popescu M, Bennett TL, Lewine JD, Drake WB, Gustafson KM. (2007) Magnetographic assessment of fetal hiccups and their effect on fetal heart rate rhythm. *Physiol Meas* 28: 665–676.

Prechtl HFR. (1958) The directed head turning response and allied movements of the human baby. *Behaviour* 13: 212–242.

Prechtl HFR. (1974) The behavioural states of the newborn infant (a review). *Brain Res* 76: 185–212.

Prechtl HFR. (1984a) Continuity and change in early neural development. In: Prechtl HFR, editor. *Continuity of Neural Functions From Prenatal to Postnatal Life. Clinics in Developmental Medicine No. 94*. London: Spastics International Medical Publications. p 1–15.

Prechtl HFR. (1984b) *Continuity of Neural Functions From Prenatal to Postnatal Life. Clinics in Developmental Medicine No. 94*. London: Spastics International Medical Publications.

Prechtl HFR. (1985) Ultrasound studies of human fetal behaviour. *Early Hum Dev* 12: 91–98.

Prechtl HFR. (1986) New perspectives in early human development. *Eur J Obstet Gynecol Reprod Biol* 21: 347–355.

Prechtl HFR. (1989) Fetal behaviour. In: Hill A, Volpe JJ, editors. *Fetal Neurology*. New York: Raven Press. p 1–16.

Prechtl HFR. (1990) Qualitative changes of spontaneous movements in fetus and preterm infants are a marker of neurological dysfunction. *Early Hum Dev* 23: 151–159.

Prechtl HFR. (1997) State of the art of a new functional assessment of the young nervous system. An early predictor of cerebral palsy. *Early Hum Dev* 50: 1–11.

Prechtl HFR. (2001a) General movement assessment as a method of developmental neurology: new paradigms and their consequences. Ronnie MacKeith lecture. *Dev Med Child Neurol* 43: 838–842.

Prechtl HFR. (2001b) Prenatal and postnatal development of human motor behaviour. In: Kalverboer AF, Gramsbergen A, editors. *Handbook of Brain and Behaviour in Human Development*. London: Kluwer Academic Publishers. p 415–428.

Prechtl HFR, Connolly KJ. (1981) Maturation and development. An introduction. In: Conolly KJ, Prechtl HFR, editors. *Maturation and Development: Biological and Psychological Perspectives. Clinics in Developmental Medicine No. 77/78*. London: Heinemann. Philadelphia: Lippincott. p 9–12.

Prechtl HFR, Einspieler C. (1997) Is neurological assessment of the fetus possible? *Eur J Obstet Gynecol Reprod Biol* 75: 81–84.

Prechtl HFR, Nijhuis JG. (1983) Eye movements in the human fetus and newborn. *Behav Brain Res* 10: 119–124.

Prechtl HFR, Fargel JW, Weinmann HM, Bakker HH. (1979) Postures, motility and respiration of low-risk preterm infants. *Dev Med Child Neurol* 21: 3–27.

Preyer W. (1885) *[Special Physiology of the Embryo]*. Leipzig: Grieben. (In German)

Preyer W. (1890) [*The Soul of the Child. Observations on the Intellectual Development of the Person in the First Year of Life.*] Leipzig: Grieben. (In German)

Pritchard JA. (1966) Fetal swallowing and amniotic fluid volume. *Obstet Gynecol* 28: 606–610.

Provine RR. (1986) Yawning as a stereotyped action pattern and releasing stimulus. *Ethology* 72: 109–122.

Provine RR, Hamernik HB, Curchack BC. (1987a) Yawning: relation to sleeping and stretching in humans. *Ethology* 76: 152–160.

Provine RR, Tate BL, Geldmacher LL. (1987b) Yawning: no effect of 3–5 % CO2, 100 % O2, and exercise. *Behav Neural Biol* 48: 382–393.

Purves D, Lichtman JW. (1980) Elimination of synapses in the developing nervous system. *Science* 210: 153–157.

Rabinowitz R, Peters MT, Vyas S, Campbell S, Nicolaides KH. (1989) Measurement of fetal urine production in normal pregnancy by real-time ultarsonography. *Am J Obstet Gynecol* 161: 1264–1266.

Rayburn WF. (1982) Antepartum fetal assessment. Monitoring fetal activity. *Clin Perinatol* 9: 231–252.

Reifferscheid K. (1911) [Intrauterine fetal breathing movements]. *Deutsch Med Wochenschr* 37: 877–880. (In German)

Reinold E. (1971) [Observation of fetal movement in the first half of pregnancy with ultrasound]. *Pädiat Pädol* 6: 274–279. (In German)

Reppert SM, Schwartz WJ. (1984) Functional activity of the suprachiasmatic nuclei in the fetal primate. *Neurosci Lett* 46: 145–149.

Ritchie JWK. (1980) The response to changes in the composition of maternal inspired air in human pregnancy. *Semin Perinatol* 4: 295–299.

Ritchie JWK, Lakhani K. (1980a) Fetal breathing movements and maternal hyperoxia. *Br J Obstet Gynaecol* 87: 1084–1086

Ritchie JWK, Lakhani K. (1980b) Fetal breathing movements in response to maternal inhalation of 5% carbon dioxide. *Am J Obstet Gynecol* 136: 386–388.

Roberts AB, Mitchell J. (1995) Pulmonary hypoplasia and fetal breathing in preterm premature rupture of membranes. *Early Hum Dev* 41: 27–37.

Roberts AB, Perrins R. (1995) Positive feedback as a general mechanism for sustaining rhythmic and non-rhythmic activity. *J Physiol Paris* 89: 241–248.

Roberts AB, Little D, Cooper DJ, Campbell S. (1979) Normal patterns of fetal activity in the third trimester. *Br J Obstet Gynaecol* 86: 4–9.

Roberts AB, Goldstein I, Romero R, Hobbins JC. (1991) Fetal breathing movements after preterm rupture of membranes. *Am J Obstet Gynecol* 164: 821–825.

Robinson HP, Shaw-Dunn J. (1973) Fetal heart rates as determined by sonar in early pregnancy. *J Obstet Gynaecol Br Commonw* 80: 805–809.

Roodenburg PJ, Wladimiroff JW, van Es A, Prechtl HFR. (1991) Classification and quantitative aspects of fetal movements during the second half of normal pregnancy. *Early Hum Dev* 25: 19–35.

Ross M, Nijland M. (1997) Fetal swallowing: relation to amniotic fluid regulation. *Clin Obstet Gynecol* 40: 352–365.

Ruano-Gil D, Nardi-Vilardaga J, Tejedo-Mateu A. (1978) Influence of extrinsic factors on the development of the articular system. *Acta Anat* 101: 36–44.

Sadovsky E, Polishuk WZ. (1977) Fetal movements in utero. Nature, assessment, prognostic value, timing of delivery. *Obstet Gynecol* 50: 49–55.

Sadovsky E, Laufer N, Allen JW. (1979) The incidence of different types of fetal movements during pregnancy. *Br J Obstet Gynaecol* 86: 10–14.

Saint-Anne Dargassies S. (1979) Normal and pathological fetal behaviour as seen through neurological study of the premature newborn. *Contrib Gynecol Obstet* 6: 42–49.

Saper CB, Chou TC, Scammell TE. (2001) The sleep switch: hypothalamic control of sleep and wakefulness. *Trends Neurosci* 24: 726–731.

Schillinger H. (1976) Detection of heart action and active movements of the human embryo by ultrasound time motion techniques. *Eur J Obstet Gynecol Reprod Biol* 6: 333–338.

Schreyer P, Bar-Natan N, Sherman DJ, Arieli S, Caspi E. (1991) Fetal breathing movements before oxytocin induction in prolonged pregnancies. *Am J Obstet Gynecol* 165: 577–581.

Schürmann M, Hesse MD, Stephan KE, Saarela M, Zilles K, Hari R, Fink GR. (2005) Yearning to yawn: the neural basis of contagious yawning. *Neuroimage* 24: 1260–1264.

Sepulveda W, Mangiamarchi M. (1995) Fetal yawning. *Ultrasound Obstet Gynecol* 5: 57–59.

Shawker TH, Schuette WH, Whitehouse W, Rifka SM. (1980) Early fetal movement: a real time ultrasound study. *Obstet Gynecol* 55: 194–198.

Sherer DM, Hearn B, Woods JR Jr. (1990) Possible intermittent umbilical cord occlusion. *J Ultrasound Med* 9: 182.

Sherer DM, Eggers PC, Smith SA, Abramowicz JS. (1991) Fetal sucking of the umbilical cord. *J Ultrasound Med* 10: 300.

Sherer DM, Metlay LA, Woods JR Jr. (1995) Lack of mandibular movement manifested by absent fetal swallowing: a possible factor in the pathogenesis of micrognathia. *Am J Perinatol* 12: 30–33.

Shirozu H, Koyanagi T, Takashima T, Horimoto N, Akazawa K, Nakano H. (1995) Penile tumescence in the human fetus at term – a preliminary report. *Early Hum Dev* 41: 159–166.

Sissons HA. (1956) The growth of the bone. In: Bourne GH, editor. *Biochemistry and Physiology of Bone*. New York: Academic Press. p 443–451.

Snyder FF. (1949) *Obstetrical Analgesia and Anesthesia*. Philadelphia: WB Saunders.

Sontag LW, Wallace RF. (1934) Preliminary report of the Fels Fund study of fetal activity. *Am J Dis Child* 48: 1050–1057.

Staras K, Kemenes I, Benjamin PR, Kemenes G. (2003) Loss of self-inhibition is a cellular mechanism for episodic rhythmic behaviour. *Curr Biol* 13: 116–124.

Stark RI, Daniel SS, Graland M, Jaille-Marti JC, Kim YI, Leung K, Myers MM, Tropper PJ. (1994) Fetal hiccups in the baboon. *Am J Physiol* 267: R1479–R1487.

Stehouwer DJ, Farel PB. (1980) Central and peripheral controls of swimming in anuran larvae. *Brain Res* 195: 323–335.

Suzue T, Shinoda Y. (1999) Highly reproducible spatiotemporal patterns of mammalian embryonic movements at the developmental stage of the earliest spontaneous motility. *Eur J Neurosci* 11: 2697–2710.

Tabak J, Senn W, O'Donovan MJ, Rinzel J. (2000) Modelling of spontaneous activity in developing spinal cord using activity-dependent depression in an excitatory network. *J Neurosci* 20: 3041–3056.

Takashima T, Horimoto N, Satoh S, Maeda H, Koyanagi T, Nakano H. (1991) Characteristics of binocular movements in the human fetus at term, assessed with real-time ultrasound. *Jap Soc Ultrason Med* 59(Suppl 2): 883–884.

Takashima T, Koyanagi T, Horimoto N, Satoh S, Nakano H. (1995) Breech presentation: is there a difference in eye movement patterns compared with cephalic presentation in the human fetus at term? *Am J Obstet Gynecol* 172: 851–855.

Tatsumura M. (1991) [Studies on features of fetal movement and development of the human fetus with use of fetal actogram]. *Nippon Sanka Fujinka Gakkai Zasshi* 43: 864–873. (In Japanese)

Taub E. (1976) Motor behavior following deafferentation in the developing and motorically mature monkey. In: Herman R, Grillner S, Stein PSG, Stuart D, editors. *Neural Control of Locomotion*. New York: Plenum. p 675–705.

ten Hof J, Nijhuis IJM, Nijhuis JG, Narayan H, Taylor DJ, Visser GHA, Mulder EJH. (1999) Quantitative analysis of fetal general movements: methodological considerations. *Early Hum Dev* 56: 57–73.

ten Hof J, Nijhuis IJ, Mulder EJ, Nijhuis JG, Narayan H, Taylor DJ, Westers P, Visser GH. (2002) Longitudinal study of fetal body movements: nomograms, intrafetal consistency, and relationship with episodes of heart rate patterns A and B. *Pediatr Res* 52: 568–575.

Tongsong T, Chanprapaph P, Khunamornpong S. (2000) Prenatal ultrasound of regional akinesia with Pena-Shokier phenotype. *Prenat Diagn* 20: 422–425.

Trudinger BJ, Knight PC. (1980) Fetal age and patterns of human fetal breathing movements. *Am J Obstet Gynecol* 137: 724–728.

Twiest M. (1974) Why the yawn? *N Engl J Med* 290: 1439.

Usiak MF, Landmesser LT. (1999) Neuromuscular activity blockade induced by muscimol and D-tubocurarine differentuially affects the survival of embryonic chick motoneurons. *J Neurosci* 19: 7925–7939.

Valentin L, Lofgren O, Maršál K, Gullberg B. (1984) Subjective recording of fetal movements. I. Limits and acceptability in normal pregnancies. *Acta Obstet Gynecol Scand* 63: 223–228.

van Dongen LGR, Goudie EG. (1980) Fetal movement patterns in the first trimester of pregnancy. *Br J Obstet Gynaecol* 87: 191–193.

van Heeswijk M, Nijhuis JG, Hollanders HM. (1990) Fetal heart rate in early pregnancy. *Early Hum Dev* 22: 151–156.

van Tol-Geerdink JJ, Sparling JW, Chescheir NC. (1995) The development of hand movements in utero. *Am J Obstet Gynecol* 172: 351.

van Woerden EE, van Geijn HPM, Caron FJM, van der Valk AW, Swartjes JM, Arts NF. (1988a) Fetal mouth movements during behavioural states 1F and 2F. *Eur J Obstet Gynecol Reprod Biol* 29: 97–105.

van Woerden EE, van Geijn HP, Swartjes JM, Caron FJ, Brons JT, Arts NF. (1988b) Fetal heart rhythms during behavioural state 1F. *Eur J Obstet Gynecol Reprod Biol* 28: 29–38.

van Woerden EE, van Geijn HP, Caron FJM, Mantel R, Swartjes JM, Arts NF. (1989) Fetal hiccups; characteristics and relation to fetal heart rate. *Eur J Obstet Gynecol Reprod Biol* 30: 209–216.

van Wulfften Palthe T, Hopkins B. (1984) Development of the infant's social competence during early face-to-face interaction: a longitudinal study. In: Prechtl HFR, editor. *Continuity of Neural Functions From Prenatal to Postnatal Life. Clinics in Developmental Medicine No. 94.* London: Spastics International Medical Publications. p 198–219.

Velazquez M, Rayburn W. (2002) Antenatal evaluation of the fetus using fetal movement monitoring. *Clin Obstet Gynecol* 45: 993–1004.

Ververs IAP, de Vries JIP, van Geijn HP, Hopkins B. (1994) Prenatal head position from 12 to 38 weeks. II. The effects of fetal orientation and placental localization. Developmental aspects. *Early Hum Dev* 39: 93–100.

Ververs IAP, van Gelder-Hasker MR, de Vries JIP, Hopkins B, van Geijn HP. (1998) Prenatal development of arm posture. *Early Hum Dev* 51: 61–70

Vintzileos AM, Campbell WA, Nochimson DJ, Conolly ME, Fuenfer MM, Hoehn GJ. (1985) The fetal biophysical profile in patients with premature rupture of the membranes: an early predictor of fetal infection. *Am J Obstet Gynecol* 152: 510–516.

Visser GHA, Prechtl HFR. (1988) Movements and behavioural states in the human fetus. In: Jones CT, editor. *Fetal and Neonatal Development.* Ithaca, New York: Perinatology Press. p 581–590.

Visser GHA, Goodman JDS, Levine DH, Dawes GS. (1982) Diurnal and other cyclic variations in human fetal heart rate near term. *Am J Obstet Gynecol* 142: 535–544.

Visser GHA, Laurini RN, de Vries JIP, Bekedam DJ, Prechtl HFR. (1985) Abnormal motor behaviour in anencephalic fetuses. *Early Hum Dev* 12: 173–182.

Vles JS, Kingma H, Caberg H, Daniels H, Casaer P. (1989) Posture of low-risk preterm infants between 32 and 36 weeks postmenstrual age. *Dev Med Child Neurol* 31: 191–195.

Walker BE, Quarles J. (1962) Palate development in mouse foetuses after tongue removal. *Arch Oral Biol* 21: 405–412.

Walusinski O. (2010) Fetal yawning. Front Neurol Neurosci 28: 32–41.

Weiss PA. (1941) Self-differentiation of the basic patterns of coordination. *Comp Psychol Monogr* 17: 1–96.

Wells LJ. (1954) Development of the human diaphragm and pleural sacs. *Contrib Embryol* 35: 107–134.

Wigglesworth JS. (1988) Lung development in the second trimester. *Br Med Bull* 44: 894–908.

Wigglesworth JS, Desai R. (1982) Is fetal respiratory function a major determinant of perinatal survival? *Lancet* 1(8266): 264–267.

Wilkinson C, Robinson J. (1982) Braxton Hicks' contractions and fetal breathing movements. *Aust NZ J Obstet Gynecol* 22: 212–214.

Windle WF. (1940) *Physiology of the Fetus. Origin and Extent of Function in Fetal Life.* Philadelphia: WB Saunders.

Windle WF. (1971) *Physiology of the Fetus. Relation to Brain Damage in the Prenatal Period.* Springfield, IL: Charles C Thomas.

Windle WF, Orr DW. (1934) The development of behaviour in chick embryos: spinal cord structure correlated with early somatic motility. *J Comp Neurol* 60: 287–307.

Witter F, DiPietro J, Costigan K, Nelson P. (2007) The relationship between hiccups and heart rate in the fetus. *J Matern Fetal Neonatal Med* 20: 289–292.

Wladimiroff JW. (1975) Effect of frusemide on fetal urine production. *Br J Obstet Gynaecol* 82: 221–224.

Wolff PH. (1986) The serial organization of sucking in the young infant. *Pediatr* 42: 943–956.

Wouldes TA, Roberts AB, Pryor JE, Bagnall C, Gunn TR. (2004) The effect of methadone treatment on the quantity and quality of human fetal movement. *Neurotoxicol Teratol* 26: 23–34.

Yan F, Dai SY, Akther N, Kuno A, Yanagihara T, Hata T. (2006) Four-dimensional sonographic assessment of fetal facial expression early in the third trimester. *Int J Gynaecol Obstet* 94: 108–113.

Yigiter AB, Kavak ZN. (2006) Normal standards of fetal behaviour assessed by four-dimensional sonography. *J Matern Fetal Neonatal Med* 19: 707–721.

Zheng YT, Sampson MB, Soper R. (1998) The significance of umbilical vein Doppler changes during fetal hiccups. *J Matern Fetal Invest* 8: 89–91.

Zimmer EZ, Divon MY, Goldstein I, Sarna Z, Paldi E. (1985) Intrauterine fetal activity in at term and prolonged pregnancies. *J Perinatal Med* 13: 201–204.

Zimmer EZ, Chao CR, Guy GP, Marks F, Fifer WP. (1993) Vibroacoustic stimulation evokes human fetal micturition. *Obstet Gynecol* 81: 178–180.

3
PRENATAL LATERALITY

Early right-to-left dominance in certain brain areas

In most right-handed adults several brain structures – such as the planum temporale, the parietal opercule or the pars opercularis of the frontal lobe (Broca region) – are larger in the left hemisphere than in the right hemisphere (Geschwind and Galaburda 1985). During early development, however, there is a right hemispheric dominance. Certain areas of the right hemisphere mature more quickly than homologous areas in the left hemisphere (de Schonen and Mathivet 1989). By 31 weeks' gestation, it becomes recognisable that the transverse temporal gyrus is larger in the right hemisphere than it is in the left (Chi et al 1977). Furthermore, auditory evoked responses reveal a side-different latency development, which suggests an earlier maturation of certain right than homologous left hemispheric brain areas (Schleussner et al 2004). Also, in infants the regional cerebral blood flow is greater in the right hemisphere, especially in the posterior associative area. This predominance only shifts to the left side after 3 years of age (Chiron et al 1997), which is due to the emergence of functions – such as certain visuospatial and language abilities – that are initially localised in the right hemisphere but later move to the left hemisphere.

When does handedness start to develop?

Handedness is the most familiar manifestation of behavioural lateralisation in everyday life. In their spontaneous movements, newborn infants already show a right-to-left arm dominance (Goodwin and Michel 1981, von Hofsten 1982). Also, preterm infants predominantly contact their mouth with their right hand (Konishi et al 1997), and they show a marked tendency to lie with the head to the right (Gesell and Ames 1947, Turkewitz and Creighton 1974, Prechtl et al 1979, Vles et al 1988, Konishi et al 1997). This can partly be explained by the fact that most caregivers are right-handed and therefore find it more convenient to turn the baby's head to the right (Cioni and Pellegrinetti 1982, Konishi et al 1986, Vles et al 1988). Clearly, a head preference by as soon as 1 hour after birth (Hopkins et al 1987) corroborates the assumption that the origin of such an asymmetry could be prenatal.

IS THE FETAL HEAD POSITION LATERALISED?

Up to the age of 26 weeks, the fetal head is preferentially positioned in the midline (van Gelder et al 1990). The preference of one side – which, in cephalic fetuses, actually tends to be the right side – only starts a few weeks before the expected date of birth (Ververs et al 1994, Fong et al 2005). By contrast, fetuses in breech presentation do not have a preferred head position. When fetuses in breech position do show a lateralised head position, the preference is not necessarily to the right (Fong et al 2005). These findings support the idea that intrauterine environmental influence might play an important role in the development of fetal lateralised behaviour. Fetuses in breech position have more freedom of head movements. This can lead to a less pronounced difference in the stimulation of the otoliths (Previc 1991), and hence to a less pronounced vestibular lateralisation. The fixed position of the head in cephalic fetuses, on the other hand, leads to an unequal sharing of the hair cells, e.g. during maternal walking, which results in a left-otolithic dominance. Consequently, the ipsilateral sternocleidomastoid muscle will be activated more, which, in turn, may lead to a head preference to the right (Previc 1991).

THE RIGHT-HANDED FETUS: A TOPIC OF DEBATE

Hepper and associates observed a right-arm preference from 10–12 weeks onwards (Hepper et al 1998); at 15 weeks, fetuses start to favour sucking on their right-hand thumb (Hepper et al 1990, 1991). This lateralisation seems to persist throughout the first two trimesters. The incidence of left-arm movements decreases earlier (after 21 weeks) than the incidence of right-arm movements (24 weeks; McCartney and Hepper 1999). Based on these findings, Hepper favours Annett's theory on a genetic basis for lateralisation (Annett 1985), since restrictions for body or head position cannot be decisive for behavioural asymmetries at such an early age.

The findings of Hepper and associates have never been replicated. By contrast, a cross-sectional study on fetuses aged 14, 20, 26 and 38 weeks showed a strikingly similar number of right- and left-hand contacts with the mouth, face and other body parts (van Tol-Geerdink et al 1995). A few years later, hand-to-head contacts were observed weekly from 12 to 38 weeks' gestation in a longitudinal study on 10 healthy fetuses (de Vries et al 2001). A strong unimanual bias was indeed observable between 12 and 32 weeks. However, such unimanual contacts do not seem to constitute a lateral preference, for neither right- nor left- side contacts establish a stable relationship with the head position. By 36 weeks, there is a shift to bimanual hand-to-head contacts. At this age, fetuses in a cephalic position show a preference for a right-sided head position (Ververs et al 1994).

All in all, there is no evidence that hand-to-head contact and head position co-develop to form a preferred ipsilateral synergy.

REFERENCES

Annett M. (1985) *Left, Right, Hand and Brain: The Right Shift Theory*. London: Lawrence Erlbaum.

Chi JG, Dooling EC, Gilles FH. (1977) Left-right asymmetries of the temporal speech areas of the human fetus. *Arch Neurol* 34: 346–348.

Chiron C, Jambaque I, Nabbout R, Lounes R, Syrota A, Dulac O. (1997) The right brain hemisphere is dominant in human infants. *Brain* 120: 1057–1065.

Cioni G, Pellegrinetti G. (1982) Lateralization of sensory and motor functions in human neonates. *Percept Mot Skills* 54: 1151–1158.

de Schonen S, Mathivet E. (1989) First come, first served: a scenario about the development of hemispheric specialization in face recognition during infancy. *Eur Bull Cogn Psychol* 9: 3–44.

de Vries JIP, Wimmers RH, Ververs IA, Hopkins B, Savelsbergh GJ, van Geijn HP. (2001) Fetal handedness and head position preference: a developmental study. *Dev Psychobiol* 39: 171–178.

Fong B, Savelsbergh GJP, van Geijn HP, de Vries JIP. (2005) Does intra-uterine environment influence fetal head-position preference? A comparison between breech and cephalic presentation. *Early Hum Dev* 81, 507–517.

Geschwind N, Galaburda AM. (1985) Cerebral lateralization. *Arch Neurol* 42: 428–459.

Gesell A, Ames LB. (1947) The development of handedness. *J Gen Psychol* 70: 155–175.

Goodwin RS, Michel GF. (1981) Head orientation position during birth and in infant neonatal period, and hand preference at 19 weeks. *Child Dev* 52: 819–826.

Hepper PG, Shahidullah S, White R. (1990) Origins of fetal handedness. *Nature* 347: 431.

Hepper PG, Shahidullah S, White R. (1991) Handedness in the human fetus. *Neuropsychologia* 29: 1107–1111.

Hepper PG, McCartey GR, Shannon EA. (1998) Lateralised behaviour in first trimester human foetuses. *Neuropsychologia* 36: 531–534.

Hopkins B, Lems YL, Janssen B, Butterworth G. (1987) Postural and motor asymmetries in newlyborns. *Hum Neurobiol* 6: 152–156.

Konishi Y, Mikawa H, Suzuki J. (1986) Asymmetrical head turning of preterm infants: some effects on later postural and functional lateralities. *Dev Med Child Neurol* 28: 450–457.

Konishi Y, Takaya R, Kimura K, Takeuchi K, Saito M, Konishi K. (1997) Laterality of finger movements in preterm infants. *Dev Med Child Neurol* 39: 248–252.

McCartney G, Hepper P. (1999) Development of lateralized behaviour in the human fetus from 12 to 27 weeks' gestation. *Dev Med Child Neurol* 41: 83–86.

Prechtl HFR, Fargel JW, Weinmann HM, Bakker HH. (1979) Postures, motility and respiration of low-risk preterm infants. *Dev Med Child Neurol* 21: 3–27.

Previc FH. (1991) A general theory concerning the prenatal origins of cerebral lateralisation in humans. *Psychol Rev* 98: 299–334.

Schleussner E, Schneider U, Arnscheidt C, Kähler C, Haueisen J, Seewald HJ. (2004) Prenatal evidence of left-right asymmetries in auditory evoked responses using fetal magnetoencephalography. *Early Hum Dev* 78: 133–136.

Turkewitz G, Creighton S. (1974) Changes in lateral differentiation of head posture in the human neonate. *Dev Psychobiol* 8: 85–89.

van Gelder RS, Dijkman MMTT, Hopkins B, van Geijn HP, Ho-Meau-Long DC. (1990) Prenatal development of head orientation preference. *Int J Prenatal Perinatal Psychol Med* 4: 201–206.

van Tol-Geerdink JJ, Sparling JW, Chescheir NC. (1995) The development of hand movements in utero. *Am J Obstet Gynecol* 172: 351.

Ververs IAP, de Vries JIP, van Geijn HP, Hopkins B. (1994) Prenatal head position from 12 to 38 weeks. I. Developmental aspects. *Early Hum Dev* 39:83–91.

Vles JSH, Oostenbrugger R, van Kingma H, Caberg H, Casaer P. (1988) Head position in low-risk premature infants: impact of nursing routines. *Biol Neonate* 54: 307–313.

von Hofsten C. (1982) Eye-hand coordination in the newborn. *Dev Psychol* 18: 450–461.

4
BEHAVIOURAL STATES

Classification of behavioural states

Behavioural states represent distinct conditions of neural activity that are mutually exclusive and stable over time. They recur repeatedly and change from one into the other during short transitions (Prechtl 1974).

In order to define a behavioural state, it is necessary that a number of variables meet clearly defined criteria at the same time. The context in which the assessment of behavioural states is applied (for example, whether or not equipment for polygraphy is available), as well as the professional background of the investigator, will determine the choice of variables – that is, whether they are purely observed (Wolff 1959, Prechtl 1974) or require electrophysiological recordings (Dreyfus-Brisac 1962, Monod and Pajot 1965, Prechtl et al 1968, 1969). In both cases, the terminology should be non-interpretative. For this reason, a descriptive classification of behavioural states has been suggested (Prechtl 1974), based on numbers in order to avoid physiological interpretation.

The great advantage of applying the state concept in behavioural observations or physiological measurements is that it facilitates understanding of an otherwise unexplained variability (Prechtl 1992). The state concept can then be used for standardisation of the conditions under which specific measurements of neural activity are carried out. This is also true for the standardisation of neurological assessment (Prechtl 1977).

Behavioural states in the neonate

In the observation of neonatal behaviour, the following four variables have been chosen to define the various behavioural states (Prechtl 1974): respiration (regular versus irregular); eyes (open versus closed); body movements (absent versus present); and crying (absent versus present). The advantage of these criteria lies in the simplicity of observational diagnosis, which does not require application of electrodes or wires. The same criteria can also be applied for polygraphic recordings, thus keeping the terminology consistent and independent from the mode of data acquisition. With these four variables, five mutually exclusive and qualitatively different states can be distinguished (Table 4.1). Other variables, the so-called state concomitants, are specific for a particular state, but since they are not continuously present during the respective state, they should not be included in the

TABLE 4.1
TABLE 4.1
Behavioural states in the newborn infant

	Respiration	Eyes	Gross movements	Vocalisation
State 1	Regular	Closed	Absent, some startles	Absent
State 2	Irregular	Closed	Incidental	Absent
State 3	Regular	Open	Absent	Absent
State 4	Irregular	Open	Continuous	Absent
State 5	Irregular	Open or closed	Present	Present, crying, fussing

From Prechtl HFR (1974) The behavioural states of the newborn infant (a review). *Brain Res* 76: 185–212, with permission.

state definition. Examples are tracé alternant electroencephalography (EEG), startles, mouthing, grimaces, smiling movements, visual scanning or stretching.

Each behavioural state has a certain duration. In the neonate, state 1 lasts for about 20 minutes and state 2 for about 30–40 minutes, while state 3 – the shortest – usually only lasts for a few minutes. The duration of states 4 and 5 is variable and depends on environmental conditions as well as on the temperament of the infant.

Behavioural states in the fetus
Several studies on preterm infants (Parmelee et al 1967, Dreyfus-Brisac 1970, Prechtl et al 1979, Curzi-Dascalova et al 1983) have shown that well-developed state cycles are present a few weeks before term. In this regard, the question arose as to whether the fetal behavioural states are similar to those of a preterm infant of the same age. For practical reasons, however, the state criteria applied in the neonate cannot be used for the fetus; where breathing movements are not continuously present, opening or closing of the eyes cannot be observed easily, and no EEG can be recorded.

In 1982, definitions of four different fetal heart-rate patterns – A to D (Figure 4.1) – were introduced to describe behavioural states in combination with the presence or absence of body and eye movements (Table 4.2; Nijhuis et al 1982). At around 30 weeks, a so-called coincidence occurs, a linkage of variables that are as yet unstable (Figure 4.2a; Visser et al 1987, Drogtrop et al 1990). Near term, their linkage is such that fetal behavioural states can be described (Table 4.2; Figure 4.2b): they are stable over time and recur every 2 hours (Visser and Mulder 1993, de Vries and Fong 2006).

RECORDING BEHAVIOURAL STATES
Since fetal behavioural states are defined on the basis of fetal heart-rate patterns as well as fetal body movements and fetal eye movements, it is necessary to record the fetal heart

	Fetal Heart Rate Pattern
State 1F	a 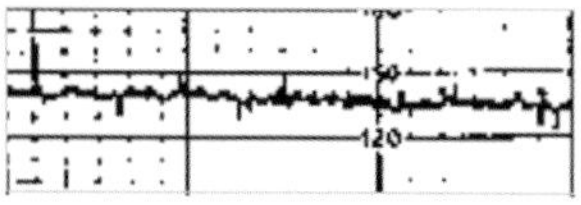 Stable heart rate with a small oscillation bandwidth; isolated accelerations (strictly related to movements) may occur.
State 2F	b 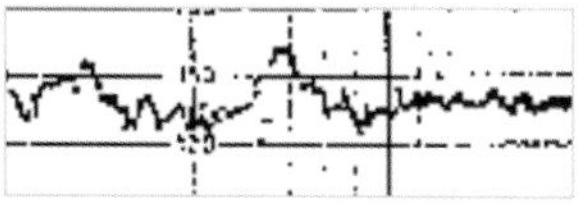 Heart rate with a wider oscillation bandwidth than fetal heart rate pattern A and with frequent accelerations during movements.
State 3F	c 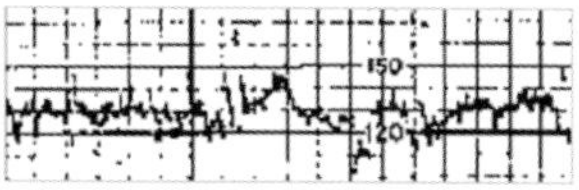 The heart rate is stable but with a wider oscillation bandwidth than fetal heart rate pattern A and with no accelerations.
State 4F	d 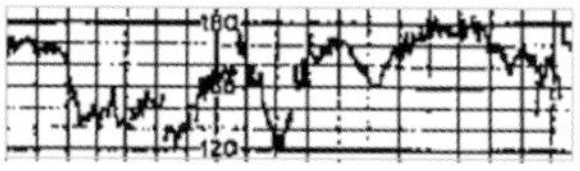 Unstable heart rate unstable with large and long-lasting accelerations, frequently fused into a sustained tachycardia.

Figure 4.1 Fetal heart-rate patterns a–d (beats per minute); duration 3 minutes. From Nijhuis JG, Prechtl HFR, Martin CB, Bots RSGM. (1982) Are there behavioural states in the human fetus? *Early Hum Dev* 6: 177–195, with permission.

rate (with a cardiotocograph) and the fetal body and eye movements (with two real-time ultrasound transducers) simultaneously. The transducer probes are positioned on the maternal abdomen in order to obtain a parasagittal section through the face of the fetus and a transverse section through the upper part of the fetal trunk. With the first probe, it is possible to verify fetal eye movements as well as other movements of the head. With the second probe, fetal body and breathing movements can be detected (Nijhuis et al 1982, Romanini and Rizzo 1995). In order to minimise the influence of diurnal variation and maternal food intake, recordings should be performed around the same time of the day,

TABLE 4.2
Behavioural states in the fetus

	Fetal heart rate pattern	Eye movements	Gross movements
State 1F	A	Absent	Incidental
State 2F	B	Present	Periodic
State 3F	C	Present	Absent
State 4F	D	Present	Continuous

From Nijhuis JG, Prechtl HFR, Martin CB, Bots RSGM. (1982) Are there behavioural states in the human fetus? *Early Hum Dev* 6: 177–195, with permission

preferably in the afternoon, 2 hours after a standardised 1000kcal lunch (Romanini and Rizzo 1995). In order to cover the complete cycle of fetal states, a recording time of 2 hours is needed.

By using a moving-window technique (3 minutes), short-lasting events are omitted during analysis (Nijhuis et al 1982). The window is shifted over each state variable. If a state variable (e.g. fetal eye movements) appears in the window, it is categorised as 'present'. A variable is scored as 'absent' if it does not appear at all in a particular window. Thus, a profile is generated for each variable and behavioural states can be identified.

Such an assessment, which facilitates recognition of the presence or absence of fetal eye and body movements, is relatively easy for expert investigators to reproduce. Fetal heart-rate patterns can be reliably classified with specific analysis systems (cf, for example, Lange et al 2009).

STATE 1F

State 1F (F = fetal) (Table 4.2; Figures 4.2b and 4.3) is similar to the neonatal state 1, i.e. non-rapid-eye-movement (NREM) sleep or quiet sleep. It represents a quiescence that can be interrupted by brief body movements, mostly startles. Eye movements are absent. The fetal heart-rate pattern A (Fig. 4.1) is stable, with a small oscillation bandwidth and no accelerations, except in combination with startles (Nijhuis et al 1982, Nijhuis 2003).

Fetal heart-rate pattern A can be observed from around 32 weeks onwards (Pillai et al 1992, ten Hof et al 2002). At term, healthy fetuses may show fetal heart-rate pattern A for as long as 60 minutes (Table 4.3), occasionally for more than 60 minutes; even values of up to 75 minutes have been recorded (Patrick et al 1982). A healthy term fetus remains in state 1F for about one-third of the time (Arabin et al 1988, Pillai and James 1990a, Nijhuis and van de Pas 1992).

Generally speaking, the organisation of behavioural states is not easily affected by external factors; actually, most stimuli fail to induce a state transition when the fetus is in state 1F (Visser and Mulder 1993): the fetus remains in state 1F in spite of Braxton Hicks

(a) Case 1, 31 weeks

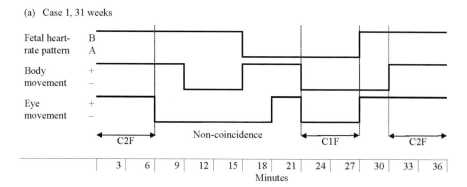

Fetal heart-   B
rate pattern A

Body   +
movement   –

Eye   +
movement   –

C2F   Non-coincidence   C1F   C2F

| 3 | 6 | 9 | 12 | 15 | 18 | 21 | 24 | 27 | 30 | 33 | 36 |

Minutes

b) Case 1, 40 weeks

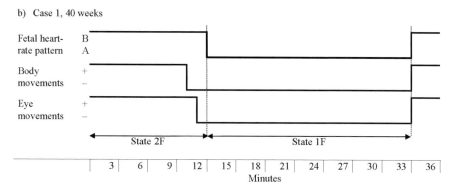

Fetal heart-   B
rate pattern A

Body   +
movements   –

Eye   +
movements   –

State 2F   State 1F

| 3 | 6 | 9 | 12 | 15 | 18 | 21 | 24 | 27 | 30 | 33 | 36 |

Minutes

Figure 4.2 Thirty-six minutes of observation in the same fetus at (a) 31 weeks' and (b) 40 weeks' gestation. Coincidences of 1F and 2F parameters at 31 weeks are indicated by C1F or C2F, respectively. At 40 weeks, there are behavioural states. The state variables appear to be relatively independent of one another at 31 weeks, as evidenced by the periods of non-coincidence, whereas at 40 weeks the relative simultaneity of the two state transitions (2 minutes, < 0.5 minutes) proves that there is a linkage between the state variables. C = coincidence; + = present; – = absent. Adapted from Nijhuis JG, Prechtl HFR, Martin CB, Bots RSGM. (1982) Are there behavioural states in the human fetus? *Early Hum Dev* 6: 177–195, with permission.

contractions (Mulder and Visser 1987), uterine contractions during labour (Griffin et al 1985), induced maternal emotions (van den Bergh et al 1989), shaking of the maternal abdomen (Visser et al 1983) or transabdominal sound stimulation (Schmidt et al 1985). Correspondingly, it is difficult to wake a newborn infant from state 1. While stimuli in the normal physiological range have little or no effect on state 1F, inappropriate stimuli, which are strong, or even painful, such as a vibroacoustic stimulation, induce excessive fetal movements and prolonged tachycardia, indicating a transition from state 1F to 4F, which is totally uncharacteristic of healthy fetuses (Timor-Tritsch 1986, Visser and Mulder 1993).

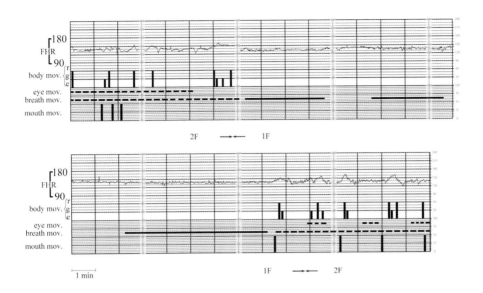

Figure 4.3 Thirty-one minutes of observation of a 38-week-old fetus. As indicated (2F→, ←2F), the recording begins and ends in state 2F (fetal heart-rate pattern B, frequent general and extremity movements, eye movements present). In between, there is a period of state 1F (fetal heart-rate pattern A, no body movements, no eye movements). Irregular breathing movements are indicated by a broken line; regular breathing movements are indicated by a solid line. Eye movements are indicated by a broken line. e = extremity movements; FHR = fetal heart rate in beats per minute; g = general movements; mov. = movements; r = rotations. From Nijhuis JG, Prechtl HFR, Martin CB, Bots RSGM. (1982) Are there behavioural states in the human fetus? *Early Hum Dev* 6: 177–195, with permission.

State 1F concomitants

Fetal breathing movements are less frequent during state 1F than during state 2F if their overall rate of occurrence is low (van Vliet et al 1985, Rizzo et al 1988, Mulder et al 1995); if their rate of occurrence is high, however, they are regular during state 1F and irregular during state 2F (Figure 4.3; Nijhuis et al 1983). Regular mouthing can only be observed during state 1F (van Woerden et al 1988, Pillai and James 1991). Yawning and grimaces rarely occur during state 1F. Fetal voiding appears to be inhibited during state 1F (Arduini et al 1985, 1991).

STATE 2F

State 2F (Table 4.2; Figures 4.2b and 4.3) is similar to the neonatal state 2, i.e. REM sleep or active sleep. Frequent body movements – mainly stretches and general movements – are present. Rapid eye movements occur. The fetal heart-rate pattern B (Figure 4.1) has a wider oscillation bandwidth than the fetal heart-rate pattern A; acceleration is frequent

TABLE 4.3
Duration (median [range]) of fetal heart rate pattern A from 32 to 42 weeks' gestation obtained on 14
306 uncomplicated pregnancies

Gestational age, weeks	Median (range), minutes
32–34	14.5 (4–32)
36	18 (9–35)
37	22 (11–41)
38	23 (14–42)
39	25 (13–44)
40	30 (15–60)
41	26 (12–52)
42	28 (15–50)

Data from Romanini and Rizzo (1995), ten Hof et al (2002).

during movements (Nijhuis et al 1982, Nijhuis 2003). The duration of state 2F increases with gestational age (Nijhuis and van de Pas 1992, Okai et al 1992).

The pulsatility index, a measure of peripheral vascular resistance, is lower during state 2F than during state 1F, which indicates an increased perfusion of the muscles to meet the energy demand of enhanced activity during state 2F (van Eyck et al 1985, Romanini and Rizzo 1995, Boito et al 2004). Other haemodynamic changes include increased right-to-left shunt at the level of the foramen ovale (van Eyck et al 1990), increased cardiac output (Rizzo et al 1990, Boito et al 2004), reduced blood flow through the ductus arteriosus (Mooren et al 1989) and a rise of venous pressure (Boito et al 2004). No haemodynamic changes occur in the umbilical artery (van Eyck et al 1990). All these changes are consistent with a redistribution of the fetal blood flow, which leads to a preferential streaming of well-oxygenated blood to the left heart and, consequently, to the brain (Gagnon 1995, Romanini and Rizzo 1995, Mirmiram et al 2003).

State 2F concomitants
During state 2F, episodes of rapid but irregular (in rate and amplitude) breathing movements occur (Figure 4.3; Nijhuis et al 1983, Cosmi et al 2001). Periodic sighs are often observed during such breathing movements. Frequently, jaw opening, tongue protrusion, yawning and grimaces occur (van Woerden et al 1988). Voiding seems to be initiated or facilitated by the transition to state 2F (Visser et al 1981a, Koyanagi et al 1992). Penile tumescence occurs more often and for longer spans during state 2F than during state 1F (Shirozu et al 1995).

STATE 3F

State 3F (Table 4.2; Figure 4.4) is similar to the neonatal state 3, or quiet wakefulness. Gross body movements are absent. Eye movements are present. The fetal heart-rate pattern C (Figure 4.1) is stable but shows a wider oscillation bandwidth than fetal heart-rate pattern A; there are no accelerations (Nijhuis et al 1982, Nijhuis 2003). With an incidence of around 3%, state 3F is rare (Nijhuis et al 1982, Schmidt et al 1985, Arduini et al 1989, van Woerden et al 1989, James et al 1995, DiPietro et al 1996).

Bursts of fetal sucking movements during state 3F may entail a sinusoidal-like heart-rate pattern, which is not to be confused with the real sinusoidal pattern observable in fetuses with severe anaemia (Nijhuis et al 1984).

STATE 4F

State 4F (Table 4.2; Figure 4.4) is similar to the neonatal state 4, or active wakefulness. There is vigorous continual activity in the fetus. Eye movements are continually present but more difficult to observe, because of the frequent positional changes of the head. The fetal heart-rate pattern D (Figure 4.1) is unstable and shows great, long-lasting accelerations, which often results in sustained tachycardia (Nijhuis et al 1982, Patrick et al 1984, Nijhuis 2003). State 4F constitutes 9–16% of the fetal states (Arabin et al 1988, Pillai and James 1990a, DiPietro et al 1996).

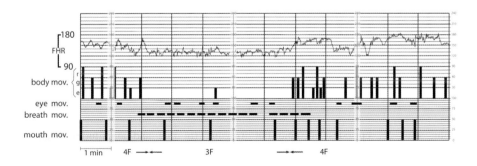

Figure 4.4 Twelve minutes of observation of a 38-week-old fetus. As indicated (4F→, ←4F), the recording begins and ends in state 4F (fetal heart-rate pattern D, frequent body movements consisting of rotations, general movements and extremity movements, eye movements present). In between there is a period of state 3F (fetal heart-rate pattern C, only one extremity movement, eye movements present). Irregular breathing movements as well as eye movements are indicated by a broken line. e = extremity movements; FHR = fetal heart rate in beats per minute; g = general movements; mov. = movements; r = rotations. From Nijhuis JG, Prechtl HFR, Martin CB, Bots RSGM. (1982) Are there behavioural states in the human fetus? *Early Hum Dev* 6: 177–195, with permission.

IS THERE A FETAL HOMOLOGUE OF CRYING (STATE 5F)?

Crying is a complex, rhythmical series of sounds that requires precise coordination of various motor systems (Hopkins and Wulffthen Palthe 1987). The most comprehensive description defines infant cry as a rhythmic repetition of an expiratory sound (lasting 0.6–1.3 seconds), followed by a brief pause (0.2 seconds), then by an inspiratory sound or whistle (0.1–0.2 second), and yet another pause (0.2 second), before the next sound is made on expiration (Wolff 1969). Fundamental to crying is vocalisation, although crying also consists of non-vocal concomitant features, which may develop before birth (Hopkins 2000).

A few years ago, a homologue of crying was elicited through vibroacoustic stimulation performed in the course of a study on the effect of exposure to tobacco and cocaine during pregnancy (Gingras et al 2005). The fetus responded to the stimulus by startling and turning the head. There was a small expiratory movement, followed by a deep inspiratory movement and a pronounced expiratory movement. This expiratory motion was accompanied by jaw opening, taut tongue and chest depression. It was immediately followed by three extended breathing movements, with a progressive increase in chest rise and head tilt. Each end-inspiratory movement was marked by chin quiver. The last extended breathing movement ended with a turn of the head into an oblique position, as well as mouthing and swallowing. Once detected, this kind of episode during vibroacoustic stimulation was also observed in other fetuses from 28 weeks onward, lasting for 15–20 seconds each (Gingras et al 2005).

Vagitus uterinus, the audible cry of the fetus

A cry of the fetus is a startling event. It is sometimes found at term, but has also been described in fetuses aged 21–22 weeks (Humphrey 1978). It is associated with ruptured membranes that allow air to enter the uterus, and by subsequent operative intervention that stimulates the fetus (Blair 1965, Thiery et al 1973). Blair (1965) described a case where it was decided to induce labour. The membranes were ruptured by means of a Drew–Smythe catheter; when liquid stopped draining, the obstetrician heard air gurgling through the catheter into the uterus, so the instrument was withdrawn. This was followed by a few cries from the fetus. Liley (1972) reported a case of air amniocentesis where a substantial volume of intra-amniotic air led to prolonged loud fetal crying. In a case like this, the fetus would swallow air, some of which would pass into the larynx since, at this stage, neuromuscular control at the entrance to the larynx is not yet perfectly developed; and a cry would be produced during the expiratory phase (Blair 1965).

The developmental course of behavioural states

FETAL QUIESCENCE

From 10 weeks' gestation onwards, the following two types of quiescence can be observed: (1) short phases of inactivity intersperse all kinds of behavioural patterns; the fetus stops whatever activity he or she is doing for almost 1 minute, only to resume the same activity or start a different one a moment later (Piontelli 2006); and (2) the fetus remains motionless for at least 3 minutes (van Dongen and Goudie 1980, de Vries et al 1985). Such resting periods increase with advancing gestation. They can last up to 15 minutes by mid-gestation (de Vries et al 1982, de Vries and Fong 2006). During the second half of pregnancy, fetal quiescence increases further (ten Hof et al 2002).

FROM COINCIDENCE TO STATE

Cycles between periods of high and low motor activity begin around mid-gestation (Swartjes et al 1990, Groome et al 1992). With progressing pregnancy, episodes of both activity and rest increasingly become linked to the specific fetal heart-rate patterns. By 25–26 weeks' gestation, the association between fetal heart-rate pattern B and the presence of body movements links with the occurrence of eye movements; however, this linkage is not yet stable over time and transitions do not occur simultaneously (Arduini et al 1986, Drogtrop et al 1990). For such short episodes of linkage between state variables, the term *'coincidence'* was coined (Nijhuis et al 1982). A coincidence of all three state variables (Figure 4.2a) typically occurs around 30 weeks' gestation (Visser et al 1987, Drogtrop et al 1990, Nijhuis and van de Pas 1992, Nijhuis et al 1999), resulting in a decrease of periods of non-coincidence, i.e. of the percentage of time during which the state criteria are not met (Nijhuis et al 1982, Arduini et al 1986, 1989). Only from 36 weeks onwards are behavioural states well developed in fetuses (Nijhuis et al 1982), or in preterm infants (Prechtl et al 1979). Now the parameters of the three state variables – the fetal heart-rate pattern, body movements and eye movements – change concurrently (over a period of 3 minutes) from one state to the other, remaining closely linked over a longer period of time (Figure 4.2b; Nijhuis et al 1982).

A *transition* is the time interval between two different and consecutive behavioural states (Figure 4.5). The onset of a transition is the beginning of loss of coincidence between the variables; the transition ends when all three state variables synchronise into a new state. There is a progressive reduction in the duration of transitions from 28 weeks of gestation onwards; prior to 32 weeks, there are virtually no transitions shorter than 3 minutes (Romanini and Rizzo 1995). The fetal heart-rate pattern is usually the first variable to change from pattern A to B, indicating a transition from state 1F to state 2F (Figure 4.5). Conversely, the fetal heart-rate pattern is the last variable to change in a transition from state 2F to state 1F (Figure 4.2b; Swartjes et al 1990, Arduini et al 1991, Groome et al 1996, Nijhuis et al 1998). The fact that the transition from state 2F to 1F lasts longer than the other way round (Figure 4.2b; Arduini et al 1991, Nijhuis et al 1999) supports the hypothesis that 1F is a better-organised state of sleep than 2F, with a higher degree of homeostatic control and more structured transitions out of this state (Groome et al 1996).

Near term, state 1F is present for about 25% of the time and state 2F for about 50% of the time, while states 3F and 4F, or episodes of non-coincidence, cover the remaining

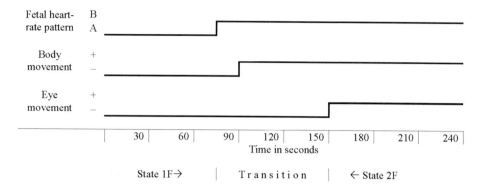

Figure 4.5 Example of a behavioural state transition (lasting 1 minute) from state 1F to state 2F. The fetal heart-rate pattern is the first variable to change, followed by the fetal body movements and the fetal eye movements. Adapted from Nijhuis JG, van de Pas M, Jongsma HW. (1998) State transitions in uncomplicated pregnancies after term. *Early Hum Dev* 52: 125–132, with permission.

25%. The mean duration of an enclosed period of state 2F is 60 minutes, and of state 1F about 30 minutes, which amounts to a complete sleep cycle of approximately 90 minutes (Visser and Mulder 1993).

After 41 weeks, the sleep states 1F and 2F decrease, mainly at the expense of state 2F, whereas wakefulness (states 3F and 4F) increases (Figure 4.6). This increase in fetal wakefulness reflects fetal distress, as the fetal heart-rate pattern D shows prolonged accelerations, resulting in a sustained tachycardia with only short periods of return to the baseline, in which it resembles tachycardia with decelerations (van de Pas et al 1994).

In fetuses of nulliparae, behavioural states appear at a somewhat later gestational age (van Vliet et al 1985). The reason for this may be related to differences in the maternal adaptation to the first pregnancy as opposed to subsequent ones. Infants of nulliparae are 150–200g lighter at birth than those of multiparae, and this difference is fairly consistent from about 32 weeks of gestation onwards. Moreover, placental weight is lower in first pregnancies. Intra-uterine nutrition can be suboptimal in first pregnancies compared with later ones, which is possibly related to immunological variations (Warburton and Naylor 1971) or to differences in the adaptation of the uterine circulation to pregnancy (Thomson et al 1968). It is thus possible that a slightly better placental function in subsequent pregnancies leads to slightly earlier maturation of some features of central nervous system function, including the appearance of behavioural states (van Vliet et al 1985).

Finally, the organisation of fetal states seems to be a stable individual attribute that is maintained across the prenatal and neonatal periods. Fetuses with high state concordance at 36 weeks have a good state regulation after birth; as neonates they are more alert, have a better orientation, and are less irritable (DiPietro et al 2002).

Duration (secs)

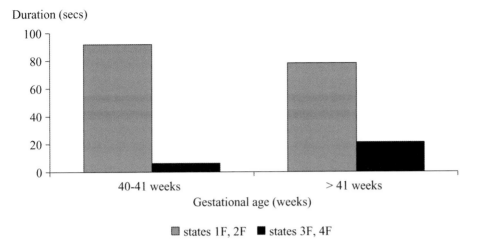

states 1F, 2F ■ states 3F, 4F

Figure 4.6 Wakefulness (states 3F and 4F; black) increases significantly from 6% (at 40–41 weeks, N=12) to 21.5% after 41 weeks (N=12; p=0.014). Sleep states 1F and 2F (grey) decrease from 92% at 40–41 weeks to 78% after 41 weeks (p=0.014). Data from van de Pas M, Nijhuis JG, Jongsma HW. (1994) Fetal behaviour in uncomplicated pregnancies after 41 weeks of gestation. *Early Hum Dev* 40: 29–38, with permission

IS THE STATE PROFILE OF A NEONATE COMPARABLE TO THAT OF A FETUS?

Theoretically, one would not necessarily expect fetal and neonatal behavioural states to be comparable, as extensive physiological changes occur at birth and afterwards. In fact, the neonatal heart rate is about 20 beats per minute lower than the fetal heart rate, but the corresponding state-specific heart-rate patterns are similar (James et al 1995). The relative ratio of state 1F to state 2F is also similar before and after birth – approximately one-third of state 1F and two-thirds of state 2F (Pillai and James 1990b). After birth, there are more transitions, albeit shorter ones (Groome et al 1999). The frequency of eye movements and body movements is similar in states 1F and 1, as well as in state 2F and 2, but body movements are less frequent in the fetal state 4F than in the neonatal state 4 (Pillai and James 1990b).

Implications for the assessment of fetal health

The continuous alteration of behavioural states changes not only fetal motility and heart rate but also fetal haemodynamics, responsiveness and metabolism (Romanini and Rizzo 1995). Therefore, any researcher studying fetal pathophysiology, and any clinician evaluating fetal health, must be familiar with behavioural states. Not taking them into account can lead to inconsistencies in the findings as well as to incorrect patient management (Visser et al 1989, Romanini and Rizzo 1995, Nijhuis 2003).

A SILENT FETAL HEART-RATE PATTERN CAN REFLECT STATE 1F

The widely used non-stress test merely focuses on recording the fetal heart rate (Spencer 1990). The main feature of normality in the interpretation of the non-stress test is the presence of a so-called reactive tracing, which represents fetal heart-rate accelerations. In the literature, the suggested ideal number of accelerations varies from one to five, over a period of 20–30 minutes (see also Chapter 8, p 158). One problem is that, in non-stress tests, the age of the fetus is not taken into account, since a clear developmental trend can be seen in both the amplitude and duration of accelerations (Visser et al 1981b). Furthermore, a silent fetal heart-rate pattern can indeed indicate fetal stress, but it sometimes also reflects a physiological condition, namely behavioural state 1F. Healthy term fetuses can show non-reactive tracings (fetal heart-rate pattern A) for up to 1 hour (Table 4.3).

HAEMODYNAMIC CHANGES DURING STATE 2F

Doppler flow-velocity measurements are used for early detection of hypertension or intrauterine growth retardation. Behavioural states are associated with substantial changes in fetal haemodynamics. A lower pulsatility index during state 2F is a normal haemodynamic adaptive response to a period of fetal activity (van Eyck et al 1987). Similarly, an increased right-to-left shunt at the level of the foramen ovale (van Eyck et al 1990), an increased left cardiac output (Rizzo et al 1990) and a reduced blood flow through the ductus arteriosus (Mooren et al 1989) are normal adaptations during state 2F.

VIBROACOUSTIC STIMULATION DURING STATE 1F CAN CAUSE HARM

If the fetal response to vibroacoustic stimulation is characterised by transient tachycardia – which sometimes lasts up to several minutes, and by an increase in fetal movements (Serafini et al 1984), this is considered an indicator of good fetal health. The ability of the fetus to react to a stimulus, however, varies according to the respective behavioural state. Responses are most evident when a vibroacoustic stimulus is applied during state 1F (Devoe et al 1990): here, tachycardia can last for up to 1 hour. Since no other kind of stimulation causes such a prolonged heart-rate response, some authors have expressed concern at its use (Romanini and Rizzo 1985, Patrick and Gagnon 1989, Visser et al 1989).

FETAL VOIDING IS INHIBITED DURING state 1F

Fetal urine production, which is analysed by serial measurements of the fetal bladder (Rabinowitz et al 1989), increases with advancing gestation. Voiding is also influenced by the behavioural states (Visser et al 1981a, Arduini et al 1985, 1991); it does not occur during state 1F but is facilitated with the transition into state 2F.

Dysfunctions of fetal behavioural states

It is assumed that behavioural states reflect fetal brain development. Hence, their analysis is used to assess the integrity of the central nervous system. In general, a state disturbance consists of a high percentage of non-coincidence of state parameters and in a lack of synchrony at state transitions (Visser and Mulder 1993, Romanini and Rizzo 1995). For example, fetuses of mothers with type 1 diabetes show a poorer concordance among indices of behavioural states, a higher frequency of asynchronous and disrupted transitions between behavioural states, and shorter rest–activity cycles than similarly aged fetuses of mothers who do not have diabetes (Visser et al 1985, Robertson and Dierker 1986, Mulder et al 1987).

Corticosteroids (betamethasone, dexamethasone) induce prolonged episodes of fetal quiescence (fetal heart-rate pattern A, absence of general movements), thus simulating a more mature fetus (Derks et al 1998). Maternal alcohol intake particularly has an effect on state 2F, with the fetal eye movements reduced and fetal breathing movements almost completely suppressed (Mulder et al 1998). Fetuses of mothers with a high caffeine consumption spend more time in state 4F, at the expenses of state 2F (Devoe et al 1993).

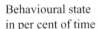

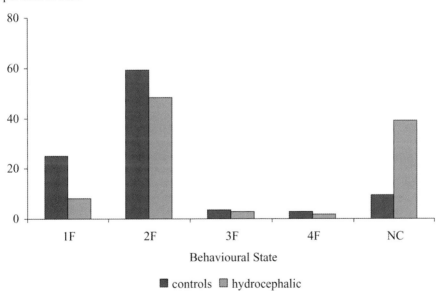

Figure 4.7 Distribution of fetal behavioural states in healthy (black) and hydrocephalic (grey) fetuses between 36 and 38 weeks of gestation. NC = non-coincidence. From Arduini D, Rizzo G, Massacesi M, Boccolini MR, Romanini C, Mancuso S. (1991) Longitudinal assessment of behavioural transitions in healthy human fetuses during the last trimester of pregnancy. *J Perinat Med* 19: 67–72, with permission.

An abnormal state organisation such as a high percentage of non-coincidence at term is also associated with developmental delay (James et al 1995), congenital abnormalities (Pillai et al 1991) or sudden infant death (Smoleniec and James 1995). Hydrocephalic fetuses also tend to show grossly abnormal behavioural states (Figure 4.7). Fetal heart-rate patterns A and B can be normal even if their clustering with body and eye movements is extremely low, thus resulting in a high percentage of non-coincidence (Arduini et al 1987).

In growth-retarded fetuses, the development of organised behavioural states is significantly delayed, which manifests in a higher frequency of periods of non-coincidence around term than in low-risk fetuses (van Vliet et al 1985, Rizzo et al 1987). This deviation sometimes precedes the occurrence of abnormal heart rate tracings – which require prompt delivery – by weeks (Arduini et al 1989, Romanini and Rizzo 1995).

The long observation period that is usually required for a behavioural-state analysis (i.e. 2 hours), together with the time-consuming off-line analysis of state variables, set a natural limit to their clinical application. Therefore, some studies are restricted to the analysis of state transitions. In intrauterine growth-retarded fetuses, for example, state variables change in random order during transition (Arduini et al 1989, Nijhuis et al 1999). We should bear in mind, though, that such a finding is normal in healthy neonates (Shirataki and Prechtl 1977).

REFERENCES

Arabin B, Riedewald S, Zacharias C, Saling E. (1988) Quantitative analysis of fetal behavioural patterns with real-time sonography and the actocardiograph. *Gynecol Obstet Invest* 26: 211–218.

Arduini D, Rizzo G, Giorlandino C, Vizzone A, Nava S, Dell'Acqua S, Valensise H, Romanini C (1985). The fetal behavioural states: an ultrasonic study. *Prenat Diagn* 5: 269–276.

Arduini D, Rizzo G, Giorlandino C, Nava S, Dell'Acqua S, Valensise H, Romanini C. (1986) The development of fetal behavioural states: A longitudinal study. *Prenat Diagn* 6: 117–124.

Arduini D, Rizzo G, Caforio L, Mancuso S. (1987) Development of behavioural states in hydrocephalic fetuses. *Fetal Ther* 2: 135–143.

Arduini D, Rizzo G, Caforio L, Boccolini MR, Romanini C, Mancuso S. (1989) Behavioural state transitions in healthy and growth retarded fetuses. *Early Hum Dev* 19: 155–165.

Arduini D, Rizzo G, Massacesi M, Boccolini MR, Romanini C, Mancuso S. (1991) Longitudinal assessment of behavioural transitions in healthy human fetuses during the last trimester of pregnancy. *J Perinat Med* 19: 67–72.

Blair RG. (1965) Vagitus uterinus. Crying in utero. *Lancet* 2(7423): 1164–1165.

Boito SM, Ursem NT, Struijk PC, Stijnen T, Wladimiroff JW. (2004) Umbilical venous volume flow and fetal behavioural states in the normally developing fetus. *Ultrasound Obstet Gynecol* 23: 138–142.

Cosmi EV, Cosmi E, La Torre R. (2001) The effects of fetal breathing movements on the utero-fetal-placental circulation. *Early Pregnancy* 5: 51–52.

Curzi-Dascalova L, Lebrun F, Korn G. (1983) Respiratory frequency according to sleep states and age in normal premature infants. *Pediatr Res* 17: 152–156.

Derks JB, Mulder EJH, Visser GHA. (1995) The effects of maternal betamethasone administration on the fetus. *Br J Obstet Gynaecol* 102: 40–46.

Devoe LD, Murray C, Faircloth D, Ramos E. (1990) Vibroacoustic stimulation and fetal behavioural state in normal term human pregnancy. *Am J Obstet Gynecol* 163: 1156–1161.

Devoe LD, Murray C, Youssif A, Arnaud M. (1993) Maternal caffeine consumption and fetal behavior in normal third-trimester pregnancy. *Am J Obstet Gynaecol* 168: 1105–1111.

de Vries JIP, Fong BF. (2006) Normal fetal motility: an overview. *Ultrasound Obstet Gynecol* 27: 701–711.

de Vries JIP, Visser GHA, Prechtl HFR. (1982) The emergence of fetal behaviour. I. Qualitative aspects. *Early Hum Dev* 7: 301–322.

de Vries JIP, Visser GHA, Prechtl HFR. (1985) The emergence of fetal behaviour. II: Quantitative aspects. *Early Hum Dev* 12: 99–120.

DiPietro JA, Hodgson DM, Costigan KA, Hilton SC, Johnson TR. (1996) Fetal neurobehavioural development. *Child Dev* 67: 2553–2567.

DiPietro JA, Bornstein MH, Costigan KA, Pressman EK, Hahn CS, Painter K, Smith BA, Yi LJ. (2002) What does fetal movement predict about behaviour during the first two years of life? *Dev Psychobiol* 40: 358–371.

Dreyfus-Brisac C. (1962) The electroencephalogram of the premature infant. *World Neurol* 3: 5–15.

Dreyfus-Brisac C. (1970) Ontogenesis of sleep in human prematures after 32 weeks of conceptional age. *Dev Psychobiol* 3: 91–121.

Drogtrop AP, Ubels R, Nijhuis JG. (1990) The association between fetal body movements, eye movements and heart-rate patterns in pregnancies between 25 and 30 weeks of gestation. *Early Hum Dev* 23: 67–73.

Gagnon R. (1995) Developmental aspects of alterations in fetal behavioural states. In: Lecanuet JP, Fifer WP, Krasnegor NA, Smotherman WP, editors. *Fetal Development. A Psychobiological Perspective*. Hillsdale, Hove: Lawrence Erlbaum Associates. p 129–148.

Gingras JL, Mitchell EA, Grattan KE. (2005) Fetal homologue of infant crying. *Arch Dis Child Fetal Neonatal Ed* 90: F415-F418.

Griffin RL, Caron FJM, van Geijn HP. (1985) Behavioural states in the human fetus during labor. *Am J Obstet Gynecol* 152: 828–833.

Groome LJ, Owen J, Singh KP, Neely CL, Gaudier FL. (1992) Spontaneous movement of the human fetus at 18 to 22 weeks of gestation: evidence of early organization of the active-rest-cycle. *J Matern Fetal Invest* 2: 27–32.

Groome LJ, Benanti JM, Bentz LS, Singh KP. (1996) Morphology of active sleep-quiet sleep transitions in normal human term fetuses. *J Perinatal Med* 24: 171–176.

Groome LJ, Swiber MJ, Holland SB, Bentz LS, Atterbury JL, Trimm RF 3rd. (1999) Spontaneous motor activity in the perinatal infant before and after birth: stability in individual differences. *Dev Psychobiol* 35: 15–24.

Hopkins B. (2000) Development of crying in normal infants: method, theory and some speculations. In: Barr RG, Hopkins B, Green JA, editors. *Crying as a Sign, a Symptom and a Signal. Clinics in Developmental Medicine No. 152*. London: Cambridge University Press. p 176–209.

Hopkins B, van Wulfften Palthe T. (1987) The development of the crying state during early infancy. *Dev Psychobiol* 20: 165–175.

Humphrey T. (1978) Function of the nervous system during prenatal life. In: Stave U, editor. *Perinatal Physiology*. New York: Plenum. p 651–683.

James DJ, Pillai M, Smoleniec J. (1995) Neurobehavioural development in the human fetus. In: Lecanuet JP, Fifer WP, Krasnegor NA, Smotherman WP, editors. *Fetal Development. A Psychobiological Perspective*. Hillsdale, Hove: Lawrence Erlbaum Associates. p 101–128.

Koyanagi T, Horimoto N, Satoh S, Inoue M, Nakano H. (1992) The temporal relationship between the onset of rapid eye movement period and the first micturition thereafter in the human fetus with advance in gestation. *Early Hum Dev* 30: 11–19.

Lange S, van Leeuwen P, Schneider U, Frank B, Hoyer D, Geue D. (2009) Heart rate features in fetal behavioural states. *Early Hum Dev* 85: 131–135.

Liley AW. (1972) The fetus as a personality. *Austral New Zealand J Psychiatr* 6: 99–105.

Mirmiran M, Maas YGH, Ariagno RL. (2003) Development of fetal and neonatal sleep and circadian rhythms. *Sleep Med Rev* 7: 321–334.

Monod N, Pajot N. (1965) The sleep of the full-term newborn and premature infant. I. Analysis of the polygraphic study (rapid eye movements, respiration and EEG) in the fullterm newborn. *Biol Neonat* 8: 281–307.

Mooren K, van Eyck J, Wladimiroff JW. (1989) Human fetal ductal flow velocity waveforms relative to behavioural states in normal term pregnancy. *Am J Obstet Gynecol* 160: 371–374.

Mulder EJH, Visser GHA. (1987) Braxton Hicks' contractions and motor behaviour in the near-term human fetus. *Am J Obstet Gynecol* 156: 543–549.

Mulder EJH, Visser GHA, Bekedam DJ, Prechtl HFR. (1987) Emergence of behavioural states in fetuses of type I diabetic mothers. *Early Hum Dev* 15: 231–252.

Mulder EJH, Leiblum DM, Visser GHA. (1995) Fetal breathing movements in late diabetic pregnancy: relationship to fetal heart-rate patterns and Braxton Hicks' contractions. *Early Hum Dev* 43: 225–232.

Mulder EJH, Morssink LP, van der Schee T, Visser GHA. (1998) Acute maternal alcohol consumption disrupts behavioural state organization in the near-term fetus. *Pediatr Res* 44: 774–779.

Nijhuis JG. (2003) Fetal behaviour. *Neurobiol Aging* 24: S41-S46.

Nijhuis JG, van de Pas M. (1992) Behavioral states and their ontogeny: human studies. *Semin Perinat* 16: 206–210.

Nijhuis JG, Prechtl HFR, Martin CB, Bots RSGM. (1982) Are there behavioural states in the human fetus? *Early Hum Dev* 6: 177–195.

Nijhuis JG, Martin CB Jr, Gommers S, Bouws P, Bots RS, Jongsma HW. (1983) The rhythmicity of fetal breathing varies with behavioural state in the human fetus. *Early Hum Dev* 9: 1–7.

Nijhuis JG, Staisch KJ, Martin CB Jr, Prechtl HFR. (1984) A sinusoidal-like fetal heart-rate pattern in association with fetal sucking – report on two cases. *Eur J Obstet Gynecol Reprod Biol* 16: 353–358.

Nijhuis JG, van de Pas M, Jongsma HW. (1998) State transitions in uncomplicated pregnancies after term. *Early Hum Dev* 52: 125–132.

Nijhuis IJ, ten Hof J, Nijhuis JG, Mulder EJ, Narayan H, Taylor DJ, Visser GH. (1999) Temporal organization of fetal behaviour from 24-weeks gestation onwards in normal and complicated pregnancies. *Dev Psychobiol* 34: 257–268.

Okai T, Kozuma S, Shinozuka N, Kuwabara Y, Mizuno M. (1992) A study on the development of sleep-wakefulness cycle in the human fetus. *Early Hum Dev* 29: 391–396.

Parmelee AH Jr, Wenner WH, Akiyama Y, Schultz M, Stern E. (1967) Sleep states in premature infants. *Dev Med Child Neurol* 9: 70–77.

Patrick J, Gagnon R. (1990) Adaptation to vibroacoustic stimulation. In: Dawes GS, Borruto F, Zacutti A, Zacutti A Jr, editors. *Fetal Autonomy and Adaptation*. Chicester: John Wiley and Sons. p 39–53.

Patrick J, Campbell K, Carmichael L, Natale R, Richardson B. (1982) Patterns of gross fetal body movements over 24-hour observation intervals during the last 10 weeks of pregnancy. *Am J Obstet Gynecol* 146: 363–371.

Patrick J, Carmichael L, Chess L, Staples C. (1984) Accelerations of the human fetal heart rate at 38–40 weeks' gestational age. *Am J Obstet Gynecol* 148: 35–41.

Pillai M, James D. (1990a) Behavioral states in normal mature human fetuses. *Arch Dis Child (Fetal & Neonatal Ed)* 65: 39–43.

Pillai M, James D. (1990b) Are the behavioural states of the newborn comparable to those of the fetus? *Early Hum Dev* 22: 39–49.

Pillai M, James D. (1991) Human fetal mouthing movements: a potential biophysical variable for distinguishing state 1F from abnormal fetal behaviour; report of 4 cases. *Eur J Obstet Gynecol Repr Biol* 38: 151–156.

Pillai M, Garrett C, James D. (1991) Bizarre fetal behaviour associated with lethal congenital anomalies: a case report. *Eur J Obstet Gynecol Reprod Biol* 39: 215–218.

Pillai M, James D, Parker M. (1992) The development of ultradian rhythms in the human fetus. *Am J Obstet Gynecol* 167: 172–177.

Piontelli A. (2006) On the onset of human fetal behaviour. In: Manca M, editor. *Psychoanalysis and Neuroscience*. Mailand: Springer. p 391–418.

Prechtl HFR. (1974) The behavioural states of the newborn infant (a review). *Brain Res* 76: 185–212.

Prechtl HFR. (1977) *The Neurological Examination of the Fullterm Newborn Infant. Second Revised and Enlarged Edition. Clinics in Developmental Medicine No. 63*. London: Heinemann.

Prechtl HFR. (1992) The organization of behavioral states and their dysfunction. *Semin Perinatol* 16: 258–263.

Prechtl HFR, Akiyama Y, Zinkin P, Kerr Grant D. (1968) Polygraphic studies of the fullterm newborn. II. Computer analysis of recorded data. In: Bax MCO, MacKeith RC, editors. *Studies in Infancy. Clinics in Developmental Medicine No. 27.* London: Spastics Society. p 22–40.

Prechtl HFR, Weinmann HM, Akiyama Y. (1969) Organization of physiological parameters in normal and neurologically abnormal infants. *Neuropediatr* 1: 101–129.

Prechtl HFR, Fargel JW, Weinmann HM, Bakker HH. (1979) Postures, motility and respiration of low-risk preterm infants. *Dev Med Child Neurol* 21: 3–27.

Rabinowitz R, Peters MT, Vyas S, Campbell S, Nicolaides KH. (1989) Measurement of fetal urine production in normal pregnancy by real-time ultrasonography. *Am J Obstet Gynecol* 161: 1264–1266.

Rizzo G, Arduini D, Pennestri F, Romanini C, Mancuso S. (1987) Fetal behaviour in growth retardation: its relationship to fetal blood flow. *Prenatal Diagn* 7: 229–238.

Rizzo G, Arduini D, Mancuso S, Romanini C. (1988) Computer assisted analysis of fetal behavioural states. *Prenatal Diagn* 8: 479–484.

Rizzo G, Arduini D, Valensise H, Romanini C. (1990) Effects of behavioural states on cardiac output in healthy human fetuses at 36–38 weeks of gestation. *Early Hum Dev* 23: 109–115.

Robertson SS, Dierker LJ. (1986) The development of cyclic motility in fetuses of diabetic mothers. *Dev Psychobiol* 19: 223–234.

Romanini C, Rizzo G. (1995) Fetal behaviour in normal and compromised fetuses. An overview. *Early Hum Dev* 43: 117–131.

Schmidt W, Boos R, Gnirs J, Auer L, Schulze S. (1985) Fetal behavioural states and controlled sound stimulation. *Early Hum Dev* 12: 145–153.

Serafini P, Lindsay MBJ, Nagey DA, Pupkin MJ, Tseng P, Crenshaw CJ. (1984) Antepartum fetal heart rate response to sound stimulation: the acoustic stimulation test. *Am J Obstet Gynecol* 48: 41–45.

Shirataki S, Prechtl HFR. (1977) Sleep state transitions in newborn infants: Preliminary study. *Dev Med Child Neurol* 19: 316–325.

Shirozu H, Koyanagi T, Takashima T, Horimoto N, Akazawa K, Nakano H. (1995) Penile tumescence in the human fetus at term – a preliminary report. *Early Hum Dev* 41: 159–166.

Smoleniec J, James D. (1995) Fetal behaviour and the sudden infant death syndrome. *Arch Dis Child Fetal Neonatal Ed* 72: 168–171.

Spencer JAD. (1990) Antepartum cardiotocography. In: Chamberlain G, editor. *Modern Antenatal Care of the Fetus.* Oxford: Blackwell Scientific Publications. p 163–188.

Swartjes JM, van Geijn HP, Mantel R, van Woerden EE, Schoemaker HC. (1990) Coincidence of behavioural state parameters in the human fetus at three gestational ages. *Early Hum Dev* 23: 75–83.

ten Hof J, Nijhuis IJ, Mulder EJ, Nijhuis JG, Narayan H, Taylor DJ, Westers P, Visser GH. (2002) Longitudinal study of fetal body movements: nomograms, intrafetal consistency, and relationship with episodes of heart-rate patterns A and B. *Pediatr Res* 52: 568–575.

Thiery M, Le Sian Yo A, Vrijens M, Janssens D. (1973) Vagitus uterus. *J Obstet Gynecol Br Commonw* 80: 183–185.

Thomson AM, Billewicz WZ, Hytten FE. (1968) The assessment of fetal growth. *J Obstet Gynaecol Br Commonw* 75: 903–916.

Timor-Tritsch IE. (1986) The effect of external stimuli on fetal behaviour. *Eur J Obstet Gynecol Reprod Biol* 21: 321–329.

van den Bergh BRH, Mulder EJH, Visser GHA, Poelmann-Weesjes G, Bekedam DJ, Prechtl HFR. (1989) The effect of (induced) maternal emotions on fetal behaviour: a controlled study. *Early Hum Dev* 19: 9–19.

van de Pas M, Nijhuis JG, Jongsma HW. (1994) Fetal behaviour in uncomplicated pregnancies after 41 weeks of gestation. *Early Hum Dev* 40: 29–38.

van Dongen LGR, Goudie EG. (1980) Fetal movement patterns in the first trimester of pregnancy. *Br J Obstet Gynaecol* 87: 191–193.

van Eyck J, Wladimiroff JW, Noordam MJ, Tonge HM, Prechtl HFR. (1985) The blood flow velocity waveforms in the fetal descending aorta; its relationship to behavioural states in normal pregnancy at 37–38 weeks of gestation. *Early Hum Dev* 14: 99–107.

van Eyck J, Wladimiroff JW, Wijngaard JAGW, Noordam MJ, Prechtl HFR. (1987) The blood flow velocity waveforms in the fetal internal carotid and umbilical artery; its relationship to behavioural states in normal pregnancy at 37–38 weeks of gestation. *Br J Obstet Gynaecol* 94: 736–741.

van Eyck J, van Stewart PA, Wladimiroff JW. (1990) Human fetal foramen ovale flow velocity waveforms relative to behavioural states in normal pregnancy. *Am J Obstet Gynecol* 163, 1239–1242.

van Vliet MAT, Martin CB Jr, Nijhuis JG, Prechtl HFR. (1985) The relationship between fetal activity, and behavioral states and fetal breathing movements in normal and growth retarded fetuses. *Am J Obstet Gynecol* 153: 582–588.

van Woerden EE, van Geijn HPM, Caron FJM, van der Valk AW, Swartjes JM, Arts NF. (1988) Fetal mouth movements during behavioural states 1F and 2F. *Eur J Obstet Gynecol Reprod Biol* 29: 97–105.

van Woerden EE, van Geijn HP, Caron FJM, Mantel R, Swartjes JM, Arts NF. (1989) Fetal hiccups; characteristics and relation to fetal heart rate. *Eur J Obstet Gynecol Reprod Biol* 30: 209–216.

Visser GHA, Mulder EJ. (1993) The effect of vibro-acoustic stimulation on fetal behavioural state organization. *Am J Industr Med* 23: 531–539.

Visser GHA, Goodman JDS, Levine DH, Dawes GS. (1981a) Micturition and the heart rate period cycle in the human fetus. *Br J Obstet Gynaecol* 88: 803–805.

Visser GHA, Dawes GS, Redman CW. (1981b) Numerical analysis of the normal human antenatal fetal heart rate. *Br J Obstet Gynaecol* 88: 792–802.

Visser GHA, Zellenberg HJ, de Vries JIP, Dawes GS. (1983) External physical stimulation of the human fetus during episodes of low heart rate variation. *Am J Obstet Gynecol* 145: 579–584.

Visser GH, Bekedam DJ, Mulder EJ, van Ballegooie E. (1985) Delayed emergence of fetal behaviour in type-1 diabetic women. *Early Hum Dev* 12: 167–172.

Visser GHA, Poelman-Weesjes G, Cohen TM, Bekedam DJ. (1987) Fetal behaviour at 30–32 weeks of gestation. *Pediatr Res* 22: 655–658.

Visser GHA, Mulder HH, Wit HP, Mulder EJH, Prechtl HFR. (1989) Vibroacoustic stimulation of the human fetus: effects on behavioural state organisation. *Early Hum Dev* 19: 285–296.

Warburton D, Naylor AF. (1971) The effect of parity on placental weight and birth weight: an immunological phenomenon? A report of the Collaborative Study of Cerebral Palsy. *Am J Hum Genet* 23: 41–54.

Wolff PH. (1959) Observations on newborn infants. *Psychosom Med* 21: 110–118.

Wolff PH. (1969) The natural history of crying and other vocalizations in early infancy. In Foss BM, editor. *Determinantes of Infant Behaviour*. London: Methuen. p 81–109.

5
FETAL RESPONSIVENESS

Introduction

Alongside the ontogeny of spontaneous motor activity, the ability of the fetus to respond to stimulation is another landmark in the development of fetal behaviour. The fetal environment is a source of continuous and adequate stimulation, especially for the auditory, olfactory and tactile senses. In addition, external stimuli (1) impinge directly on the fetus by transmission through the maternal body, uterus and amniotic fluid; and (2) are indirectly transferred through maternal reactions and thus through the mother's haemodynamic and endocrinological system. Consequently, the developing brain permanently interacts with a variety of sensory stimuli.

Most interestingly, the various sensory systems respond to stimulation before they are fully developed (Ronca and Alberts 1995). This mechanism is actually necessary for maturation of the sensory pathways. Another interesting aspect is the question of whether and when responsiveness includes conscious perception, and, in this context, whether perception can elicit emotion. Since thalamocortical fibres only begin to form between 22 and 26 weeks (Kostovic and Rakic 1990), fetal responses before or around this time should be interpreted with caution.

Fetal responsiveness is also clinically important. As early as in 1871, fetal responsiveness was considered a sign of fetal well-being: a midwifery textbook recommended placing one hand on one side of the maternal abdomen, and tapping the opposite side with the other hand. As a sign of normality, this should stimulate a brisk movement of the fetus (Bullock 1871). We know today that the probability of obtaining a fetal response with the same or similar stimuli depends on a number of factors such as gestational age, behavioural state, concurrent stimulation or individual history.

Typically, changes in fetal movements and/or in the fetal heart rate are used to document prenatal responsiveness. While reactivity refers to the magnitude of a motor or heart-rate response, habituation relates to the ease with which a response to successive stimulation declines (Sherrington 1904). For a fetus to be assessed with motor reactivity, he or she must move within 3 seconds after cessation of the stimulus. In view of the fact that the fetus often moves spontaneously (Chapter 2), and that such movements are associated with heart-rate accelerations (Chapter 4), care must be taken not to misinterpret the findings during, or immediately after, stimulation.

The auditory system: the most extensively studied prenatal sensory system
The German paediatrician Albrecht Peiper was the first to suggest that fetuses could hear. Based on complaints of expectant mothers about increased fetal activity during symphonic concerts, he carried out experiments with a car horn and indeed managed to elicit strong fetal movements (Peiper 1925). Two years later, Forbes and Forbes (1927) also reported on a pregnant mother who had actually experienced painful fetal activity following the applause after a symphonic concert.

THE DEVELOPMENT OF THE AUDITORY SYSTEM
The peripheral auditory system develops from an ectodermal thickening that forms the auditory placode (Altmann 1950), which invaginates into the surrounding mesenchyme and forms a vesicular shaped pit, the otocyst. At 4 weeks, the otocyst divides into two lobes; one lobe becomes the cochlea, the other one the labyrinth (Figure 5.1). The organ of Corti, where the auditory receptors are located, begins to develop at 8 weeks and opens around 20 weeks (Bibas et al 2008). By that time, the cochlea seems to function (Pujol et al 1991, Morlet et al 1995). However, thresholds are very high and way beyond the range of naturally occurring acoustic events. Hair-cell differentiation, synaptogenesis and ciliogenesis are only completed at 24 weeks, forming the basis for the frequency-related displacement of the cochlear partition (Nakai 1970, Pujol et al 1991). Two weeks later, the auditory nerve is myelinated, and yet another week later the central auditory pathways are myelinated as well (Figure 5.1; Moore et al 1995, Moore 2002). By now (26–28 weeks), thalamic fibres have reached the auditory cortical plate (Krmpotic-Nemanic et al 1983). From this age onwards, auditory evoked responses are detectable in preterm infants (Rotteveel et al 1987). Magnetoencephalographic (MEG) recordings of fetal auditory evoked fields can be successfully performed at a mere 28–29 weeks (Lengle et al 2001, Schleussner et al 2001, Zappasodi et al 2001), with a response rate of about 65% (Eswaran et al 2005). During the following weeks, the latency of the auditory evoked response declines from 300ms to nearly 150ms at term (Schleussner et al 2001, Holst et al 2005). At term, functional magnetic resonance imaging (fMRI) provides evidence that one or both temporal lobes are activated (Moore et al 2001).

HOW DOES THE SOUND REACH THE FETAL EAR?
The sound environment of the fetus is determined by the noise floor, the attenuation of external signals provided by the tissues and fluids surrounding the fetal head, the route of sound transmission into the fetal inner ear, and the sensitivity of the hearing mechanism (Gerhardt and Abrams 2000). The fact that – unlike after birth – the fetal inner ear is hypoxic, leads to a reduction of the endocochlear potential, to a depression of cochlear transduction and amplification, and consequently to an additional sensorineural component of threshold elevation in the fetus (Sohmer and Freeman 2001). The pathway

- The otocyst divides into two lobes: one becomes the cochlea, the other the labyrinth
    - The cochlea starts to curl
        - The organ of Corti develops
            - The cochlea reaches its full morphological development: it measures 3mm and creates 2.5 coils
            - The external ear can be visualised by means of ultrasound
                - The inner hair cells and the three rows of outer hair cells can be recognised but do not yet function
                    - The tunnel of Corti opens
                        - Thalamocortical fibres begin to emerge
                            - Hair-cell differentiation and ciliogenesis are completed
                                - The auditory nerve is myelinated
                                    - The central auditory pathways are myelinated
                                    - Thalamic afferents reach the auditory cortical plate

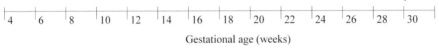

Gestational age (weeks)

Figure 5.1 Anatomical and functional development of the auditory system (Nakai 1970, Krmpotic-Nemanic et al 1983, Kostovic and Rakic 1990, Pujol et al 1991, Arabin 2002, Moore 2002, Bibas et al 2008).

by which sound reaches and activates the fetal inner ear has been the subject of controversy. There are basically two hypotheses:

1. Acoustic stimuli pass through the fluid-filled external auditory canal and the middle ear system to the inner ear (Querleu et al 1989, Lecanuet and Schaal 1996). The fetal middle ear transmission differs from the postnatal one: postnatally, the middle ear adapts to the amplification of acoustic stimuli from the aerial environment of the outer ear to the liquid environment of the cochlea. Prenatally, sound energy can reach the cochlear receptors without the need of amplification, since the amniotic fluid, tissues and bones have similar conduction properties

2. Bone conduction is the dominant mechanism for fetal hearing, with little or no contribution from the external and middle ears (Bradley and Mistretta 1975, Gerhardt and Abrams 2000, Sohmer et al 2001). The bone conduction route implies that sound energy is diminished by 10–20dB for frequencies lower than 250Hz, and by 40–50dB for frequencies between 250 and 500Hz (Arabin 2002).

Basically, acoustic stimuli arise from two environments: firstly, the 'intrauterine world' provides stimuli caused by maternal circulation and digestion, but also by the

93

mother's voice; and secondly, as birth approaches, sound stimuli from the 'extrauterine world' are increasingly responded to.

THE INTRAUTERINE NOISE LEVEL
The fetal environment clearly contains an impressive array of sounds that vary in pitch and loudness and are associated with maternal respiratory, cardiovascular and intestinal activity, as well as with the mother's body movements. Depending on the frequency, sound pressure levels of 60–95dB were measured by means of microphones after rupture of the membranes, or by hydrophones positioned in a pocket of fluid (Walker et al 1971, Gagnon et al 1992). Low frequency (<100Hz), which dominates the intrauterine noise floor, correlates with the maternal systole, reaching levels as high as 90–95dB (Bradley and Mistretta 1975). Owing to habituation, the fetus does not react to this background noise (Sadovsky et al 1986).

Maternal vocalisation and externally generated noise sometimes exceed this internal background. External, environmentally generated noise is usually attenuated in such a way that it does not exceed the intrauterine noise level. The fetus is only exposed to low-frequency environmental noise in exceptional situations – when, for example, an underground train passes by the pregnant woman. Stimuli of such an intensity, and so different in nature from the usual maternal stimuli, can cause fetal response (Bradley and Mistretta 1975, Gerhardt and Abrams 2000).

FETAL RESPONSE TO EXOGENOUS SOUNDS
Observations of fetuses responding to natural external noises are scarce. Apart from the historical and rather anecdotal reports mentioned above (Peiper 1925, Forbes and Forbes 1927), there is, to our knowledge, only one report on three term fetuses who responded to an air-raid alarm with severe fetal bradycardia (less than 60 beats per minute). It took 2 minutes for the fetal heart rate to return to a normal pattern (Yoles et al 1993). It seems most probable, however, that the fetuses had responded to maternal stress rather than to the auditory stimulus.

Since the beginning of studies on fetal responsiveness, various types of stimuli have been emitted in a variety of administration modes (airborne, air coupled or vibratory): pure tones, various bandwidth frequency noises, high-pass filtered or unfiltered pink or white noises, and the electro-acoustic larynx. The way a stimulus is sensed by the fetus is different from the way it is perceived ex utero. Owing to frequency-dependent attenuation (Richards et al 1992), the fetus has a sensation as though the bass control were turned up, and the treble control turned down (Gagnon et al 1992, Gerhardt and Abrams 2000), as this is how sounds are modified by the tissues and fluids of the womb before reaching the fetus' head.

The primary purpose of most auditory experiments on human fetuses was not to study the development of the auditory sense but to test fetal well-being and/or find possible hearing defects before birth. Such studies usually employ sine wave stimuli of 500–5000Hz at intensities of 90–120dB, which cause motor responses and fetal heart-rate accelerations of at least 15 beats per minute, sustained for at least 2 minutes (Trudinger and Boylan 1980, Birnholz and Benacerraf 1983, Kisilevsky et al 2000).

As responsiveness depends on the behavioural state (Prechtl 1974, Schmidt et al 1985, Timor-Tritsch 1986), there are, in general, fewer responses during the sleep states (1F, 2F) than during state 4F, which only represents 9–16% of the fetal states (see Chapter 4). In state 1F, there is hardly any response. The fact that researchers often disregard these physiological changes constitutes a serious limitation to a significant number of studies.

What levels of sound pressure levels and frequencies elicit fetal reaction?
The auditory system of the fetus does not automatically react to any stimulus, regardless of the frequency range. Its development follows a consistent pattern. The fetus starts hearing in the frequency range of 250–500Hz (as opposed to 20–20000Hz in adults). With progressing gestation, the fetal hearing range increases (Figure 5.2). The fetus does not exhibit responsiveness to a wider range of frequencies until 37–38 weeks. At that age, the sound-pressure level required to evoke a fetal response is 20–30dB lower than it was 10 weeks earlier (Hepper and Shahidulla 1994a, Kisilevsky et al 2000), which indicates that the fetal auditory system becomes more sensitive with increasing age. Similarly, the sound-pressure level required to elicit an auditory evoked brainstem response decreases by 20dB from 30 to 40 weeks, as shown by studies on preterm infants (Lary et al 1985).

When does sound discrimination start?
One- to 2-month-old infants are able to discriminate between voiced and voiceless forms of plosives (e.g. [t] versus [d]), different vowels (e.g. [a] versus [i]), the place of articulation (e.g. [ba] versus [ga]), and different vowel–consonant clusters (e.g. [ad] versus [ag]; Morse 1972, Trehub 1973).

It is of major interest whether fetuses are also able to differentiate between sound variations, since this fundamental competence is a prerequisite for the development of a functional auditory system, and consequently of a proper speech and language. As verified by means of fetal heart-rate decelerations, which Sokolov considered to be an orienting response (Sokolov 1963), term fetuses discriminate between different vowels (Groome et al 1999), between [babi] and [biba] (Lecanuet et al 1989), and between a female and male speaker (Lecanuet et al 1993). Typically, such discrimination occurs at a sound-pressure level of 85–90dB. If the sound-pressure level increases, the fetal heart beat accelerates (Groome et al 1997), which is interpreted as a defensive reaction (Sokolov 1963).

Preterm fetuses, too, distinguish between different phonemes, like, for example between [baba] and [bibi], but they need a higher sound pressure (110dB) than term fetuses (Shahidullah and Hepper 1994). By means of fetal MEG and the oddball paradigm, sound differentiation has even been found in fetuses as young as 28 weeks (Draganova et

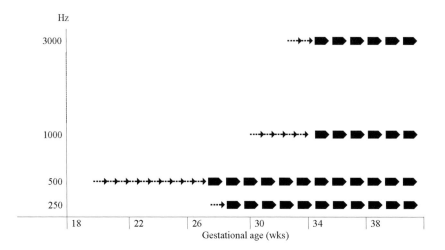

Figure 5.2 Development of fetal responsiveness to increasing frequency levels in Hz (related to the pitch of the sound), from a study on 450 fetuses. ⋯➤= some fetuses respond, others do not; ➡ = all assessed fetuses respond. Created using data from Hepper PG, Shahidullah S. (1994) Development of fetal hearing. *Arch Dis Child* 71: F81–F87.

al 2007), although it usually starts at around 35 weeks. A discriminative response to deviant versus standard sounds occurs at an average latency of 330ms, which could be a fetal analogy to the adult mismatch negativity (Draganova et al 2005, Huotilainen et al 2005). A serious deficiency of these results is that none of the studies they are based on takes into account the behavioural state of the fetus.

Acoustic stimulation increases fetal swallowing: a word of caution
Acoustic stimulation is associated with increased fetal swallowing activity (Petrikovsky et al 1993). This can lead to a diminution of amniotic fluid. Yet if amniotic fluid is low, acoustic stimulation must be used with extreme caution! Petrikovsky and colleagues (1993) reported on seven patients with borderline amniotic fluid indices who developed oligohydramnios after acoustic stimulation experiments; two fetuses even needed acute obstetric intervention.

THE MOTHER'S VOICE, A SALIENT STIMULUS FROM PRENATAL TO POSTNATAL LIFE
The sensitivity of the fetus to low-frequency sound includes the exposure to voice. The average fundamental frequency of an adult male's voice is 125Hz, which is approximately

one octave below middle C on the piano keyboard. The average fundamental frequency of the female's voice is 220Hz. Speech produced during normal conversation has a sound-pressure level of 65–75dB (Gerhardt and Abrams 1996). In the uterus, the sound-pressure level of the mother's voice is enhanced by an average of 5dB, whereas external male and female voices are attenuated by an average of 2dB and 3dB respectively (Richards et al 1992).

Voicing information – the term refers to the presence or absence of vocal-fold vibrations (e.g. [p] versus [b]) – is better transmitted to the fetus than place or manner information. Place information relates to the place of articulation of a particular sound (e.g. lips versus alveolar ridge); manner information describes the way in which a specific speech sound is produced (e.g. plosive versus fricative; Gerhardt and Abrams 2000). Experiments on sheep fetuses show that the intelligibility of (meaningless) phonemes recorded in utero is reduced (Griffiths et al 1994), although a male voice is more intelligible (55%) than a female one (34%). These results place a question mark over the assumption that the neonate is devoid of experience with speech. Moreover, considerable attention should be given to the possibility that the fetus actually perceives speech and forms memories of it, which enables him/her as a newborn infant to distinguish between sounds and voices.

Indeed, it seems to be the case that term fetuses differentiate between their mother's voice and a female stranger's voice (Kisilevsky et al 2003), in fact even between the mother's tape-recorded voice and her natural voice (Hepper and Shahidullah 1994a). However, familiar nursery rhymes – as opposed to unfamiliar ones – elicit negligible heart-range changes (DeCasper et al 1994) or ambiguous responses (Krueger et al 2004), although a fMRI study revealed a temporal lobe activation in two of three term fetuses in response to a tape recording of the mother reciting a rhyme (Hykin et al 1999).

WHAT IS MUSIC TO THE FETUS?
The fetus can sense rhythms and male or female singing (Woodward and Guidozzi 1992, Gerhardt and Abrams 1996, Abrams et al 1998). Any alteration in the fetus's heart rate depends on the loudness of the music, on how abruptly the music crescendos, on the frequency range that a specific piece of music covers, and, of course, on the fetus' behavioural state (Lind 1980). By the end of pregnancy, fetal movements become more lively when exposed to music – for instance to Brahms' lullaby (Kisilevsky et al 2004) or the theme song of a television soap opera (Hepper 1991). A fMRI study has shown that exposure to Spanish guitar music – with its wide dynamic range of frequency and intensity – activates both the frontal and temporal lobes (Moore et al 2001).

A topic of discussion is whether fetal responsiveness is directly related to the presentation of music or only a secondary reaction to the mother's emotion (Sontag et al 1969, Zimmer et al 1982). When the mother listens to her favourite type of music with headphones, inaudible to the fetus, fetal breathing movements decrease and body movements increase, although the fetal heart rate does not react consistently (Olds 1985).

On the other hand, by a mere 28 weeks' gestation (Kisilevsky et al 2004), the fetal heart rate increases immediately when the fetus is presented with a different piece of music from the mother, who uses headphones (Lind 1980).

Does the newborn remember prenatal experiences with music?
Hicks (1995) suggested that, in order to create a familiar atmosphere for the newborn baby, the same piece of music should be played during delivery that had been played during the last weeks of pregnancy. However, there is little evidence of newborn infants recognising music that had been played to them during late pregnancy (Damstra-Wijmenga 1991), and there are only a few reports to confirm that the newborn infant – unlike the fetus – reduces his or her movements, but also cries less and becomes more alert when listening to a familiar tune (Hepper 1988, James et al 2002).

There is no evidence of a long-term benefit after fetal exposure to voice or music
During the 1970s, numerous psychological and nursing reports expressed concern about stimulus deprivation in hospitalised infants. This aroused clinical and parental interest in possible beneficial effects of stimulation by means of sounds such as heart beats, lullabies, white noise and human speech. Many of the studies were flawed, while others had not been designed to evaluate clinical interventions. Even so, the clinicians', parents' and manufacturers' interest in exposing the fetus or the preterm infant to a variety of mechanically or electronically produced sounds and other sensory stimuli has not ceased to this day (Gardner et al 1984, Philbin et al 2000). Mothers have been recommended to wear commercial products such as little bells on chains throughout pregnancy, in order to supposedly 'enhance neural maturation', although there is no proof of effect or long-term benefit to the child's intelligence or general development (Arabin 2002). It is, however, obvious that talking, singing or playing music to the fetus automatically creates a caring relationship, and this, in turn, may cause postnatal behaviour to be more balanced (Lind 1980).

Intense noise exposure has an adverse effect
Excessive acoustic stimulation – for instance by means of unphysiological frequencies and intensities of audio-speakers or megaphones, with the sole aim to obtain a reaction – can even pose a risk to the auditory development and behavioural state regulation in the unborn child. For one thing, it directly affects the developing fetus; but then it also affects the mother, and hence the fetus by neuroendocrine effects. In addition, maternal noise exposure during pregnancy significantly increases the risk of having a hearing-impaired child (exposure to 95dB for 8 hours per day, for example, increases the risk by a factor of three; Lalande et al 1986). Fifty per cent of those children whose mothers have been exposed to noise levels of more than 85dB (for example in the weaving industry) show a

significant hearing loss at an age of 4–7 years (Daniel and Laciak 1982, Lalande et al 1986). Hence, prevention of hearing loss in the unborn is a crucial issue. Although the fetus is more aquatic than terrestrial, and the patterns of hearing loss caused by noise are quite different from those in an adult (Gerhardt and Abrams 2000), great care must be taken while the auditory system is still developing, to avoid exposure of the fetus and neonate to noise levels (sustained or impulsive) that might cause impairment of hearing.

Vibroacoustic stimulation: a harmful procedure
Seventy-five years ago, Sontag and Wallace from the Fels Institute (see Chapter 1, p 21) gave the following precise description of how the fetus reacts to vibroacoustic stimulation: when a small block of wood is placed on the abdomen of a woman who is 8 months pregnant, and a doorbell clapper is permitted to strike at the rate of 120 vibrations per second, there is, in approximately 90% of cases, an immediate convulsive response on the part of the fetus. The response is in the form of violent kicking and moving as well as a sudden increase in fetal heart rate. The heart rate remains high for a while before decreasing to the previous baseline (Sontag and Wallace 1934).

Such a response to vibroacoustic stimuli can sometimes be observed at a mere 24–25 weeks' gestation (Birnholz and Benaceraff 1983); by 26–27 weeks, every second fetus responds in this way (Kuhlman and Depp 1988, Kisilevsky et al 1992). The response to vibroacoustic stimulation is considered to be indicative of fetal activity; the elicited accelerations of fetal heart rate are used clinically for fetal monitoring (Goodlin and Schmidt 1972, Smith 1995, Hoh et al 2009, Petrović et al 2009), although it has been shown that such heart-rate accelerations are not instrumental in distinguishing between low-risk and high-risk fetuses (Kisilevsky et al 1990).

The term vibroacoustic refers to stimuli applied to the maternal abdomen, usually above the fetal head. There are no standards of application regarding stimulus intensity, duration or rate of repetition (DiPietro 2005). An artificial, electric larynx with an output of approximately 110dB in a frequency range of 250–850Hz is usually fixed to the maternal abdomen. When the stimulus is applied for at least 3 seconds during state 1F, observers expect a healthy fetus to respond (Fox and Badalian 1993), which, in actual fact, not even all term fetuses do (Devoe et al 1985). Moreover, in the case of a vibroacoustic stimulation, the pregnant woman cannot be masked during the application of the stimulus, because she would definitely feel the stimulus. And lastly, when the stimulus appears to be applied but is not actually activated, there is sometimes still a fetal response, which indicates that fetal response can even be triggered by maternal anticipation (Visser et al 1989, DiPietro et al 1996).

The response consists of an increase of fetal movements (Gagnon et al 1986, Dirix et al 2009), usually initiated by startles (Divon et al 1985, Kuhlman and Depp 1988); an increase of the fetal heart rate (Ohel et al 1987), which may even last up to 1 hour (Visser et al 1989); a decrease of fetal breathing movements, which remain irregular for up to 1 hour after stimulation (Gagnon et al 1986); an increase of eye movements (Gagnon et al

1989) and eye blinks (Birnholz and Benacerraf 1983); an increase of fetal hiccups (Kiuchi et al 2000); and an onset of voiding (Zimmer et al 1993). Occasionally, fetal heart-rate decelerations are seen in normally grown fetuses near term (Visser et al 1989). Long-lasting continuous tachycardia may even occur without accompanying body or eye movements, resulting in disorganised behavioural states (Visser et al 1989, Kiuchi et al 2000).

The mechanism by which vibroacoustic stimulation affects the fetus is unknown. It is probable that the vibratory component is more important than acoustics (Grimwade et al 1971). Fetal sensitivity could be related to the maturation of sensory pathways that involve Meissner corpuscles, since the incidence and intensity of the response are related to progressing gestation (Gagnon et al 1987). The response may well reflect a sudden release of fetal catecholamines and an increase of fetal blood pressure (Gagnon et al 1986, Visser and Mulder 1993). fMRI shows an activation within the temporal region (Fulford et al 2004).

The fetal behavioural state achieved after the application of vibroacoustic stimulation depends on the pre-existing state: from state 2F, a fetus proceeds to 4F, but the effect is not consistent and is generally shorter (Visser et al 1989, Devoe et al 1990, Kiuchi et al 2000). By contrast, responses are more evident when the stimulus is applied during state 1F (Visser et al 1989, Petrović et al 2009): once again the fetus changes into state 4F (Gagnon et al 1989, Visser et al 1989, Devoe et al 1990, Bartnicki and Dudenhausen 1995), but such a transition is never seen physiologically, since state 4F is normally preceded by states 2F or 3F (Nijhuis et al 1982, Prechtl 1989). As in neonates, a transition from state 1 to state 4 can only be brought about by means of painful stimuli (Visser et al 1989); the fetal response to vibroacoustic stimulation is similar to that caused by pain (Prechtl 1989, Visser et al 1989, Rayburn 1995) and unphysiological stress (Zimmer et al 1993). Since the sudden profound tachycardia that can be induced is alarming, vibroacoustic stimulation should not be used in a routine clinical setting (Prechtl 1989, Visser and Mulder 1993).

Sense of touch: the first sense to function prenatally

In 1952, Hooker used a series of touch stimuli to demonstrate that exteriorised embryos and fetuses responded to cutaneous stimulation by a mere 8 weeks. Stroking the upper or lower lip caused the first reflex response. It takes another 5–6 weeks for the rest of the body surface to become sensitive to stroking (Figure 5.3). Interestingly, at the time of the first response to touch, the growing nerve fibres are still some distance from the basement membrane (Hooker 1952, Humphrey 1966). This suggests that the growing nerve fibres must be sensitive to tactile stimulation transmitted mechanically through the fetal skin. It takes 9 weeks for the first nerve tips to make contact with the basement membrane of the cutaneous epithelium (Figure 5.3). From 11 weeks to almost mid-gestation, Pacinian corpuscles develop in the entire body, with a greater density than in adults, especially in the free-ending nerves (Humphrey 1964, Bradley and Mistretta 1975). As the hands and fingers grow, the nerve endings do not increase in number but become more widely spaced (Bradley and Mistretta 1975).

Fetal life is marked by constant exteroceptive contact: fetuses toss and turn frequently, and by doing so they touch the uterus or umbilical cord or other parts of the intrauterine environment. When at rest, the fetal body usually lies against the uterus, thus coming into physical contact with the environment.

A SPECIAL SITUATION FOR THE EXTEROCEPTIVE SENSE: THE MULTIPLE PREGNANCY
The first contact between twins – usually between their arms or legs – occurs at 8 weeks' gestation (Arabin et al 1996). This contact appears to be gentle and smooth. A week later, the co-twin begins to react to tactile stimuli. Leg contacts become more forceful from 10 weeks onwards (Arabin et al 1996). Another 2 weeks later, prolonged contacts between the bodies occur. From 13 weeks onwards, twins touch each other's head with the lips, which is sometimes followed by an obvious reaction.

The contact between monochorionic monoamniotic twins emerges a few days earlier and occurs more often than in dichorionic dizygotic twins (Arabin et al 1996, Piontelli et al 1997).

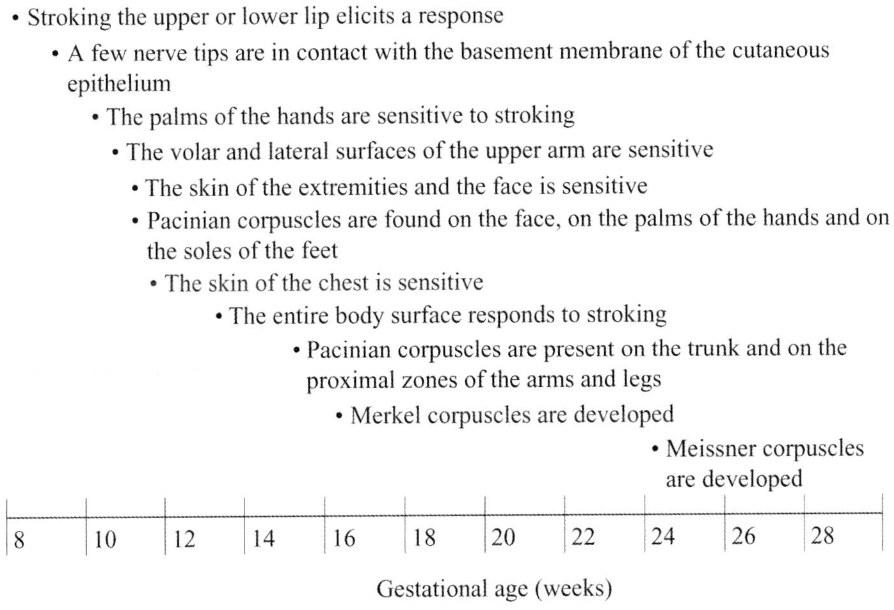

• Stroking the upper or lower lip elicits a response
  • A few nerve tips are in contact with the basement membrane of the cutaneous epithelium
    • The palms of the hands are sensitive to stroking
     • The volar and lateral surfaces of the upper arm are sensitive
      • The skin of the extremities and the face is sensitive
      • Pacinian corpuscles are found on the face, on the palms of the hands and on the soles of the feet
       • The skin of the chest is sensitive
        • The entire body surface responds to stroking
         • Pacinian corpuscles are present on the trunk and on the proximal zones of the arms and legs
          • Merkel corpuscles are developed
            • Meissner corpuscles are developed

| 8 | 10 | 12 | 14 | 16 | 18 | 20 | 22 | 24 | 26 | 28 |

Gestational age (weeks)

Figure 5.3 Development of the cutaneous receptors and responsiveness to exteroceptive stimulation (Hooker 1952, Humphrey 1964, 1966, Bradley and Mistretta 1975).

It is important to be aware that both the initiating movement and the so-called reacting movement might be part of a general movement and might hence be endogenously generated rather than an actual reaction. Furthermore, 'reactions' can also be passive responses to touch, because even dead twins sometimes move after a forceful touch from the living co-twin.

Does the fetus react to external displacement?
Proprioception includes sensitivity of the body to its own motion, based on stimulation of neuromuscular spindles, Golgi tendon receptors and deep tactile sensors, but also on vestibular sensors, which report the head posture and head movements. Shaking or swinging displacement of the maternal abdomen can activate some of these sensors – a circumstance that was made clinical use of during the 1980s to elicit fetal movements and consequently fetal heart-rate accelerations (Evertson et al 1979, Reinold 1979, Issel 1983). Other studies, on the other hand, came to the conclusion that fetal behaviour did not change even after vigorous external physical stimulation (Richardson et al 1981, Rayburn 1982, Visser et al 1983, Lecanuet and Jacquet 2002). Lateral shaking of the uterus or gentle swinging in a rocking chair or porch swing is absolutely pointless: it does not induce a state shift to 2F or 4F when the fetus is in a non-reactive fetal heart-rate episode (state 1F), and thus has no useful purpose (Visser et al 1983, Lecanuet and Jacquet 2002).

There is little knowledge about fetal sensitivity to temperature
The intrauterine temperature permanently ranges between 0.5°C and 1.5°C above the maternal core temperature (Bradley and Mistretta 1975). Mothers have reported increased fetal movements during hot baths (Hepper and Shahidullah 1994b), but it is not known if such enhanced movement is a response to the increase in temperature.

Fetal hiccups have been induced by irrigating the amniotic cavity with cold solutions (Liley 1972). During labour, injections of cold water through the dilating cervix and ruptured membranes produce heart-rate accelerations (Bradley and Mistretta 1975), although the benefit of such an experiment is doubtful.

Does the fetus feel pain?
Fetal pain is a delicate issue in public debate – especially regarding late abortion, but also the ever-increasing number of intrauterine interventions. A justification of the administration of fetal analgesia and anaesthesia lies not only in the moral obligation to prevent suffering, but also in the possibility of long-term neurodevelopmental sequelae due to pain and stress (Smith et al 2000). There is increasing evidence that early painful or stressful events can sensitise an individual to later pain or stress (Lowery et al 2007).

The International Association for the Study of Pain has defined pain as an unpleasant sensory and emotional experience associated with actual or potential tissue damage (Merskey and Bogduk 1994). Pain consists of two components: (1) nociception, the sensation of the stimulus, frequently accompanied by a movement in response to a noxious stimulus, but without cortical involvement or conscious perception; and (2) pain perception as a conscious emotional reaction – in short, the unpleasant feeling following a noxious stimulus. Nociception often – but not always – causes pain. When, for example, a noxious stimulus is administered below the level at which a spinal cord has been transected, the pain stays away. On the other hand, pain may occur in the absence of nociception, as happens when a person complains of pain but has no tissue damage and has received no prior peripheral stimulus (Benatar and Benatar 2001, Rokyta 2008, Derbyshire 2010).

Nociception and pain perception occur in two anatomically and physiologically separate neural systems (Vanhatalo and van Nieuwenhuizen 2000). Nociception involves peripheral sensory receptors, whose afferent fibres synapse on interneurones in the substantia gelatinosa of the spinal cord, which in turn synapse on motor neurones that also reside in the spinal cord. These motor neurones trigger muscle contraction, causing the fetus to pull the limbs away from the stimulus. In contrast, pain perception requires cortical recognition of the stimulus as unpleasant. Afferents of the peripheral sensory receptors synapse on spinal cord neurones; their axons project to the thalamus, which sends afferents to the cerebral cortex, activating a number of cortical regions. Pain impulses are also processed in a number of subcortical structures, such as the hypothalamic-pituitary system, amygdala and basal ganglia and the brainstem (Fitzgerald 2005). These brain areas account for the subconscious feeling of painfulness and for a number of pain-triggered autonomic and hormonal reactions, which do not require cortical level of activity (Vanhatalo and van Nieuwenhuizen 2000).

DEVELOPMENTAL CONSIDERATIONS

The first afferent pathways to the cortical plate (at 16 weeks' gestation) are monoaminergic and do not pass through the thalamus (Kostovic and Rakic 1990, Zecevic and Verney 1995). Thalamic fibres do not penetrate the subplate zone until 20 weeks (Figure 5.4). The subplate is a transient structure, one layer deeper than the cortical plate. It serves as a waiting compartment for various afferents on their way to the cortical plate. Subplate neurones can synapse with cortical plate neurones and thus direct the outgrowth of thalamic afferents to their synaptic targets in the cortical plate (Kostovic and Judas 2002). From 22 weeks onwards, thalamocortical fibres begin to form (Figure 5.4; Kostovic and Rakic 1990), but they are only functional by 24–26 weeks' gestation (Hrbek et al 1973, Klimach and Cooke 1988, Vanhatalo and van Nieuwenhuizen 2000, Clancy et al 2003).

Based on these findings, some researchers have concluded that fetuses feel no pain before the third trimester (Derbyshire and Furedi 1996, Wise 1997, Derbyshire 2010). Others, however, consider neuroendocrine or haemodynamic reactions to noxious stimuli – which occur from 16 weeks onwards – to be a good enough reason for the administration of analgesia during potentially painful interventions (van de Velde et al 2006).

• Development of cutaneous receptors
• Afferent fibres connect peripheral receptors with the dorsal horn
    • C-fibres grow into the fetal spinal cord
        • Neural elements containing substance P and its receptors appear in the dorsal root ganglia and dorsal horn of the spinal cord
        • Development of the afferent system located in the substantia gelatinosa of the dorsal horn
            • Monoamine fibres reach the cortex; they do not pass through the thalamus
                • Neurones for nociception are present in the dorsal root ganglion
                    • Thalamic afferents reach the somatosensory subplate zone
                        • Direct thalamocortical fibres that are not specific for pain begin to emerge
                            • Mediodorsal thalamic afferents, which will project to the anterior cingulate cortex and will become relevant to pain perception, are present in the cortical plate
                                • Thalamic fibres reach the developing prefrontal cortex

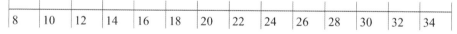

 8   10   12   14   16   18   20   22   24   26   28   30   32   34

Gestational age (weeks)

Figure 5.4 Anatomical and functional development of the nociceptive and pain systems (Humphrey 1964, Okado 1981, Charnay et al 1983, Kostovic and Goldman-Rakic 1983, Rizvi et al 1987, Mrzljak et al 1988, Kostovic and Rakic 1990, Fitzgerald 1993, Konstantinidou et al 1995, Zecevic and Verney 1995).

The scientific discourse as to whether the fetus feels pain includes the issue of physiological stress response, which may or may not be associated with pain. Thanks to the outstanding work of Anand and collaborators (Anand and Hickey 1987, Anand et al 1987), it became increasingly clear that preterm infants experience stress during invasive procedures and that, as a consequence, their long-term development might be affected. Also, from 16–18 weeks' gestation onwards, the fetus undergoes circulatory and hormonal changes in response to invasive procedures (Teixeira et al 1996, Glover and Fisk 1999, Smith et al 2000, Fisk et al 2001, van de Velde et al 2006, Lowery et al 2007).

Haemodynamic responses

Fetal cerebral blood flow increases during venipuncture or transfusion that accesses the fetal hepatic vein through the innervated fetal abdominal wall, but no increase is seen if such procedures are carried out through the non-innervated umbilical cord (Teixeira et al 1996, 1999).

Neuroendocrine responses

Piercing the fetal abdomen to access the intrahepatic vein for transfusion substantially increases levels of beta-endorphin (increase by 590%), cortisol (increase by 183%) and fetal noradrenaline (increase by 196%; Giannakoulopoulos et al 1994, 1999). It is important to bear in mind, however, that these hormones also increase during maternal exercise or umbilical cord transfusion, or after repeated cordocenteses.

Behavioural reactions

Inadvertent contact between the amniocentesis needle and the fetus increases the number of fetal movements (Hill et al 1979) and elicits brisk withdrawals of the fetus (Petrikovsky and Kaplan 1995). During invasive procedures such as heel lancing, 25-week-old preterm infants show facial and body movements. They screw up the eyes, open the mouth, clench the hands and withdraw the limbs, just as older infants do when in pain (Grunau and Craig 1987).

Early development of chemosensation

Amniotic fluid is the most direct mediator substance of potential chemical stimulation. The fraction of the fluid that is in contact with the oral and nasal chemical receptors changes continuously, due to frequent inhaling and swallowing bursts. Its composition shows daily variation, depending on maternal food intake and fetal micturition.

Oral chemoreception is both tactochemical (via the trigeminal nerve) and specifically gustatory (through the activation of taste buds). Taste buds can be found by a mere 12 weeks' gestation, reaching morphological maturity by 13 weeks (Beidler 1961). At first, they are spread all over the oral cavity, before becoming concentrated on the tongue and the anterior hard and soft palates by birth (Bradley and Mistretta 1975).

Of the four subsystems of nasal chemoreception, the trigeminal system is the earliest to function (Table 5.1). The vomeronasal system's function is to detect the non-volatile compounds of an aqueous medium. It may have evolved as a 'water olfactory organ' to act as a device for smelling dissolved compounds (Broman 1920). From 20 weeks' gestation onwards – perhaps even earlier – it fulfils an important task for the fetus (Schaal et al 1995).

WHAT DOES THE FETUS TASTE AND SMELL?

Preyer (1885) wrongly assumed – as did Carmichael almost a century later, in 1970 – that there could be no fetal olfactory sensation, since the olfactory cavity was filled with amniotic fluid. However, in some amphibians, such as the tortoise, electrophysiological responses were the same whether odorants were dissolved in water or in air (Tucker 1963). Hence, if odorants are present in the amniotic fluid, they could stimulate fetal receptors. Such a stimulation is enhanced by frequent swallowing and breathing movements of the fetus. Breathing movements make the fetus 'inhale' no less than twice the volume of fluid that he/she swallows (Duenholter and Pritchard 1976). In addition,

TABLE 5.1
TABLE 5.1 The four subsystems of the nasal chemoreceptive system

	Description	Appearance	Onset of function
Main olfactory system	It is composed of the main olfactory epithelium situated at the apical part of each nasal cavity, linked by the olfactory nerve to the primary olfactory centre, the main olfactory bulbs, and then to higher diencephalic and telencephalic centres.	11 weeks	Last trimester
Trigeminal system	It comprises a network of free nerve endings diffusely distributed in the respiratory and olfactory mucosae lining the nasal cavities.	4 weeks	7 weeks
Vomeronasal system	It is formed by symmetrical invaginations on each side of the lower nasal septum, lined with bipolar sensory cells sending their axons to the accessory olfactory bulb.	5–8 weeks	? 20 weeks
Nervus terminalis system	It comprises free nerve endings in the anterior part of the nasal septum and in the main olfactory epithelium.	?	?

From Humphrey (1940), Schaal et al (1995).

106

breathing movements displace the fluid in the nasal fossae and are thus seen as a kind of amniotic sniffing (Schaal et al 1995). The release of urine can be interpreted as a short-term modification of the chemosensory milieu, since it avoids sensory adaptation.

Indeed, human amniotic fluid contains a wide range of chemical compounds. A gas chromatographic mass spectrometric analysis brought to light no less than 390 distinct compounds in a pool of amniotic fluid samples collected from 10 women at mid-gestation (Antoshechkin et al 1989). Among others, there were several derivates of short-chain fatty acids with very pungent rancid or goaty odours (proprionic, butyric, valeric, caproic acids), long-chain fatty acids with faint waxy odours (lauric, oleic, maleic, linoleic, stearic acids), indole derivates with a strong faecal note, and polyenes with a mild oily odour (Ng et al 1982, Hoffmann et al 1989, Coude et al 1990).

A more passive putative access of odorants to the nasal chemoreceptors might be through the fetal blood itself, that is, through the haematogenic pathway (Mistretta and Bradley 1986). This mechanism of stimulation is presumed to work by diffusion of bloodborne odorants from the capillary vessels running close to the olfactory mucosa.

The profiles of constituents present in both the fetal blood and the amniotic fluid depend on the maternal diet: ingestion of cumin, fenugreek or garlic, for example, alters the odour of amniotic fluid (Hauser et al 1985, Mennella et al 1995, 2001). Near term, the placenta is permeable to high-molecular-weight solutes. Because of structural (increased exchange surface and reduced thickness of the placenta) and functional (increased uteroplacental blood flow) modification in late gestation, the placental permeability is enhanced, thus increasing the influence of the maternal diet on the fetus (Schaal et al 1995). Highly lipophilic substances, which food flavours tend to be, are rapidly transferred to the fetal blood pool, but enter slowly into the amniotic pool (Seeds et al 1980). The variation range of the fetal chemical ecology is thus set by (1) the chemical inputs provided by the mother's diet; (2) their passage through the placental barrier; and (3) the metabolic processing in the fetus. What we do not know, however, is whether the fetus is able to distinguish between odours from the amniotic fluid or those from the blood.

IS THERE A PREFERENCE FOR SPECIFIC ODOURS?

It has been observed that mammalian neonates show interest in or even feel attracted to particular odours that are present at birth. One first hint of the human newborn's preference for certain odours was provided by Steiner (1979) in his search for selective neonatal responsiveness to contrastive odorants: the presentation of fruity or milky odours, which adults found to be pleasant, triggered neonatal facial responses that blinded raters interpreted as neutral or positively valenced. Conversely, the presentation of fishy or rotten odours elicited facial expressions of deprecation or dislike in the neonate. The precocity of this differential response (the test was carried out before postnatal hour 12), its independence from future postnatal experience (the test was carried out before the first feeding), and the fact that it was also observed in an anencephalic infant made Steiner conclude that there was an innate, possibly inherited, selective responsiveness to odours or odour categories (Schaal et al 1995).

On the other hand, there is evidence that the type of food eaten by women during pregnancy and, hence, the flavour principles of their respective culture could be experienced by the fetuses in a similar way as in breastfeeding. Fetuses and young infants who are accustomed to specific flavours such as carrot, cumin, garlic or anise in either the amniotic fluid or breast milk retain a stable preference for this flavour or odour (Schaal and Orgeur 1992, Hepper 1995, Schaal et al 2000, Mennella et al 2001). It has even been speculated that these early flavour experiences may provide the foundation for cultural and ethnic preferences in cuisine (Schaal et al 2000).

BEHAVIOURAL DATA ON FETAL GUSTATION AND OLFACTION ARE VAGUE

Since the newborn has a preference for sweet solutions and certain smells, it is unlikely that the chemosensitive receptors suddenly begin to function at birth. Injection of a saccharine solution into the amniotic fluid of women with chronic hydramnios led to a reduction of the maternal abdominal volume, which had been attributed to increased fetal swallowing (de Snoo 1937). On the other hand, it was also observed that some fetuses drank less after a saccharine injection (Liley 1972), which, according to the author, was hardly surprising since he personally found the saccharine tasted bitter rather than sweet. After injecting the contrast medium Lipiodol, an iodinated poppy seed oil, fetal swallowing markedly decreased (Liley 1972). Lipiodol tastes foul to both children and adults, and makes a neonate grimace or cry.

Responsiveness to external light stimulation

The development of the eye begins with outpocketing of the optic vesicle from the forebrain. The vesicle invaginates, forming a double-walled cup destined to become the retina. The optic nerve develops from the retina and grows back along the optic stalk to the brain. As the optic cup is forming, the ectoderm opposite the cup develops a thickening to form a placode. This then invaginates into the optic cup and forms the lens vesicle (Bradley and Mistretta 1975). By 6 weeks' gestation, an inner and outer neuroblastic layer can be distinguished. Bipolar and horizontal cells, as well as rods and cones, develop from the outer layer. By 13–14 weeks, identifiable rods and cones are present. It is assumed that, beginning with their differentiation, both rods and cones migrate centripetally, that is, toward the centre of the developing fovea (Spira and Hollenberg 1973, Diaz-Araya and Provis 1992). At the beginning of the third trimester, the fetal eyelids open and the macula starts to develop. By that time (23–27 weeks), the thalamic projections reach the visual cortex (Kostovic and Rakic 1984). The development of the photoreceptors of the highly specialised fovea is only completed at term. The macula even continues to differentiate during the first few months after birth (Timor-Tritsch 1986, Hevner 2000).

Unlike with other sensory modalities, there is normally no prenatal visual stimulation – regardless of the organism's level of precocity – except for spontaneous neural firing, which is essential for normal neural development (Katz and Shatz 1996).

Under experimental conditions – including, for example, flashlight stimulation applied directly to the maternal abdomen – fetal movements sometimes increase, startles may occur more frequently, and the fetal heart rate can accelerate. These reactions may be observed from 26–28 weeks onwards, although they are not consistent (Polishuk et al 1975, Peleg and Goldman 1980, Ianniruberto and Tajani 1981, Birnholz 1985, Kiuchi et al 2000). A fetus in state 1F, or even in state 2F, cannot be wakened by flashlight stimulation (Kiuchi et al 2000).

The same inconsistency – in the sense that some fetuses respond while others do not – occurs when a flash stimulus is applied to elicit visual evoked brain activity (Eswaran et al 2002). If a fetal P200 is detectable, it occurs as early as 28 weeks (Eswaran et al 2005). This latency component decreases with advancing gestational age (Eswaran et al 2004) – an effect that is known from longitudinal studies of visually evoked responses in preterm infants (Birch and O'Connor 2001) – thus reflecting the various stages in the development of myelination of the visual pathway (Tsuneishi and Casaer 2000).

fMRI studies that use a bright light source of constant intensity for several seconds have revealed an activation in the frontal cortex, which seems to correspond to the frontal eye fields and dorsolateral prefrontal cortex. Interestingly, there is no activation in the occipital region, as one would have expected (Fulford et al 2003).

Is there any evidence of fetal memory?
Prenatal learning and memory can be found throughout the animal kingdom. Rat fetuses are capable of habituation (Smotherman and Robinson 1992), which provides evidence for short-term memory; but they also appear to have a long-term memory, as classical conditioning suggests (Smotherman 1982, Hepper 1993). An example of exposure learning – and hence of long-term memory – is the fact that avian embryos are able to learn the calls of their parents (e.g. Lickliter and Stoumbos 1992). Tadpoles show a greater preference for familiar than for unfamiliar odours, and maintain this preference even after metamorphosis into frogs (Hepper and Waldman 1992).

The human fetus is certainly able to habituate, but the results of studies on classical conditioning are ambiguous. There is no evidence that memory processes in embryos and fetuses are similar to those evidenced after birth. It would be off the mark to interpret the fetuses' learning ability as an adult-like performance, or even to train them with the objective of increasing their abilities and producing superbabies (Logan 1989, Arabin 2002).

And yet the question remains: what is the function of fetal memory? Perhaps the simple answer is that there is no such function beyond the fact that, at one time or another, memory must get going. But then again, fetal memory might have an adaptive function such as to enable breastfeeding after birth. We know that the mother's diet flavours both the amniotic fluid and her breast milk (see p 107). Mothers who change their diet frequently before birth have difficulties establishing breastfeeding (Hepper 1996). Another possible function of fetal memory is the acquisition of language via the prosodic features of speech. However, all of this is a matter of mere conjecture.

HABITUATION

Habituation – the decrease in and eventual cessation of response to repeated stimulation (Jeffrey and Cohen 1971) – seems to be essential in making it possible for an individual to ignore familiar stimuli and attend to new stimuli (Bornstein 1989). It is important to ascertain whether such a response decrement is due to habituation (where memory may be involved) or to effector fatigue or receptor adaptation (where memory is not involved). Therefore, habituation studies must include the recovery response on presentation of a new stimulus – the so-called dishabituation – and subsequent re-presentation of the original stimulus with faster habituation than in the first presentation.

In what may have been the first report on habituation, Peiper (1925) noted that a shrill car horn elicited fetal movements, which decreased when the fetus was repeatedly exposed to the noise. Most of the studies on fetal habituation deal with acoustic or vibroacoustic stimulation (e.g. Sontag and Wallace 1934, Ianniruberto and Tajani 1981, Madison et al 1986, Hepper and Shahidullah 1992, Doherty and Hepper 2000, van Heteren et al 2000, Bellieni et al 2005, Dirix et al 2009). In fact, fetuses are able to habituate from 22–23 weeks' gestation onwards (Leader et al 1982), although their habituation rate is longer then (Kuhlmann et al 1988, Groome et al 1993, Morokuma et al 2004, 2008).

Testing fetal habituation was proposed as a means of assessing the fetal nervous system, since compromised or chromosomally abnormal fetuses show different habituation patterns from normal fetuses (Leader and Baillie 1988, Leader et al 1982, Hepper and Shahidullah 1992). It should be borne in mind, however, that an abnormal habituation pattern can also result from physiological factors such as varying behavioural states (Mulder et al 2001). Therefore, it is not legitimate to interpret fetal failure to habituate, or exceedingly rapid habituation, as signs of fetal distress or adverse outcome. There appear to be normal fetuses in whom it is impossible to determine habituation because of an irregular response pattern (van Heteren et al 2001).

CLASSICAL CONDITIONING

Classical conditioning involves the pairing of two stimuli – the conditioned and the unconditioned stimulus. The unconditioned stimulus elicits a response when presented alone. The conditioned stimulus elicits no reaction when presented alone. After repeated pairing with the unconditioned stimulus, however, the conditioned stimulus also elicits a response (Pavlov 1906). The first report on classical conditioning in the human fetus was by Ray (1932). Vibration, serving as a conditioned stimulus, was paired with a loud noise, the unconditioned stimulus. No results are reported for this study, other than the comment that the subject had no adverse effects from her prenatal learning. Similarly, Spelt (1938) paired vibration with a loud noise and reported that after 15–20 pairings some fetuses responded to the vibration alone. Experimental extinction, spontaneous recovery and retention of the response over a 3-week interval were also observed. We know today that the use of vibration as a conditioned stimulus places a question mark over the results of both studies. Hepper (1996, 1997) replicated Spelt's study, but used vibroacoustic stimulation – although as an unconditioned stimulus – paired with a pure tone as a conditioned stimulus. He found some evidence of conditioning in 31- to 39-week-old fetuses, but noted that half the group showed no conditioning whatsoever. In a side note, he referred to the fact that he had managed to demonstrate classical conditioning in an anencephalic fetus (Hepper 1997).

REFERENCES

Abrams RM, Griffiths SK, Huang X, Sain J, Langford G, Gerhardt KJ. (1998) Fetal music perception: the role of sound transmission. *Music Percept* 15: 307–317.

Altmann E. (1950) Normal development of the ear and its mechanics. *Arch Otolaryngol* 52: 725–766.

Anand KJ, Hickey PR. (1987) Pain and its effects in the human neonate and fetus. *N Engl J Med* 317: 1321–1329.

Anand KJ, Sippel WG, Aynsley-Green A. (1987) Randomised trial of fentanyl anaesthesia in preterm babies undergoing surgery: effects on the stress response. *Lancet* 2(8569): 62–66.

Antoshechkin AG, Golovkin AB, Maximova LA, Bakharev VA. (1989) Screening of amniotic fluid metabolites by gas chromatography-mass spectrometry. *J Chromatography* 489: 353–358.

Arabin B. (2002) Music during pregnancy. Opinion. *Ultrasound Obstet Gynecol* 20: 425–430.

Arabin B, Bos R, Rijlaarsdam R, Mohnhaupt A, van Eyck J. (1996) The onset of inter-human contacts: Longitudinal ultrasound observations in early twin pregnancies. *Ultrasound Obstet Gynecol* 8: 166–173.

Bartnicki J, Dudenhausen JW. (1995) Antepartum vibroacoustic stimulation in patients with low fetal heart rate variability. *Int J Gynaecol Obstet* 48: 173–177.

Beidler LM. (1961) Taste receptor stimulation. *Proc Biophys Biochem* 12: 107–151.

Bellieni CV, Severi F, Bocchi C, Caparelli N, Bagnoli F, Buonocore G, Petraglia F. (2005) Blink-startle reflex habituation in 30–34-week low-risk fetuses. *J Perinat Med* 33: 33–37.

Benatar D, Benatar M. (2001) A pain in the fetus: toward ending confusion about fetal pain. *Bioethics* 15: 57–76.

Bibas AG, Xenellis J, Michaels L, Anagnostopoulou S, Ferekidis E, Wright A. (2008) Temporal bone study of development of the organ of Corti: correlation between auditory function and anatomical structure. *J Laryngol Otol* 122: 336–342.

Birch EE, O'Connor AR. (2001) Preterm birth and visual development. *Semin Neonatol* 6: 487–497.

Birnholz JC. (1985) Ultrasonic fetal ophthalmology. *Early Hum Dev* 12: 199–209.

Birnholz JC, Benacerraf BR. (1983) The development of human fetal hearing. *Science* 222: 516–518.

Bornstein MH. (1989) Stability in early mental development: From attention and information processing in infancy to learning and cognition in childhood. In: Bornstein MH, Krasnegor NA, editors. *Stability and Continuity in Mental Development*. Hillsdale (NJ): Erlbaum. p 147–170.

Bradley RM, Mistretta CM. (1975) Fetal sensory receptors. *Physiol Rev* 55: 352–382.

Broman I. (1920) [The organon vomero nasale Jacobsoni – a water smell organ!]. *Anat Embryol* 58: 137–191. (In German)

Bullock WR, editor. (1871) *A Theoretic and Practical Treatise on Midwifery*. Philadelphia: Lindsay and Balkiston.

Carmichael L. (1970) Onset and early development of behaviour. In: Mussen PH, editor. *Carmichael's Manual of Child Psychology*. 3rd edition. Vol 1. New York: Wiley. p 447–563.

Charnay Y, Paulin C, Chayvialle JA, Dubois PM. (1983) Distribution of substance P-like immunoreactivity in the spinal cord and dorsal root ganglia of the human foetus and infant. *Neuroscience* 10: 41–55.

Clancy RR, Bergqvist AGC, Dlugos DJ. (2003) Neonatal electroencephalography. In: Ebersole JS, Pedley TA, editors. *Current Practice of Clinical Electroencephalography*. 3rd edition. Philadelphia, PA: Lippincott Williams & Wilkins. p 160–234.

Coude M, Chadefaux B, Rabier D, Kamoun P. (1990) Early amniocentesis and amniotic fluid organic acid levels in the prenatal diagnosis of organic acidemias. *Clin Chimica Acta* 187: 329–332.

Damstra-Wijmenga SM. (1991) The memory of the newborn baby. *Midwives Chron* 104: 66–69.

Daniel T, Laciak J. (1982) [Clinical observations and experiments on the state of the cochleovestibular system of subjects exposed to noise during fetal life]. *Rev Laryngol* 103: 313–318. (In French)

DeCasper AJ, Lecanuet JP, Busnel MC, Granier-Deferre C, Maugeais R. (1994) Fetal reactions to recurrent maternal speech. *Infant Behav Dev* 17: 159–164.

Derbyshire SW. (2010) Foetal pain? *Best Pract Res Clin Obstet Gynaecol* 24: 647–655.

Derbyshire SWG, Furedi A. (1996) Fetal pain is a misnomer. *BMJ* 313: 795.

de Snoo K. (1937) [The drinking child in the uterus]. *Monatsschr Geburtsh Gynaekol* 105: 88–97. (In German)

Devoe LD, Castillo RA, Sherline DM. (1985) The nonstress test as diagnostic test: A critical reappraisal. *Am J Obstet Gynecol* 152: 1047–1053.

Devoe LD, Murray C, Faircloth D, Ramos E. (1990) Vibroacoustic stimulation and fetal behavioural state in normal term human pregnancy. *Am J Obstet Gynecol* 163: 1156–1161.

Diaz-Araya C, Provis JM. (1992) Evidence of photoreceptor migration during early foveal development: a quantitative analysis of human fetal retinae. *Vis Neurosci* 8: 505–514.

DiPietro JA. (2005) Neurobehavioural assessment before birth. *Ment Retard Dev Disabil Res Rev* 11: 4–13.

DiPietro JA, Hodgson DM, Costigan KA, Johnson TR. (1996) Fetal antecedents of infant temperament. *Child Dev* 67: 2568–2583.

Dirix CEH, Nijhuis JG, Jongsma HW, Hornstra G. (2009) Aspects of fetal learning and memory. *Child Dev* 80: 1251–1258.

Divon MY, Platt LD, Cantrell CJ, Smith CV, Yeh SY, Paul RH. (1985) Evoked fetal startle response: A possible intrauterine neurological examination. *Am J Obstet Gynecol* 153: 454–456.

Doherty NN, Hepper PG. (2000) Habituation in fetuses of diabetic mothers. *Early Hum Dev* 59: 85–93.

Draganova R, Eswaran H, Lowery CL, Murphy P, Huotilainen M, Preissel H. (2005) Sound frequency change detection in fetuses and newborns – a magnetoencephalographic study. *Neuroimage* 28: 354–361.

Draganova R, Eswaran H, Murphy P, Lowery C, Preissl H. (2007) Serial magnetoencephalographic study of fetal and newborn auditory discriminative evoked responses. *Early Hum Dev* 83: 199–207.

Duenholter JH, Pritchard JA. (1976) Fetal respiration: Quantitative measurements of amniotic fluid inspired near term by human and rhesus fetuses. *Am J Obstet Gynecol* 125: 306–309.

Eswaran H, Wilson JD, Preissl H, Robinson SE, Vrba J, Murphy P, Rose DF, Lowery CL. (2002) Magnetoencephalographic recordings of visual evoked brain activity in the human fetus. *Lancet* 360: 779–780.

Eswaran H, Lowery CL, Wilson JD, Murphy P, Preissl H. (2004) Functional development of the visual system in human fetus using magnetoencephalography. *Exp Neurol* 190: S52–S58.

Eswaran H, Lowery CL, Wilson JD, Murphy P, Preissl H. (2005) Fetal magnetoencephalography – a multimodal approach. *Dev Brain Res* 154: 57–62.

Evertson LR, Gauthier RS, Schrifin BS, Paul RH. (1978) Antepartum fetal heart rate testing: I. The nonstress test. *Am J Obstet Gynecol* 133: 29–35.

Fisk NM, Gitau R, Teixeira JM, Giannakoulopoulos X, Cameron AD, Glover VA. (2001) Effect of direct fetal opioid analgesia on fetal hormonal and haemodynamic stress response to intra-uterine needling. *Anesthesiology* 95: 828–835.

Fitzgerald M. (1993) Development of pain pathways and mechanisms. In: Anand KIS, McGrath PJ, editors. *Pain Research and Clinical Management. Vol 5. Pain in Neonates.* Amsterdam: Elsevier. p 19–38.

Fitzgerald M. (2005) The development of nociceptive circuits. *Nat Rev Neurosci* 6: 507–520.

Forbes HS, Forbes HB. (1927) Fetal sense reactions: hearing. *J Comp Physiol Psychol* 7: 353–355.

Fox HE, Badalian SS. (1993) Fetal movement in response to vibroacoustic stimulation: a review. *Obstet Gynecol Surv* 48: 707–713.

Fulford J, Vadeyar SH, Dodampahala SH, Moore RJ, Young P, Baker PN, James DK, Gowland PA. (2003) Fetal brain activity to a visual stimulus. *Hum Brain Mapp* 20: 239–245.

Fulford J, Vadeyar S, Dodampahala SH, Ong S, Moore RJ, Baker PN, James DK, Gowland P. (2004) Fetal brain activity and hemodynamic response to a vibroacoustic stimulus. *Hum Brain Mapp* 22: 116–121.

Gagnon R, Patrick J, Foreman J, West R. (1986) Stimulation of human fetuses with sound and vibration. *Am J Obstet Gynecol* 155: 848–851.

Gagnon R, Hunse C, Carmichael L, Fellows F, Patrick J. (1987) Human fetal responses to vibratory acoustic stimulation from twenty-six weeks to term. *Am J Obstet Gynecol* 157: 1375–1381.

Gagnon R, Hunse C, Forman J. (1989) Human fetal behavioural states after vibratory stimulation. *Am J Obstet Gynecol* 161: 1470–1476.

Gagnon R, Benzaquen S, Hunse C. (1992) The fetal sound environment during vibroacoustic stimulation in labour: effect on fetal heart rate response. *Obstet Gynecol* 79: 550–555.

Gardner JM, Karmel BZ, Down JM. (1984) Relationship of infant psychobiological development to infant intervention programs. *J Child Contemp Soc* 17: 93–108.

Gerhardt KJ, Abrams RM. (1996) Fetal hearing: characterization of the stimulus and response. *Semin Perinatol* 20: 11–20.

Gerhardt KJ, Abrams RM. (2000) Fetal exposure to sound and vibroacoustic stimulation. *J Perinatol* 20: S20–S29.

Giannakoulopoulos X, Sepulveda W, Kourtis P, Glover V, Fisk NM. (1994) Fetal plasma cortisol and beta-endorphin response to intrauterine needling. *Lancet* 344: 77–81.

Giannakoulopoulos X, Teixeira J, Fisk N, Glover V. (1999) Human fetal and maternal noradrenaline responses to invasive procedures. *Pediatr Res* 45: 494–499.

Glover V, Fisk NM. (1999) Fetal pain: implications for research and practice. *Br J Obstet Gynaecol* 106: 881–886.

Goodlin RC, Schmidt W. (1972) Human fetal arousal levels as indicated by heart rate recordings. *Am J Obstet Gynecol* 114: 613–621.

Griffiths SK, Brown WS Jr, Gerhardt KJ, Abrams RM, Morris RJ. (1994) The perception of speech sounds recorded within the uterus of a pregnant sheep. *J Acoust Soc Am* 96: 2055–2063.

Grimwade J, Walker DW, Bartlett M, Gordon S, Wood C. (1971) Human fetal heart rate change and movement in response to sound and vibration. *Am J Obstet Gynecol* 109: 86–90.

Groome LJ, Gotlieb SJ, Neely CL, Waters MD. (1993) Developmental trends in fetal habituation to vibroacoustic stimulation. *Am J Perinatol* 10: 46–49.

Groome LJ, Mooney DM, Holland SB, Bentz LS, Atterbury JL, Dykman RA. (1997) The heart rate deceleratory response in low-risk human fetuses: effect of stimulus intensity on response topography. *Dev Psychobiol* 30: 103–113.

Groome LJ, Mooney DM, Holland SB, Smith LA, Atterbury JL, Dykman RA. (1999) Behavioural state affects heart rate response to low-intensity sound in human fetuses. *Early Hum Dev* 54: 39–54.

Grunau RVE, Craig KD. (1987) Pain expression in neonates: facial action and cry. *Pain* 28: 395–410.

Hauser GJ, Chitayat D, Berns L, Braver D, Muhlhauser B. (1985) Peculiar odours in newborns and maternal prenatal ingestion of spicy foods. *Eur J Pediatr* 144: 403.

Hepper PG. (1988) Fetal 'soap' addition. *Lancet* 1(8598): 1347–1348.

Hepper PG. (1991) An examination of fetal learning before and after birth. *Ir J Psychol* 12: 95–107.

Hepper PG. (1993) In utero release from a single transient hypoxic episode: a positive reinforcer? *Physiol Behav* 53: 309–311.

Hepper PG. (1995) Human fetal' olfactory learning. *Int J Prenat Perinat Psychol Med* 7: 147–151.

Hepper PG. (1996) Fetal memory: Does it exist? What does it do? *Acta Pediatr* 416: 16–20.

Hepper PG. (1997) Fetal habituation: another Pandora's box? *Dev Med Child Neurol* 39: 274–278.

Hepper PG, Shahidullah S. (1992) Habituation in normal and Down's syndrome fetuses. *Q J Exp Psychol* 44: 305–317.

Hepper PG, Shahidullah S. (1994a) Development of fetal hearing. *Arch Dis Child* 71: F81–F87.

Hepper PG, Shahidullah S. (1994b) The beginning of mind – evidence from the behaviour of the fetus. *J Reprod Inf Psychol* 12: 143–154.

Hepper PG, Waldman B. (1992) Embryonic olfactory learning in frogs. *Q J Exp Psychol* 44B: 179–197.

Hevner RF. (2000) Development of connections in the human visual system during fetal mid-gestation: a Dil-tracing study. *J Neuropathol Exp Neurol* 59: 385–392.

Hicks F. (1995) The role of music therapy in the care of the newborn. *Nurs Times* 91: 31–33.

Hill LM, Platt LD, Manning FA. (1979) Immediate effect of amniocentesis on fetal breathing and gross body movements. *Am J Obstet Gynecol* 135: 689–690.

Hoffmann G, Aramaki S, Blum-Hoffmann E, Nyhan W, Sweetman L. (1989) Quantitative analysis for organic acids in biological samples: Batch isolation followed by gas chromatographic-mass spectrometric analysis. *Clin Chemistry* 35: 587–595.

Hoh JK, Park YS, Cha KJ, Park MI. (2009) Fetal heart rate after vibroacoustic stimulation. *Int J Gynecol Obstet* 106: 14–18.

Holst M, Eswaran H, Lowery C, Murphy P, Norton J, Preissl H. (2005) Development of auditory evoked fields in human fetuses and newborns: a longitudinal MEG study. *Clin Neurophysiol* 116: 1949–1955.

Hooker D. (1952) *The Prenatal Origin of Behavior*. Lawrence: University of Kansas Press.

Hrbek A, Karlberg P, Olsson T. (1973) Development of visual and somatosensory evoked response in preterm newborn infants. *Electroenceph Clin Neurophysiol* 34: 225–232.

Humphrey T. (1940) The development of the olfactory and the accessory formations in human embryos and fetuses. *J Comp Neurol* 73: 431–478.

Humphrey T. (1964) Some correlations between the appearance of human fetal reflexes and the development of the nervous system. *Prog Brain Res* 4: 93–135.

Humphrey T. (1966) The development of the trigeminus nerve fibers to the oral mucosa compared with their development of cutaneous surfaces. *J Comp Neurol* 126: 91–108.

Huotilainen M, Kujala A, Hotakainen M, Parkkonen L, Taulu S, Simola J, Nenonen J, Karjalainen M, Näätänen R. (2005) Short-term memory functions of the human fetus with magnetoencephalography. *NeuroReport* 16: 81–84.

Hykin J, Moore R, Duncan K, Clare S, Baker P, Johnson I, Bowtell R, Mansfield P, Gowland P. (1999) Fetal brain activity demonstrated by functional magnetic resonance imaging. *Lancet* 354: 645–646.

Ianniruberto A, Tajani E. (1981) Ultrasonographic study of fetal movements. *Semin Perinatol* 5: 175–181.

Issel EP. (1983) Fetal response to external mechanical stimuli. *J Perinatal Med* 11: 232–242.

James DK, Spencer CJ, Stepsis BW. (2002) Fetal learning: a prospective randomized controlled study. *Ultrasound Obstet Gynecol* 20: 431–438.

Jeffrey WE, Cohen LS. (1971) Habituation in the human infant. *Adv Child Dev Behav* 6: 63–97.

Katz LC, Shatz CJ. (1996) Synaptic activity and the construction of cortical circuits. *Science* 274: 1133–1138.

Kisilevsky BS, Muir DW. (1991) Human fetal and subsequent newborn responses to sound and vibration. *Inf Behav Dev* 14: 1–26.

Kisilevsky BS, Muir DW, Low JA. (1990) Maturation of responses elicited by a vibroacoustic stimulus in a group of high-risk fetuses. *Matern Child Nurs J* 19: 239–250.

Kisilevsky BS, Muir DW, Low JA. (1992) Maturation of human fetal responses to vibroacoustic stimulation. *Child Dev* 63: 1497–1508.

Kisilevsky BS, Pang LH, Hains SMJ. (2000) Maturation of human fetal responses to airborne sound in low- and high-risk fetuses. *Early Hum Dev* 58: 179–195.

Kisilevsky BS, Hains SMJ, Lee K, Xie X, Huang H, Ye HH, Zhang K, Wang Z. (2003) Effects of experience on fetal voice recognition. *Psycholog Sci* 14: 220–224.

Kisilevsky BS, Hains SMJ, Jacquet AY, Granier-Deferre C, Lecanuet JP. (2004) Maturation of fetal responses to music. *Dev Sci* 7: 550–559

Kiuchi M, Nagata N, Ikeno S, Terakawa N. (2000) The relationship between the response to external light stimulation and behavioural states in the human fetus: how it differs from vibroacoustic stimulation. *Early Hum Dev* 58: 153–165.

Klimach VJ, Cooke RW. (1988) Maturation of the neonatal somatosensory evoked response in preterm infants. *Dev Med Child Dev* 30: 208–214.

Konstantinidou AD, Silos-Santiago I, Flaris N, Snider WD. (1995) Development of the primary afferent projection in human spinal cord. *J Comp Neurol* 354: 11–12.

Kostovic I, Goldman-Rakic PS. (1983) Transient cholinesterase staining in the mediodorsal nucleus of the thalamus and its connections in the developing human and monkey brain. *J Comp Neurol* 219: 431–447.

Kostovic I, Judas M. (2002) Correlation between the sequential ingrowth of afferents and transient patterns of cortical lamination in preterm infants. *Anat Rec 267*: 1–6.

Kostovic I, Rakic P. (1984) Development of prestriate visual projections in the monkey and human fetal cerebrum revealed by transient cholinesterase staining. *J Neurosci* 4: 25–42.

Kostovic I, Rakic P. (1990) Developmental history of the transient subplate zone in the visual and somatosensory cortex of the macaque monkey and human brain. *J Comp Neurol* 297: 441–470.

Krmpotic-Nemanic J, Kostovic I, Kelovic Z, Nemanic D, Mrzljak L. (1983) Development of the human fetal auditory cortex: growth of afferent fibres. *Acta Anat Basel* 116: 69–73.

Krueger C, Holditch-Davis D, Quint S, DeCasper A. (2004) Recurring auditory experience in the 28- to 34-week-old fetus. *Infant Behav Dev* 27: 537–543.

Kuhlman KA, Depp R. (1988) Acoustic stimulation testing. *Obstet Gynecol Clin North Am* 15: 303–319.

Kuhlman KA, Burns KA, Depp R, Sabbagha RE. (1988) Ultrasonic imaging of normal fetal response to external vibratory acoustic stimulation. *Am J Obstet Gynecol* 158: 47–51.

Lalande NM, Hetu R, Lambert J. (1986) Is occupational noise exposure during pregnancy a high-risk factor of damage to the auditory system of the fetus? *Am J Ind Med* 10: 427–435.

Lary S, Briassoulis G, de Vries L, Dubowitz LM, Dubowitz V. (1985) Hearing response threshold in preterm and term infants by auditory brainstem response. *J Pediatr* 107: 593–599.

Leader LR, Baillie P. (1988) The changes in fetal habituation patterns due to a decrease in inspired maternal oxygen. *Br J Obstet Gynaecol* 95: 664–668.

Leader LR, Baille P, Martin B, Vermeulen E. (1982) The assessment and significance of habituation to a repeated stimulus by the human fetus. *Early Hum Dev* 7: 211–219.

Lecanuet JP, Jacquet AY. (2002) Fetal responsiveness to maternal passive swinging in low heart arte variability state: effects of stimulation direction and duration. *Dev Psychobiol* 40: 57–67.

Lecanuet JP, Schaal B. (1996) Fetal sensory competencies. *Eur J Obstet Gynecol Reprod Biol* 68: 1–23.

Lecanuet JP, Granier-Deferre C, Busnel MC. (1989) Differential fetal auditory reactiveness as a function of stimulus characteristics and state. *Semin Perinatol* 13: 421–429.

Lecanuet JP, Granier-Deferre C, Jacquet AY, Capponi I, Ledru L. (1993) Prenatal discrimination of a male and female voice uttering the same sentence. *Early Dev Parenting* 2: 217–228.

Lengle JM, Chen M, Wakai RT. (2001) Improved neuromagnetic detection of fetal and neonatal auditory evoked responses. *Clinical Neurophysiol* 112: 785–792.

Lickliter R, Stoumbos J. (1992) Modification of prenatal auditory experience alters postnatal auditory preference of bobwhite quail chicks. *Q J Exp Psychol* 44B: 199–214.

Liley AW. (1972) The fetus as a personality. *Aust N Z J Psychiatr* 6: 99–105.

Lind J. (1980) Music and the small human being. *Acta Paediatr Scand* 69: 131–136.

Logan B. (1989) Project prelearn: the efficacy of in utero teaching. *Int J Prenatal Perinatal Stud* 1: 365–380.

Lowery CL, Hardman MP, Manning N, Hall RW, Anand KJS. (2007) Neurodevelopmental changes of fetal pain. *Semin Perinatol* 31: 275–282.

Madison LS, Madison JK, Adubato SA. (1986) Infant behaviour and development in relation to fetal movement and habituation. *Child Dev* 57: 1475–1482.

Mennella JA, Johnson A, Beauchamp GK. (1995) Garlic ingestion by pregnant women alters the odor of amniotic fluid. *Chem Senses* 20: 207–209.

Mennella JA, Jagnow CP, Beauchamp GK. (2001) Prenatal and postnatal flavor learning by human infants. *Pediatr* 107: E88.

Merskey H, Bogduk N. (1994) International Association for the Study of Pain. *Part III: Pain Terms. A Current List with Definitions and Notes on Usage.* Seattle: IASP Press.

Mistretta CM, Bradley RM. (1986) Development of the sense of taste. In: Blass ME, editor. *Handbook of Behavioral Neurobiology. Vol 8. Developmental Psychobiology and Developmental Neurobiology.* New York: Plenum Press. p 163–203.

Moore JK. (2002) Maturation of human auditory cortex: Implications for speech perception. *Ann Oto Rhino Laryngol Suppl* 189: 7–10.

Moore JK, Perazzo LM, Braun A. (1995) Time course of axonal maturation in the human brain stem auditory pathway. *Hear Res* 87: 21–31.

Moore JR, Vadeyar S, Fulford J, Tyler DJ, Gribben C, Baker PN, James D, Gowland PA. (2001) Antenatal determination of fetal brain activity in response to acoustic stimulus using functional magnetic resoncance imaging. *Hum Brain Mapping* 12: 94–99.

Morlet T, Lapillonne A, Ferber C, Duclaux R, Sann L, Putet G, Salle B, Collet L. (1995) Spontaneous oto-acoustic emissions in preterm neonates: prevalence and gender effects. *Hear Res* 90: 44–54.

Morokuma S, Fukushima K, Kawai N, Tomonaga M, Satoh S, Nakano H. (2004) Fetal habituation correlates with functional brain development. *Behav Brain Res* 153: 459–463.

Morokuma S, Doria V, Ierullo A, Kinukawa N, Fukushima K, Nakano H, Arulkumaran S, Papageorghiou AT. (2008) Developmental change in fetal response to repeated low-intensity sound. *Dev Sci* 11: 47–52.

Morse PA. (1972) The discrimation of speech and nonspeech stimuli in early infancy. *J Exp Child Psychol* 14: 477–492.

Mrzljak L, Uylings HB, Kostovic I, van Eden CG. (1988) Prenatal development of neurons in the human prefrontal cortex. I: A qualitative Golgi study. *J Comp Neurol* 271: 355–386.

Mulder EJH, Robles de Medina PG, Beekhuijzen M, Wijnberger DE, Visser GHA. (2001) Fetal stimulation and activity state. *Lancet* 357: 478–479.

Nakai Y. (1970) An election microscopic study of the human fetus cochlea. *Pract Otol Rhinol Laryngol* 32: 257–267.

Ng KJ, Andresen BD, Bianchine JR, Iams JD, O'Shaugnessy RW, Stempel LE, Zuspan FP. (1982) Capillary gas chromatographic-mass spectrometric profiles of trimethylsilyl derivates of organic acids from amniotic fluids of different gestational age. *J Chromatogr* 228: 43–50.

Nijhuis JG, Prechtl HFR, Martin CB, Bots RSGM. (1982) Are there behavioural states in the human fetus? *Early Hum Dev* 6: 177–195.

Ohel G, Birkenfeld A, Rabinowitz R, Sadovsky E. (1987) Fetal response to vibratory acoustic stimulation in periods of low heart rate reactivity and low activity. *Am J Obstet Gynecol* 154: 619–621.

Okado N. (1981) Onset of synapse formation in the human spinal cord. *J Comp Neurol* 201: 211–219.

Olds C. (1985) Fetal response to music. *Midwives Chron Nurs Notes* 98: 202–203.

Pavlov I. (1906) Scientific study of the so-called psychical processes in the higher animals. *Lancet* ii: 911–915.

Peiper A. (1925) [Sensory perceptions of the child before birth]. *Monatsschr Kinderheilk* 29: 237–241. (In German)

Peleg D, Goldman JA. (1980) Fetal heart rate acceleration in response to light stimulation as a clinical measure of fetal well-being. A preliminary report. *J Perinat Med* 8: 38–41.

Petrikovsky BM, Kaplan GP. (1995) Fetal responses to inadvertent contact with the needle during amniocentesis. *Fetal Diagn Ther* 10: 83–85.

Petrikovsky BM, Schifrin B, Diana L. (1993) The effects of acoustic stimulation on fetal swallowing and amniotic fluid index. *Obstet Gynecol* 81: 548–550.

Petrović O, Finderle A, Prodan M, Skunca E, Prpić I, Zaputović S. (2009) Combination of vibroacoustic stimulation and acute variables of mFBP as a simple assessment method of low-risk fetuses. *J Matern Fetal Neonatal Med* 22: 152–156.

Philbin MK, Lickliter R, Graven SN. (2000) Sensory experience and the developing organism: a history of ideas and view of the future. *J Perinatol* 20: S2–S5.

Piontelli A, Bocconi L, Kustermann A, Tassis B, Zoppini C, Nicolini U. (1997) Patterns of evoked behaviour in twin pregnancies during the first 22 weeks of gestation. *Early Hum Dev* 50: 39–45.

Polishuk WZ, Laufer N, Sadovsky E. (1975) Fetal reaction to external light. *Harefuah* 89: 395–397.

Prechtl HFR. (1974) The behavioural states of the newborn infant (a review). *Brain Res* 76: 185–212.

Prechtl HFR. (1989) Fetal behaviour. In: Hill A, Volpe JJ, editors. *Fetal Neurology*. New York: Raven Press. p 1–16.

Preyer W. (1885) [*Special Physiology of the Embryo*]. Leipzig: Grieben. (In German)

Pujol R, Lavigne-Rebillard M, Uziel A. (1991) Development of the human cochlea. *Acta Otolaringol* 482: 7–12.

Querleu D, Renard X, Boutteville C, Crepin G. (1989) Hearing by the human fetus? *Semin Perinatol* 13: 409–420.

Ray WS. (1932) A preliminary report on a study of fetal conditioning. *Child Dev* 3: 175–177.

Rayburn WF. (1982) Antepartum fetal assessment. Monitoring fetal activity. *Clin Perinatol* 9: 231–252.

Rayburn WF. (1995) Fetal movement monitoring. *Clin Obstet Gynecol* 38: 59–67.

Reinold E. (1979) Identification and differentiation of fetal movements. *Contrib Gynecol Obstet* 6, 29–32.

Richards DS, Frentzen B, Gerhardt KJ, McCann ME, Abrams RM. (1992) Sound levels in the human uterus. *Obstet Gynecol* 80: 186–190.

Richardson BS, Campbell K, Carmichael L, Patrick J. (1981) Effects of external physical stimulation on fetuses near term. *Am J Obstet Gynecol* 139: 344–352.

Rizvi T, Wadhwa S, Bijlani V. (1987) Development of spinal substrate for nociception. *Pain* 4: S195.

Rokyta R. (2008) Fetal pain. *Neuro Endocrinol Lett* 29: 807–814.

Ronca AE, Alberts JR. (1995) Maternal contributions to fetal experience and the transition from pernatal to postnatal life. In: Lecanuet JP, Fifer WP, Krasnegor NA, Smotherman WP, editors. *Fetal Development. A Psychobiological Perspective*. Hillsdale, Hove: Lawrence Erlbaum Associates. p 331–349.

Rotteveel JJ, de Graf R, Stegeman DF, Colon EJ, Visco YM. (1987) The maturation of the central auditory conduction in preterm infants until three months postterm. V. The auditory cortical response (ACR). *Hearing Res* 27: 95–110.

Sadovsky E, Samueloff A, Sadovsky Y, Ohel G. (1986) Incidence of spontaneous and evoked fetal movements. *Gynecol Obstet Invest* 21: 177–181.

Schaal B, Orgeur P. (1992) Olfaction in utero: can the rodent model be generalized? *Q J Exp Psychol* 44B: 245–278.

Schaal B, Orgeur P, Rognon C. (1995) Odor sensing in the human fetus: anatomical, functional, and chemoecological bases. In: Lecanuet JP, Fifer WP, Krasnegor NA, Smotherman WP, editors. *Fetal Development. A Psychobiological Perspective*. Hillsdale, Hove: Lawrence Erlbaum Associates. p 205–237.

Schaal B, Marlier L, Soussignan R. (2000) Human foetuses learn odour from their pregnant mother's diet. *Chem Senses* 25: 729–737.

Schleussner E, Schneider U, Kausch S, Kähler C, Haueisen J, Seewald HJ. (2001) Fetal magnetoencephalography: a non-invasive method for the assessment of fetal neuronal maturation. *Br J Obstet Gynecol* 108: 1291–1294.

Schmidt W, Boos R, Gnirs J, Auer L, Schulze S. (1985) Fetal behavioural states and controlled sound stimulation. *Early Hum Dev* 12: 145–153.

Seeds AE, Leung LS, Stys SJ, Clark KE, Russell PT. (1980) Comparison of human and sheep chorion leave permeability to glucose, beta-hydroxybutyrate, and glycerol. *Am J Obstet Gynaecol* 138: 604–608.

Shahidullah S, Hepper PG. (1994) Frequency discrimination by the fetus. *Early Hum Dev* 36: 13–26.

Sherrington CS. (1904) The correlation of reflexes and the principle of the common path. *Report Br Assoc Adv Sci* 74: 1–14.

Smith RP. (1995) Vibroacoustic stimulation. *Clin Obstet Gynecol* 38: 68–77.

Smith RP, Gitau R, Glover V, Fisk NM. (2000) Pain and stress in the human fetus. *Eur J Obstet Gynecol Reprod Biol* 92: 161–165.

Smotherman WP. (1982) Odor aversion learning by the rat fetus. *Physiol Behav* 29: 769–771.

Smotherman WP, Robinson SR. (1992) Habituation in the rat fetus. *Q J Exp Psychol* 44B: 215–230.

Sohmer H, Freeman S. (2001) The pathway for the transmission of external sounds into the fetal inner ear. *J Basic Clin Physiol Pharmacol* 12 (Suppl 2): 91–99.

Sohmer H, Perez R, Sichel JY, Priner R, Freeman S. (2001). The pathway enabling external sounds to reach and excite the fetal inner ear. *Audiol Neurootol* 6: 109–116.

Sokolov EN. (1963) *Perception and the Conditioned Reflex.* New York: Macmillan.

Sontag LW, Wallace RF. (1934) Preliminary report of the Fels Fund study of fetal activity. *Am J Dis Child* 48: 1050–1057.

Sontag LW, Steele WG, Lewis M. (1969) The fetal and maternal cardiac response to environmental stress. *Hum Dev* 12: 1–9.

Spelt DK. (1938) Conditioned response of the human fetus in utero. *Psychol Bull* 35: 712–713.

Spira AW, Hollenberg MJ. (1973) Human retinal development: ultrastructure of the inner retinal layers. *Dev Biol* 31: 1–21.

Steiner JE. (1979) Human facial expressions in response to taste and smell stimulations. In: Lipsitt LP, Reese HW, editors. *Advances in Child Development. Vol 13*. New York: Academic Press. p 257–295.

Teixeira J, Fogliani R, Giannakoulopoulos X, Glover V, Fisk NM. (1996) Fetal haemodynamic stress response to invasive procedures. *Lancet* 347: 624.

Teixeira JMA, Glover V, Fisk NM. (1999) Acute cerebral redistribution in response to invasive procedures in the human fetus. *Am J Obstet Gynecol* 181: 1018–1025.

Timor-Tritsch IE. (1986) The effect of external stimuli on fetal behaviour. *Eur J Obstet Gynecol Reprod Biol* 21: 321–329.

Trehub SE. (1973) Infant's sensitivity to vowel and tonal contrasts. *Dev Psychol* 9: 91–96.

Trudinger BJ, Boylan P. (1980) Antepartum fetal heart rate monitoring: Value of sound stimulation. *Obstet Gynecol* 55: 265–268.

Tsuneishi S, Casaer P. (2000) Effects of preterm extrauterine visual experience on the development of the human visual system: a flash VEP study. *Dev Med Child Neurol* 42: 663–668.

Tucker D. (1963) Physical variables in the olfactory stimulation process. *J Gen Physiol* 46: 453–489.

van de Velde M, Jani J, de Buck F, Deprest J. (2006) Fetal pain perception and pain management. *Semin Fetal Neonat Med 11*: 232–236.

Vanhatalo S, van Nieuwenhuizen O. (2000) Fetal pain? *Brain Dev* 22: 145–150.

van Heteren CF, Boekkooi PF, Jongsma HW, Nijhuis JG. (2000) Fetal learning and memory. *Lancet* 356: 1169–1170.

van Heteren CF, Boekkooi PF, Jongsma HW, Nijhuis JG. (2001) Fetal habituation to vibroacoustic stimulation in relation to fetal states and fetal heart rate parameters. *Early Hum Dev* 61: 135–145.

Visser GHA, Mulder EJ. (1993) The effect of vibro-acoustic stimulation on fetal behavioural state organization. *Am J Industr Med* 23: 531–539.

Visser GHA, Zellenberg HJ, de Vries JIP, Dawes GS. (1983) External physical stimulation of the human fetus during episodes of low heart rate variation. *Am J Obstet Gynecol* 145: 579–584.

Visser GHA, Mulder HH, Wit HP, Mulder EJH, Prechtl HFR. (1989) Vibroacoustic stimulation of the human fetus: effects on behavioural state organisation. *Early Hum Dev* 19: 285–296.

Walker D, Grimwade J, Wood C. (1971) Intrauterine noise: a component of the fetal environment. *Am J Obstet Gynecol* 109: 91–95.

Wise J. (1997) Fetuses cannot feel pain before 26 weeks. *Br Med J* 315: 1112.

Woodward SC, Guidozzi F. (1992) Intrauterine rhythm and blues? *Br J Obstet Gynecol* 199: 787–789.

Yoles I, Hod M, Kaplan B, Ovadia J. (1993) Fetal 'fright-bradycardia' brought on by air-raid alarm in Israel. *Int J Gynaecol Obstet* 40: 157–160.

Zappasodi F, Tecchio F, Pizzella V, Cassetta E, Romano GV, Filligoi G, Rossini PM. (2001) Detection of fetal auditory evoked responses by means of magnetoencephalography. *Brain Res* 917: 167–173.

Zecevic N, Verney C. (1995) Development of the catecholamine neurons in human embryos and fetuses, with special emphasis on the innervation of the cerebral cortex. *J Comp Neurol* 351: 509–535.

Zimmer EZ, Divon MY, Vilensky A, Sarna Z, Peretz BA, Paldi E. (1982) Maternal exposure to music and fetal activity. *Eur J Obstet Gynecol Reprod Biol* 13: 209–213.

Zimmer EZ, Chao CR, Guy GP, Marks F, Fifer WP. (1993) Vibroacoustic stimulation evokes human fetal micturition. *Obstet Gynecol* 81: 178–180.

6
FETAL BEHAVIOUR IN TWINS

Introduction

Monozygotic twins share all their genes, whereas, from a genetic point of view, dizygotic twins are like ordinary siblings. Dizygotic twins always have separate placentas and amniotic sacs. Monozygotic twins can have two placentas, depending on when the twinning division takes place. The majority (70%) of monozygotic twins share the same placenta but inhabit two different amniotic sacs, which is why they are called monochorionic-diamniotic twins (Piontelli 2006). Although monozygotic twins initially show more intra-pair similarities in spontaneous and reactive activity, they are not behaviourally identical from the start. By halfway through pregnancy, they reach the same degree of behavioural individuality as dizygotic twins (Piontelli et al 1999, Piontelli 2006). There has been no comparative study, so far, on the onset of spontaneous movements in twins and singletons. What we do know is that the activity level is higher in twins than in singletons, and more so in triplets or quadruplets (Samueloff et al 1983, Ohel et al 1985). Until 15 weeks' gestation, the relatively high activity level is similar in monozygotic and dizygotic twins. Thereafter, spontaneous movements diminish in both groups, but more significantly in monozygotic twins (Piontelli et al 1999). Quickening is observed somewhat later than in singletons, namely at 18–20 weeks (Piontelli 2002).

Behavioural recordings in twin fetuses

Simultaneous sonographic visualisation of both fetuses in their entirety is only possible until approximately 15 weeks' gestation. After this time, twins can only be observed separately. The use of two independent probes is not feasible, since the probes would interfere with each other due to the complex spatial positioning of the two bodies. Hence, one fetus is usually observed for 20–30 consecutive minutes, after which the probe is moved to the other twin. However, care should always be taken to include parts of the co-twin in the ultrasonic field of one twin.

Inter-pair contact, myths and facts

There are many popular beliefs about the intrauterine activities of twins, such as reports on twins stimulating each other in all sorts of ways (Hepper 1996, Piontelli 2002, 2006).

Even kissing and boxing matches have been described 'scientifically' (Ianniruberto and Tajani 1981, Arabin et al 1996). Apart from other objections, it is difficult to imagine that behavioural and emotional patterns as complex as kissing could possibly be performed through the membranes that, in 99% of all twin pregnancies, separate the two amniotic sacs (Piontelli 2002, 2006).

Even though direct contacts between the twins are clearly not an expression of an intense and lively fetal social life, they are nonetheless an active and distinctive feature of their intrauterine environment. By 13 weeks' gestation, twins seem to react to physical contact caused by the co-twin's spontaneous movements (Arabin et al 1996, Piontelli et al 1997, 1999). For a description of the movements elicited by the contact, see Chapter 5, p 101. As stated before, some 'reactions' are actually part of a general movement and are therefore spontaneously generated rather than being reactions in the proper sense (Video 25). During the first half of pregnancy, only about 5% of all movements seem to be elicited (Samueloff et al 1991). There are also periods in which a fetus appears to be indifferent to physical contact: the body is displaced by the co-twin within the amniotic fluid – often quite far from the original position – only to fall back into an inactive state, seemingly unperturbed (Piontelli 2002).

Identical twins are not identical from a behavioural point of view

Twin fetuses have separate umbilical cords and an unequal placental share; they float in different amounts of amniotic fluid and have individual blood circuits. Their environments – including potential maternal stressors – can hardly be regarded as equal (Piontelli 2006). Consequently each twin, regardless of zygosity, develops an individual style of acting and reacting within the broader range of behavioural patterns (Piontelli et al 1999, Nijhuis and Visser 2003). One twin may be more 'dominant' in the sense of being more active, but less reactive, which could be attributed to a decrease of stimuli from the co-twin. Similar to singletons, there is a high intra-fetal consistency in the scope of activity: the fetus who is more active at a particular point of observation remains more active during all subsequent observations (Piontelli et al 1999). Interestingly, active twins tend to be heavier at birth than their (more passive) co-twins (Piontelli 2006), and they remain more active after birth (Degani et al 2009). Reactivity levels, however, are equally distributed, regardless of birth weight (Piontelli et al 1999).

Monozygotic twins show greater similarities in their activity and reactivity levels than dizygotic twins, although the similarity decreases with increasing age. By 22 weeks, their differences in activity and reactivity are almost the same as in dizygotic twins (Piontelli et al 1999). Hence, so-called identical twins are never really identical from a behavioural point of view, not even in early pregnancy (Piontelli et al 1999).

Only half of the breathing movements and 25% of the body movements occur simultaneously (Zimmer et al 1988). There is, however, a remarkable synchronicity of fetal heart rate (Devoe and Azor 1981, Sherer et al 1990, 1994, Gallagher et al 1992, Lunshof et al 1997), which cannot be explained by monozygosity, as it also holds true for

Fetal heart-rate patterns in per cent of time

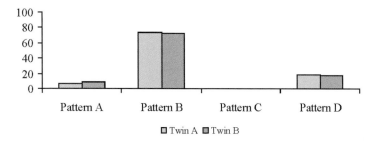

Figure 6.1 Percentage of state related fetal heart rate patterns in (A-D beats per minute) in 15 pairs of twins median age 34 weeks. Created from data using Galagher et al. 1992 which are base on 35 minutes of observation

dizygotic twins (Piontelli 2006). Near term, when behavioural states are present, the variation in the fetal heart-rate patterns is almost the same in both twins (Figure 6.1); hence, sleep or awake states occur in synchrony, whereby dichorionic, dizygotic twins are less synchronised (90%) than monochorionic, monozygotic twins (95%; Gallagher et al 1992).

REFERENCES

Arabin B, Bos R, Rijlaarsdam R, Mohnhaupt A, van Eyck J. (1996) The onset of inter-human contacts: longitudinal ultrasound observations in early twin pregnancies. *Ultrasound Obstet Gynecol* 8: 166–173.

Degani S, Leibovitz Z, Shapiro I, Ohel G. (2009) Twin's temperament: early prenatal sonographic assessment and postnatal correlation. *J Perinatol* 29: 337–342.

Devoe LD, Azor H. (1981) Simultaneous nonstress fetal heart rate testing in twin pregnancy. *Obstet Gynecol* 58: 450–455.

Gallagher MW, Costigan K, Johnson TRB. (1992) Fetal heart rate accelerations, fetal movement, and fetal behaviour patterns in twin gestations. *Am J Obstet Gyncecol* 167: 1140–1144.

Hepper PG. (1996) Fetal behaviour: why so sceptical? *Ultrasound Obstet Gynecol* 8: 145–148.

Ianniruberto A, Tajani E. (1981) Ultrasonographic study of fetal movements. *Semin Perinatol* 5: 175–181.

Lunshof S, Boer K, van Hoffen G, Wolf H, Mirmiran M. (1997) The diurnal rhythm in fetal heart rate in a twin pregnancy with discordant anencephaly: comparison with three normal twin pregnancies. *Early Hum Dev* 48: 47–57.

Nijhuis JG, Visser GHA. (2003) Discussion of 'fetal behaviour' and 'fetal behaviour: a commentary'. *Neurobiol Aging* 24: S51–S52.

Ohel G, Samueloff A, Navot D, Sadovsky E. (1985) Fetal heart rate accelerations and fetal movements in twin pregnancies. *Am J Obstet Gynecol* 152: 686–687.

Piontelli A. (2002) *Twins. From Fetus to Child*. London and New York: Routledge

Piontelli A. (2006) On the onset of human fetal behaviour. In: Manca M, editor. *Psychoanalysis and Neuroscience*. Mailand: Springer. p 391–418.

Piontelli A, Bocconi L, Kustermann A, Tassis B, Zoppini C, Nicolini U. (1997) Patterns of evoked behaviour in twin pregnancies during the first 22 weeks of gestation. *Early Hum Dev* 50: 39–45.

Piontelli A, Bocconi L, Boschetto C, Kustermann A, Nicolini U. (1999) Differences and similarities in the intra-uterine behaviour of monozygotic and dizygotic twins. *Twin Res* 2: 264–273.

Samueloff A, Evron S, Sadovsky E. (1983) Fetal movements in multiple pregnancy. *Am J Obstet Gynecol* 146: 789–792.

Samueloff A, Younis JS, Strauss N, Baras M, Sadovsky E. (1991) Incidence of spontaneous and evoked fetal movements in the 1st-half of twin pregnancy. *Gynecol Obstet Invest* 31: 200–203.

Sherer DM, Nawrocki MN, Peco NE, Metlay LA, Woods JR Jr. (1990) The occurrence of simultaneous fetal heart rate accelerations in twins during nonstress testing. *Obstet Gynecol* 76: 817–821.

Sherer DM, D'Amico ML, Cox C, Metlay LA, Woods JR Jr. (1994) Association of in utero behavioural patterns of twins with each other as indicated by fetal heart rate reactivity and nonreactivity. *Am J Perinatol* 11: 208–212.

Zimmer EZ, Goldstein I, Alglay S. (1988) Simultaneous recording of fetal breathing movements and body movements in twin pregnancy. *J Perinat Med* 16: 109–112.

7
DETERMINANTS OF FETAL BEHAVIOUR

It was assumed for a long time that the fetus lived utterly isolated from the bustle of the outside world (Preyer 1885, Windle 1940, Reynolds 1962). More recently, however, it has become clear that pregnancy-related and maternal factors affect fetal behaviour. Even the fetus's sex has an influence on some behavioural features.

Behavioural similarities and differences between female and male fetuses
Compared with females, newborn males are less responsive to auditory and social stimuli; they cry more, are more irritable and easier to arouse, have a higher heart rate and exhibit more startles but fewer mouth and sucking movements (Korner 1969, Collaer and Hines 1995, Weinberg et al 1999, Hafström and Kjellmer 2000, Nagy et al 2001). Given these findings, the idea of continuity suggests that sex differences do not appear at birth but have their developmental origin in the prenatal period.

Male fetuses are indeed more vulnerable to teratogenicity, including hypoxia (Spinillo et al 1994). Regarding their skeletal and respiratory development, they are less mature than female fetuses of comparable gestational age (Khoury et al 1985), although their higher birthweight suggests a higher degree of maturation.

Several studies set out to detect sex differences in specific aspects of fetal behaviour, but failed to do so: throughout pregnancy, female and male fetuses have an equal number of movement patterns (Valentin et al 1984, de Vries et al 1985, 1988, Pillai and James 1990, Rayburn 1990); this is also true for female and male twins (Zimmer et al 1988a). The heart-rate patterns and behavioural states are equal in both sexes, as is the basal fetal heart rate and its variability, or the rate of occurrence of general movements during the various behavioural states (Petrie and Segalowitz 1980, Dawes et al 1982, Rayburn 1982, Pillai and James 1990, Pillai et al 1992, DiPietro et al 1996, 2004, Nijhuis et al 1998, Oguch and Steer 1998, Robles de Medina et al 2003). Moreover, the gestational age at which a fetus first shows heart-rate accelerations in response to vibroacoustic stimulation is the same in males and females (DiPietro et al 1996).

In some studies, however, male fetuses had a higher heart-rate variability throughout gestation, and a somewhat earlier emergence of behavioural-state organisation (Di Pietro et al 1998, Pressman et al 1998, Bernardes et al 2008). They also moved their legs more than their female counterparts (Almli et al 2001).

Female fetuses, on the other hand, move their jaws more than males (Hepper et al 1997, Miller et al 2006). Hepper and colleagues considered this to be a sign of advanced development, since jaw movements enable the neonate to suck, to ingest nourishment – and hence to survive. Indeed, male preterm infants show fewer and less-intense sucking movements than preterm females (Hafström and Kjellmer 2000); as term newborns, males show fewer rhythmical mouthing and fewer lingual movements during bottle feeding (Korner 1973, Lundqvist and Hafström 1999).

Regarding fetal responsiveness, females react more maturely to vibroacoustic stimulation (Buss et al 2009), to which they also habituate 2 weeks earlier than males (Leader et al 1982).

Fetal behaviour during uterine contractions
Braxton Hicks contractions are not influenced by fetal behavioural states; nor are they related to state transitions. Fetal body movements do not trigger Braxton Hicks contractions, but the latter coincide with a specific cluster of body movements during the ascending phase of the contractions (Mulder and Visser 1987). Breathing movements are clustered during the descending phase of short-lasting contractions, but decrease gradually during the long-lasting phase (Wilkinson and Robinson 1982). Diabetes in pregnancy is a condition in which Braxton Hicks contractions do not affect fetal breathing movements (Mulder et al 1995).

A different picture is presented during labour: normally the fetus moves more during contractions than between them (Wittmann et al 1979, Sadovsky et al 1984, Zimmer et al 1988b, Reddy et al 1991). If accompanied by fetal movements, contractions last twice as long (Reddy et al 1991).

With the fetus in breech position, the environment changes fundamentally
At 30–32 weeks' gestation, 10–15% of all fetuses are in breech position. At term delivery, the majority of fetuses assume the vertex position, with the head being the lowest part of the fetus. Only 3% of fetuses remain in breech around term (Takashima et al 1995, Fong et al 2008). This means that, especially towards the end of pregnancy, the fetal parts in the lower segment of the uterus are surrounded by the bony maternal pelvis, thus being more restricted in their movements than the fetal parts in the upper segment of the uterus, which are surrounded by muscular tissue (Fong et al 2005).

EFFECTS ON FETAL BEHAVIOUR
Breech presentation has no influence on the quantity of movements (Luterkort and Maršál 1985, Kean et al 1999, van der Meulen et al 2008). However, breech fetuses spend more time with their knees extended than cephalic fetuses, who cross their legs more often (Fong et al 2009a).

Although the overall number of eye movements is more or less the same in breech fetuses and in cephalic fetuses (see Chapter 2, p 45), the former show fewer horizontal eye movements and more vertical and oblique eye movements, which suggests a difference in neural control of oculomotor activity (Takashima et al 1995).

As mentioned in Chapter 3 (p 70), the intrauterine environment plays an important role in the development of side preferences. With advancing age, cephalic fetuses increasingly abandon the midline head position and develop a preference to the right (Ververs et al 1994). This is not the case in breech fetuses: if they have a lateral preference at all, it is not necessarily to the right (Fong et al 2005). These findings support the hypothesis that breech fetuses can move their head more freely, which obviously leads to a less pronounced difference in stimulation of the right or left otoliths and hence to a less pronounced vestibular lateralisation (Previc 1991).

Breech and cephalic fetuses are similar in the number of heart-rate accelerations, but breech fetuses exhibit more behavioural-state transitions than cephalic fetuses (Kean et al 1999).

Their different sensory experience may be the reason why breech fetuses move less than cephalic fetuses in response to vibroacoustic stimuli, but more in response to airborne sound stimuli (van der Meulen et al 2008).

POSTNATAL CONSEQUENCES OF THE FETAL BREECH POSITION

The constriction of the lower part of the fetal body can have mechanical consequences, namely enhancement of hip flexion and reduction of hip extension (Fong et al 2009b); dysplasia of the hip (Hinderaker et al 1994a, Ruhmann et al 1999, Andersson and Odén 2001, Omeroglu and Koparal 2001); hip dislocation of the newborn (Hsieh et al 2000); and even hip deformation (Hjelmstedt and Asplund 1983). Fetuses in breech have a 10 degree greater anteflexion of the femoral neck than fetuses in the vertex position (Hinderaker et al 1994b), and their popliteal angle at birth is more open (Bartlett et al 2000, Sekulić et al 2009). At the age of 6 weeks, they score lower on the Alberta Infant Motor Scale than the normative sample (Bartlett et al 2000). Up to 6 months of age, the magnet response and the withdrawal reflex are abnormal: in infants born after complete breech position (with hips and knees flexed, the feet protruding first during vaginal delivery), the magnet response consists of a weak leg extension or is absent altogether (Figure 7.1b top), whereas in infants born in incomplete breech position (with the hips flexed and the knees extended, the buttocks being the first part to present itself during vaginal delivery), leg extension is more pronounced (Figure 7.1c top). Eliciting the withdrawal reflex in infants born after complete breech presentation results in exaggerated flexion of the legs (Figure 7.1b bottom), whereas in infants born after incomplete breech presentation the response is weak, or absent, or with the legs abnormally extended (Figure 7.1c bottom; Prechtl and Knol 1958, Prechtl 1977, Sival et al 1993). Normally, the magnet response results in a moderate extension (Figure 7.1a top), while the withdrawal reflex elicits a moderate flexion (Figure 7.1a bottom; Prechtl 1977). The prenatal breech position has an adverse effect on the functional hip dynamics during early walking – mainly with support – at the age of 12–18 months (Sival et al 1993); by 2.5 years of age, however, the deficiency is gone (Fong et al 2008).

Abnormalities in the amniotic fluid volume alter the intrauterine space

THE EFFECTS OF OLIGOHYDRAMNIOS: FETAL BREATHING MOVEMENTS DECREASE, GENERAL MOVEMENTS CHANGE THEIR QUALITY

Prolonged premature rupture of the membranes, especially before 24 weeks' gestation, is associated with a high prenatal mortality rate due to complications of preterm birth such as infection and pulmonary hypoplasia (Nimrod et al 1984, Rotschild et al 1990). The debate over the cause of pulmonary hypoplasia revolves around two main theories: (1) loss of lung fluid (Adzick et al 1984, Roberts and Mitchell 1995); and (2) inhibition of fetal breathing movements (Wigglesworth and Desai 1982).

In a normal course of development, fetal breathing movements increase gradually (Figure 7.2) from 5% at mid-gestation to 25% at the age of 32 weeks (Roodenburg et al 1991). As discussed in Chapter 2 (p 35), lung development depends on the presence of normal fetal breathing movements. In pregnancies complicated by oligohydramnios, by contrast, the percentage of fetal breathing movements is constantly low (Figure 7.2), showing no positive correlation with advancing gestational age (Sival et al 1992). This reduction of breathing movements is associated with pulmonary hypoplasia secondary to premature rupture of membranes (Kivikovski et al 1988, Roberts et al 1991, Thompson et al 1992, Roberts and Mitchell 1995). Interestingly, if breathing movements are normal – in spite of oligohydramnios – lung development is also normal (Goldstein et al 1988, Blott et al 1990,).

Since oligohydramnios is not associated with a decrease in the general activity of the fetal trunk, a rupture of membranes does not result in a decrease of fetal body movements (Roberts et al 1991). There is, however, a change in the quality of general movements: a moderate reduction of amniotic fluid is associated with a decrease in movement amplitude, while a severe reduction of amniotic fluid also causes a decrease in movement speed (Ianniruberto and Tajani 1981, Sival et al 1992, Rosier-van Dunné et al 2010).

POLYHYDRAMNIOS DOES NOT SPECIFICALLY ALTER FETAL BEHAVIOUR

If fetal swallowing is grossly impaired – especially in late pregnancy – or if there is an overproduction of amniotic fluid, polyhydramnios is the outcome. The resultant enlarged intrauterine space can increase fetal activity, especially in state 1F (Vindla et al 1997). A cessation of fetal activity in the presence of polyhydramnios, on the other hand, is highly suggestive of a fetal malformation (Sadovsky and Perlman 1978, Jones 1988). Vindla and associates (1997) described a fetus with distal arthrogryposis and an unusually high rate of fetal activity, which the authors attributed to the fact that polyhydramnios was present. When oesophageal atresia is the cause of polyhydramnios, fetuses may regurgitate or

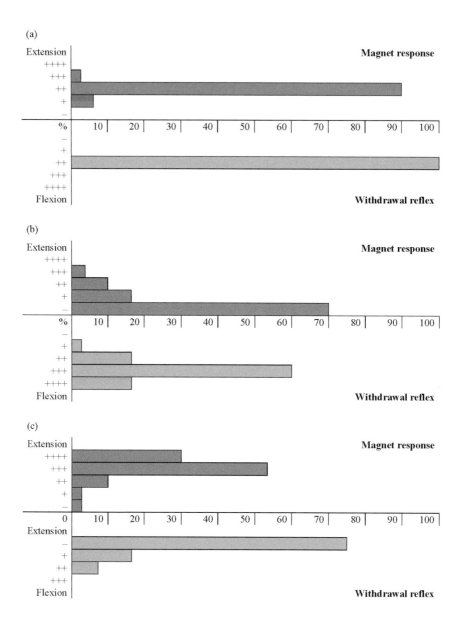

Figure 7.1 Percentage of response patterns in (a) 116 newborns delivered after uncomplicated cephalic presentation; (b) 18 newborns delivered after complete breech presentation with hips and knees flexed, the feet presenting as the first part during vaginal delivery; and (c) 35 newborns delivered after incomplete breech presentation with hips flexed and knees extended, the buttocks presenting as the first part during vaginal delivery. − = no response; + = weak response; ++ = moderate response; +++ = exaggerated response; ++++ = very exaggerated response. Created using data from Prechtl and Knol 1958; and from Prechtl 1977, with permission.

Fetal breathing movements in per cent of time

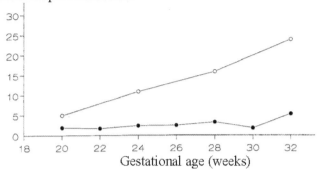

Figure 7.2 Median values of the percentage of fetal breathing movements in 11 uncomplicated pregnancies (–○–) and in 11 complicated pregnancies (–●–) in terms of oligohydramnios due to premature rupture of the membranes. From Sival DA, Visser GHA, Prechtl HFR. (1992) Fetal breathing movements are not a good indicator of lung development after premature rupture of membranes and oligohydramnios – a preliminary study. *Early Hum Dev* 28: 133–143, with permission.

vomit (Bowie and Clair 1982). Nevertheless, there are also reports of fetuses who move normally in spite of polyhydramnios (Ianniruberto and Tajani 1981).

Is the mother's physical exercise stressful for the fetus?
Many women exercise regularly during pregnancy. Thereby, the metabolic demands of the active muscles can interfere with those of the gravid uterus, which may in turn result in a poorer physical performance and/or fetal distress. Fetal growth retardation as a result of repeated stress associated with daily exercise has even been reported (Lotgering et al 1984). During maternal exercise, the blood flow in the main uterine artery decreases (Lotgering et al 1984, Clapp 1991, Erkkola et al 1992); the catecholamines increase; sometimes hypoglycaemia occurs; and, most notably, fetal temperature increases (Artal et al 1981, Jones et al 1985, Winn et al 1994).

Moderate to demanding maternal exercise (>60% increase in maternal heart rate) clearly affects the fetus and is associated with signs of transient fetal impairment: body and breathing movements decrease significantly, as does the fetal heart rate; fetal bradycardia can also occur (Dale et al 1982, Rayburn 1982, Artal et al 1984, Gorski 1985, Rauramo 1987, Winn et al 1994, Hatoum et al 1997, Manders et al 1997).

The effects of maternal physical exercise on the fetal heart rate depend on the type and intensity of exercise: in general, there is no alteration or only a slight increase in the fetal heart rate during non-exhaustive workout like, for example, relaxed swimming (Maršál et al 1979, Platt et al 1983, Artal et al 1986, Katz et al 1988); a progressive increase is associated with moderate exercise such as cycling or jogging (Collings and Curet 1985);

during strenuous exercise the fetal heart rate decreases significantly (see above). Regular maternal exercise throughout gestation (e.g. 30 minutes of aerobics, three times a week) results in a lower fetal heart rate, but also in an increased heart-rate variability during behavioural state 4F (May et al 2010).

Maternal emotions and their effects on the fetus

The impact of maternal emotions on the fetus is a keenly debated topic among psychologists and psychoanalysts, who concentrate especially on negative emotions such as anxiety and stress, while, in fact, maternal relaxation can also have an influence on fetal behaviour.

Prolonged stress reduction – by means such as yoga, progressive relaxation protocols or hypnosis intervention – has a moderate but positive effect on the gestational age and/or birthweight (Janke 1999, Narendran et al 2005). It can further improve the blood flow in the umbilical artery (Reinhard et al 2009) and reduce the maternal heart rate (Teixeira et al 2005) as well as the fetal heart rate (DiPietro et al 2008a). The effect of relaxation on fetal movements, however, is inconclusive (Field et al 1985, Zimmer et al 1988c, DiPietro et al 2008a, Reinhard et al 2009).

Stimulation of specific acupuncture points is believed to activate pathways that may trigger the release of neurotransmitters and neurohormones. Fetal movements tend to increase after acupuncture to the mother's fifth toe, the acupoint BL-67 (Cardini and Weixin 1998). Massage of highly innervated areas such as the mother's feet and hands can stimulate fetal activity (Diego et al 2002) – a phenomenon that is common knowledge among midwifes, although its underlying cause is as yet unclear.

Maternal anxiety

Whitehead (1867), observed for the first time that fetuses of anxious or emotionally stressed mothers tend to be very active (Sontag 1941, Ferreira 1965, McDonald 1968, Wolkind 1981). However, these case histories were not confirmed in controlled studies (van den Bergh et al 1989, Sjöström et al 2002). Apart from fetal hiccups, there is no certified correlation between maternal state anxiety and the fetal movement patterns (Bartha et al 2003). However, anxiety does seem to influence fetal wakefulness: state 4F lasts longer in fetuses of anxious mothers (Sjöström et al 2002).

Whereas there is little evidence for fetal behavioural changes due to maternal anxiety, there does seem to be an effect on fetal cerebral and umbilical artery haemodynamics. Fetuses of women with higher trait anxiety have a higher pulsatility index in the umbilical artery and a lower index in the fetal middle cerebral artery, which suggests a change in blood distribution in favour of brain circulation (Sjöström et al 1997, Teixeira et al 1999).

Although an immediate effect on the behaviour of the fetus is doubtful, maternal anxiety, especially from 12 to 22 weeks' gestation, appears to be associated with a reduction of grey matter volume during school age (Buss et al 2010), as well as with a number of behavioural deviations in infancy, childhood and even adolescence: irritability and difficult temperament, attention-deficit–hyperactivity disorder, externalising problems, impulsivity, self-report anxiety, slower processing speed and reaction time in cognitive and attention tasks, and even symptoms of depression (van den Bergh and Marcoen 2004, Austin et al 2005, van den Bergh et al 2005, 2008, Mennes et al 2006, van den Bergh et al 2006, DiPietro et al 2008b). We must not forget, however, that a mother with high trait anxiety will probably remain anxious after birth. In view of this, it is all the more surprising that there has so far been no study scrutinising the effects of an insecure and anxious upbringing and contrasting them with possible long-term effects of prenatal maternal anxiety.

MATERNAL STRESS INCREASES FETAL ACTIVITY
Every day we are confronted with countless situations that require adaptation. If we find it very hard or even impossible to cope with a difficulty, we feel stress. Our whole system of stress regulation is activated, namely the hypothalamus-pituitary-adrenal system and the sympathetic nervous system; various stress hormones are released into the blood in large quantities. By increasing energy substrates and stimulating the cardiovascular tone, corticoids play an invaluable part in the acute response of the organism to stress. However, prolonged effects are deleterious to the developing brain because of their catabolic action. Normally, the human fetus is relatively – albeit not completely – protected against maternal glucocorticoids by the placental enzyme 11-beta-hydroxysteroid-dehydrogenase. However, under specific conditions, maternal cortisol can actually reach the fetus: if (1) the maternal cortisol is highly concentrated; (2) the activity of 11-beta-hydroxysteroid-dehydrogenase is reduced; (3) the placenta is immature (early pregnancy); or (4) the placental function is poor, as in the case of some pregnancy complications (Benediktsson et al 1993, Mulder et al 2002). If maternal stress hormones enter the fetal circulation, they will affect the fetal hippocampal ontogeny by downregulating glucocorticoid receptors and/or exerting neurotoxic effects on hippocampal cells (Sapolsky et al 1990).

It is not the daily problems but severe maternal stress during pregnancy – such as marital discord, serious illness, death of a close relation, disruption of economic security or rape – that is associated with an adverse obstetric outcome, as reflected in increased risk for preterm delivery, low birthweight relative to the gestational age, reduced head circumference, and reduced neonatal neurological optimality (Rothberg and Lits 1991, Lou et al 1994, Copper et al 1996). There is a body of literature – although mainly based on animal experiments – on how maternal stress, acute or chronic, may affect fetal behaviour.

'When a pregnant mother falls, the baby in the womb answers' is a Yoruba saying in Western Nigeria. It is sonographically proven that fetal movements increase dramatically for a few minutes after a pregnant woman falls, even if she is not hurt but is merely embarrassed (Hepper and Shahidullah 1990).

The best documented spontaneous observation of acute stress during pregnancy and its effect on the fetus is by Ianniruberto and Tajani (1981). On 23 November 1980, they had the opportunity to observe 28 pregnant women immediately after the Maternity Hospital in Bari, Southern Italy, had been shaken by severe earthquake tremors. None of the women had a physical trauma, but they were all panic-stricken. During the following 2–8 hours, all fetuses were hyperactive, showing disordered and vigorous movements. In 20 cases, this phase was followed by a period of reduced motility, lasting from 24 to 72 hours, while eight fetuses recovered immediately.

The Fels Study (see Chapter 1, p 2) also reported on vigorous fetal activity in mothers undergoing acute stress (Sontag and Wallace 1934).

By contrast, in the case of a mother who had had an electric shock, the fetus remained motionless and was tachycardic (Ianniruberto and Tajani 1981). The state of paralysis lasted for 48 hours, before movements normalised. A severe road traffic accident elicited similar transient fetal abnormalities (Nordstrom and Ingemarsson 1998).

Severe fetal bradycardia was elicited by an air-raid alarm, albeit during labour (Yoles et al 1993).

Higher fetal activity is also recorded in expectant mothers who are very emotional, appraise their lives as very stressful and report frequent pregnancy-specific complications (DiPietro et al 2008b).

The impact of maternal stress elicited, for example, by an arithmetic test or by the Stroop colour-word matching test is not so clear. Here, fetuses responded with a decrease in motor activity (DiPietro et al 2003) or with increased heart rate, provided the mother had high anxiety scores as well (Monk et al 2000).

Finally, prolonged prenatal stress – which, by definition, is caused by a high amount of daily problems – is associated with a difficult temperament during infancy as well as early childhood behavioural problems such as a restless and quick-tempered character or externalising behaviour (Sontag and Wallace 1934, Huizink et al 2002, de Weerth et al 2003, Niederhofer 2004, Gutteling et al 2005). Again, as in the studies on the impact of maternal anxiety, none of the studies on maternal stress have taken into account the fact that daily concerns do not necessarily stop after a child is born. It seems problematic, therefore, to conclude that adverse long-term behavioural effects are solely based upon prenatal stress.

Maternal depression

The hypothesis that maternal mood has a formative influence on the fetus has survived with little empirical support. Two studies, each based on a mere 5 minutes of observation, revealed that fetuses of depressed mothers are more active than fetuses of non-depressed mothers (Dieter et al 2001, Field et al 2001). Their heart rates also tend to be higher than they normally are (Allister et al 2001, Monk et al 2004), but as none of the studies was focused on the behavioural state, no firm conclusion can be drawn on the influence of depression on fetal activity.

Substance abuse

Substance abuse by pregnant women is a serious public health problem, as its impact extends far beyond maternal health, namely to the population that is yet unborn. Intrauterine exposure to social drugs such as nicotine, alcohol or cocaine may cause structural and/or functional developmental deficits that can be lifelong. But what is the immediate effect of drugs on the fetus' behaviour?

SMOKING DURING PREGNANCY

Up to 20% of pregnant women continue to smoke throughout gestation (Slotkin 1998, Boyle 2002). It would be simplistic to limit its toxicity to nicotine alone. Lead – whose level in the cord blood increases by 15% for every 10 cigarettes smoked – and carbon monoxide are another two well-documented neuroteratogens (Rhainds and Levallois 1997, Ferriero and Dempsey 1999, Blood-Siegfried and Rende 2010). Other chemical constituents of smoke that affect the developing brain include ammonia, nitrogen oxide, hydrogen cyanide, hydrogen sulphide, methanol, pyridine, phenol, aniline and cadmium (Newnham 1991). Nicotine passes through the placenta rapidly and completely, with fetal concentrations that are generally 15% above maternal levels (Walker et al 1999), and stimulates nicotine acetylcholine receptors (Hellström-Lindahl et al 1998). This may cause target cells to switch from proliferation to differentiation too early (Ernst et al 2001). Vasoconstriction in the uterine circulation results in a decreased uteroplacental blood flow and a potentially decreased delivery of oxygen and nutrients to the fetus (Huisman et al 1997, Coppens et al 2001). Carbon monoxide binds to fetal haemoglobin, which has a higher affinity to carbon monoxide than maternal haemoglobin, and produces carboxyhaemoglobin, which in turn inhibits oxygen delivery to the tissues. Secondary to vasoconstriction and ischaemia, placental pathology shows decidual necrosis, microinfarcts, fibrinoid changes, and hypovascular and atrophic villi (Boyle 2002). In the fetal brain, the activity of the enzyme-mediated antioxidative system decreases (Li and Wang 2004) and the resulting oxidative stress may cause deficits in both behaviour and development (Rougemont et al 2002).

Maternal smoking – active or passive – has a dose-dependent negative effect upon birthweight and the newborn's length and head circumference (Ferriero and Dempsey 1999). Intrauterine growth retardation is often observed in infants of smoking mothers (Huizink and Mulder 2006). Language impairment, difficulties coping with stress, decreased ability to get along with peers, and an increase of tantrums are also associated with maternal smoking during pregnancy (Faden and Graubard 2000).

Exposure to tobacco smoke temporarily reduces the activity of the fetus (Table 7.1; Wood et al 1979, Thaler et al 1980, Rayburn 1982, Goodman et al 1984, Graça et al 1991, Coppens et al 2001). Head and arm movements in particular are reduced (Habek 2007); fetal breathing movements also decrease (Gennser et al 1975, Manning et al 1975, Manning and Feyerabend 1976, Ianniruberto and Tajani 1981, Warner et al 2002), with short intervals between the inspiratory movements (Thaler et al 1980, Eriksen et al 1983).

This effect is most apparent half an hour after smoking, but disappears another hour later (Ritchie 1980). The decrease of fetal breathing movements is directly related to the rise in plasma nicotine but unrelated to the rise in carboxyhaemoglobin, as smoking non-nicotine (herbal) cigarettes, which significantly increases carboxyhaemoglobin concentration, does not alter the incidence of breathing movements. A nicotine chewing gum, however, results in an increase of maternal plasma nicotine concentration similar to that observed after tobacco smoking, and is also associated with a reduction of fetal breathing movements (Gennser et al 1975, Manning and Feyerabend 1976).

Fetuses who are chronically exposed to cigarette smoke spend more time in state 1F and show a decrease of activity in all behavioural states (Coppens et al 2001). Their heart rate temporarily increases (Hellman et al 1961, Ritchie 1980, Sørensen and Børlum 1987, Habek 2007), whereas heart-rate variability is lower (Zeskind and Gingras 2006).

Research into the acute and chronic effects of maternal smoking on fetal responsiveness and habituation has yielded conflicting results: whereas Gingras and colleagues (2004) did not find any influence on fetal reactivity, others reported delayed response to acoustic and vibroacoustic stimulation (Graça et al 1991, Cowperthwaite et al 2007) as well as abnormally prolonged habituation rates (Leader 1987, 1995).

TWO CUPS OF COFFEE

Maternal blood pressure does not change when a habitual coffee drinker consumes more coffee than usual, but maternal heart rate does increase slightly (Huisman et al 1997). Although caffeine rapidly crosses the placenta (Goldstein and Warren 1962), neither the pulsatility index of the umbilical artery nor the baseline fetal heart rate changes (Huisman et al 1997). However, fetal swallowing decreases after maternal coffee consumption (Huisman et al 1997). The effect of caffeine on fetal breathing movements is inconclusive, and studies are difficult to compare (Lewis et al 1978, McGowan et al 1987, Salvador and Koos 1989, Etherton and Kochar 1993, Huisman et al 1997). It seems, though, that fetuses of mothers who consume a lot of coffee are more awake (state 4F), and that this is at the expense of state 2F (Devoe et al 1993, Mulder et al 2010).

TABLE 7.1
TABLE 7.1 The effect of substance abuse on fetal behaviour

	Total activity	Breathing movements	Behavioural states	Responsiveness
Smoking	Reduced	Reduced	Disorganised	Inconclusive
Coffee	Not assessed	Inconclusive	Disorganised	Not assessed
Alcohol	Reduced	Reduced	Disorganised	Not assessed
Cocaine	Exaggerated	Not assessed	Disorganised	Normal
Methadone	Reduced	Reduced	Not assessed	Not assessed

Alcohol is one of the most teratogenic substances voluntarily consumed by women during pregnancy (Pratt 1981). Approximately 10% of pregnant women drink alcohol, and approximately 2% engage in binge drinking (Centers for Disease Control and Prevention 2004). Alcohol is freely distributed from the mother's blood to the fetus. It rapidly and easily crosses both the placenta and the fetus' blood–brain barrier and disturbs the functions and interactions of maternal and fetal hormones (Huizink and Mulder 2006). Alcohol particularly impairs the functionality of the hypothalamic-pituitary-adrenal axis, but also that of the hypothalamic-pituitary-thyroid axis, which regulates the metabolism of almost all tissues (Gabriel et al 1998). It further has an adverse effect on cellular energy metabolism, neuronal migration, apoptosis and neurotransmitter production (Day and Richardson 1991, Boyle 2002). Structural consequences of heavy prenatal exposure to alcohol are disproportional reductions of the basal ganglia (Archibald et al 2001), corpus callosum thinning (Sowell et al 2001), reduced cerebellar size (Sowell et al 1996) and volume asymmetries in the hippocampus (Riikonen et al 1999). The major functional deficits are observed in the form of motor abnormalities, behavioural disorders, cognitive deficits (Ferriero and Dempsey 1999) and fetal alcohol syndrome – the most serious consequence.

Although it is still a subject of debate whether or not moderate alcohol consumption during pregnancy is harmful to the fetus, in most countries total abstinence is recommended during pregnancy (Lasegreid et al 2005).

The behaviour of a fetus exposed to alcohol is clearly deviant. Immediately after an alcoholic drink, the fetal movements decrease significantly (Table 7.1); the remaining movements are slow (Ianniruberto and Tajani 1981, Castillo et al 1989). The frequency of startles, on the other hand, is higher than in fetuses who are not exposed to alcohol (Little et al 2002, Hepper et al 2005). Fetal eye movements are reduced (Mulder et al 1998) and fetal breathing movements are suppressed (Fox et al 1978, McLeod et al 1983, 1984, Brien and Smith 1991, Mulder et al 1998).

After a mere two glasses of wine, the organisation of behavioural states is tremendously disturbed (Mulder et al 1986, 1998). State 2F is frequently interrupted, resulting in a high proportion of non-coincidence; spontaneous awakening (into state 4F) follows stable periods of state 1F (Figure 7.3) – a phenomenon that is not found in healthy fetuses but sometimes occurs after vibroacoustic stimulation during state 1F (see Chapter 5, p 99). Similar disturbances of state regulation can last up to the neonatal period (Sander et al 1977, Rosett et al 1979).

PRENATAL EXPOSURE TO COCAINE

The prevalence of cocaine abuse among pregnant women is between 1% and 10% (Pagliaro and Pagliaro 1997). The problem is that cocaine crosses the placenta by simple diffusion. Once in the fetal compartment, circulating cocaine directly blocks the reuptake of catecholamines (Ward et al 1991), but also of other biogenic amines such as serotonin,

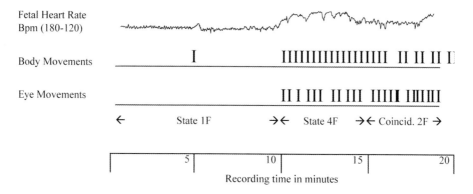

Figure 7.3 Actogram of fetal behaviour showing one of the synchronous transitions of all state variables from state 1F to state 4F. The pregnant mother drank around 10 glasses of beer per day during the first 3 months of pregnancy, and between 2 and 10 glasses of beer per day during the following months; she smoked about 10 cigarettes per day. Coincid. = coincidence. Adapted from Mulder EJ, Kamstra A, O'Brien MJ, Visser GHA, Prechtl HFR. (1986) Abnormal fetal behavioural state regulation in a case of high maternal alcohol intake during pregnancy. *Early Hum Dev* 14: 321–326, with permission.

dopamine and noradrenaline (Ronnekliev and Naylor 1995, Clarke et al 1996), thereby increasing the availability of these transmitters to bind with their receptor sites. Increased receptor binding acutely increases neuronal excitability, thus causing the cocaine 'high' (Gingras et al 1992), but at the same time it leads to deviant neuronal and astroglial development (Benveniste et al 2010).

The fetus is seldom exposed to cocaine alone. Almost 90% of cocaine-consuming pregnant women drink alcohol and smoke as well. Other confounders are poor maternal nutrition and lack of, or inadequate, pregnancy examinations (Chasnoff et al 1990, Gingras et al 1992). All of this may result in an increased incidence of placental abruption, spontaneous abortions, preterm delivery and intrauterine growth retardation, but also in microcephaly, brain malformations or vascular abnormalities (Zuckerman et al 1989, Hume et al 1994, Chiriboga et al 1995, Ferriero and Dempsey 1999). Moderate sequelae are transient generalised hypertonia, irritability or sleeping and feeding difficulties (Gingras et al 1992, Morrow et al 2001).

During exposure to cocaine (intravenous or nasal), fetal movements become excessive (Table 7.1), the quality of eye movements changes, and fetal breathing movements alter (Hume et al 1989), whereas fetal responsiveness and habituation to vibroacoustic stimulation remain within a normal range (Gingras et al 2004). The development of behavioural states is delayed (Hume et al 1989). Affected fetuses spend less time in state 1F but more time in state 4F and show fewer state transitions (Gingras et al 1998). Interestingly, all these behavioural alterations are found not only in acutely intoxicated fetuses but also in fetuses who were only exposed to cocaine during early pregnancy.

The benefits of methadone for narcotic-dependent women are well documented, but they are still inconclusive in fetuses or infants. Especially at peak methadone levels, the fetus displays a slower heart rate, a reduced heart-rate variability, and a decrease in heart-rate accelerations (Levine and Rebarber 1995, Cejtin et al 1996, Jansson et al 2005, 2009). Fetal breathing movements alter, regardless of how much time has passed since the mother's latest dose: they decrease and become slower (Archie et al 1989, Wouldes et al 2004, Jansson et al 2009). By one hour post dose, total fetal activity decreases, whereas before dose it is the same as in normally developing fetuses (Wouldes et al 2004). Body movements and breathing rate decrease less in fetuses of women on a split dose than in those whose mothers receive one single dose (Wittman and Segal 1991, Jansson et al 2009).

Maternal poisoning

There is one case history of a pregnant woman with ciguatera poisoning during the second trimester. Ciguatoxin is taken in by eating fish that have consumed toxic single-celled marine organisms. In the case mentioned above, fetal movements increased dramatically an hour after the meal, although the infant developed normally later on. This is in contrast with another report of a mother who had been exposed to ciguatoxin shortly before parturition and delivered an infant with facial palsy and myotonia of the hands. Such differences might be due to varying doses and gestational timing (Senecal and Osterloh 1991).

The effect of therapeutic drugs

Sedating medications such as barbiturates or benzodiazepines can easily cross the placenta and reduce fetal activity (Sadovsky and Polishuk 1977, Ianniruberto and Tajani 1981, Rayburn 1982), even in the first trimester of pregnancy (Jørgensen and Maršál 1988). Ianniruberto and Tajani (1981) observed some fetuses between 14 and 22 weeks who had a self-limiting epileptiform fit following maternal diazepam administration.

Intravascular injection of the non-depolarising curare-mimetic muscle relaxant pancuronium causes a pseudo-abolition of fetal movements as perceived by the mother, but no change in fetal heart rate (Spencer et al 1994).

An increase of fetal movements – assessed by maternal perception – may occur when the mother is administered the beta-adrenergic agent isoxsuprine to suppress premature labour (Samueloff et al 1984). However, a recent 5-day study has shown that the tocolytic agents atosiban (an oxytocin receptor antagonist) and nifedipine (a calcium antagonist) have no effect on either movement parameters or the fetal heart rate (de Heus et al 2009).

Aminophylline causes prompt and sustained regular fetal breathing movements, that are increased in both frequency and amplitude (Cosmi et al 2001). Conjugated estrogens, hexoprenaline, terbutaline and indometacin also enhance fetal breathing movements

(Hallak et al 1992, Cosmi et al 2001), whereas morphine administration reduces them (Kopecky et al 2000). None of these drugs have an influence on fetal body movements.

The possible effect of medication against hypertension or epilepsy is discussed later in this chapter (p 141-143).

THE EFFECT OF PRENATAL CORTICOSTEROID THERAPY

Prenatal glucocorticoid therapy (betamethasone, dexamethasone) is widely used to boost fetal lung maturation when signs are pointing to preterm delivery. As a side effect, there are considerable, albeit transient, changes in fetal behaviour: 1–3 days after betamethasone administration, fetal heart-rate variability, breathing movements and body movements decrease, resulting in a suppression of diurnal rhythms (Dawes et al 1994, Mulder et al 1994, 2004a, 2009, Derks et al 1995, Magee et al 1997, Kelly et al 2000, Cosmi et al 2001, Mushkat et al 2001, Jackson et al 2003, Koenen et al 2005, de Heus et al 2008). These changes are more pronounced in fetuses who are older than 29 weeks (Mulder et al 2004a, Lunshof et al 2005). As these alterations are similar in twins, the betamethasone level achieved is obviously high enough to reach the compartment of each twin (Ville et al 1995, Cosmi et al 2001, Mulder et al 2004b).

The described effects of betamethasone are mainly believed to be mediated in the brainstem, by functional glucocorticoid receptors (Mulder et al 1994, Derks et al 1995, Mulder et al 1997, 2004a). The prolonged time interval between drug administration and behavioural alteration is concordant with (1) the fact that corticoids enter the brain slowly, and (2) the involvement of cytosolic glucocorticoid receptors, whose range of action lasts from hours to days (Ullian 1999). Whether the behavioural changes are due to a temporary betamethasone-induced hypoxaemia is inconclusive, since the reports on Doppler flow indices of various blood vessels are controversial (Cohlen et al 1996, Cosmi et al 2001).

The therapeutic effect of betamethasone is probably more beneficial than that of dexamethasone (Roberts and Dalziel 2006), but it also has more side effects on fetal behaviour and fetal heart-rate variation (Mulder et al 2009). Dexamethasone does not influence fetal body movements (Mushkat et al 2001) and it reduces fetal breathing movements only 24 hours after administration (Mushkat et al 2001); however, it appears to increase short-term fetal heart-rate variability (Magee et al 1997, Mulder et al 1997).

Because of the obvious, albeit transient, effects of glucocorticoids on fetal behaviour, and because of some evidence that prenatal exposure to corticosteroids can increase the risk of hypertension and diabetes throughout life (Seckl 2001), repeated administration of corticosteroids faced increasing criticism (Visser et al 2001) and stricter guidelines are now in place (Visser and Anceschi 2001).

Maternal food intake and fetal behaviour

LA GRANDE BOUFFE

During the Christmas period, after 48 hours of eating at least three times as much as on normal days, fetal movements were reported to be eight times less frequent and seven times shorter than before Christmas (Hepper and Shahidulla 1991). None of the revelling pregnant women smoked, and all of them abstained from alcohol, so apparently the fetus, too, was affected by their mothers' over indulgence in food during festivities.

GLYCAEMIC LOAD AND FETAL BEHAVIOUR

Fetal breathing movements increase after maternal glucose intake

From mid-gestation onwards, the incidence of fetal breathing movements increases after a meal that is rich in carbohydrates (de Vries et al 1987), and it triples after glucose injection (Goodman 1980, Bocking et al 1982, Divon et al 1985, Meis et al 1985, Nijhuis et al 1986). Breathing movements climax 90–120 minutes after the intake of glucose (Patrick et al 1978, 1980, Nijhuis et al 1986).

Conflicting reports on the quantity of fetal body movements

Whereas fetal breathing movements are clearly associated with maternal glucose intake, it is difficult to establish such a link for total fetal activity. Some studies have revealed an increase in fetal body movements after oral glucose ingestion, especially if the intake exceeded 100mg (Miller et al 1978, Aladjem et al 1979, Gelmen et al 1980, Goldstein et al 2003), while others found no alteration whatsoever (Lewis et al 1978, Bocking et al 1982, Patrick et al 1982, Natale et al 1983, 1988), or even recorded reduced fetal activity (Edelberg et al 1987) – notably regarding hiccups, isolated leg movements, and startles (Bartha et al 2003). Differences in the amount of glucose intake and its administration, as well as the brevity of recording times – whereby the episodic nature of fetal movements is disregarded – make such studies difficult to interpret.

FASTING DECREASES FETAL BREATHING MOVEMENTS

Fetal breathing movements decrease during maternal fasting, like, for instance, during Ramadan (Mirghani et al 2003, Abd El Aal et al 2009). The same observation has been made in fetuses of mothers who eat very little or abstain from food altogether for several hours (Fox et al 1982, Harper et al 1987). When a fasting mother receives a glucose drink, fetal breathing movements increase immediately (Lewis et al 1978).

Type 1 diabetes and fetal behaviour

Maternal diabetes, though well controlled, alters the maternal metabolic milieu and can thus influence fetal growth and brain function (Romanini and Rizzo 1995). With the exception of breathing movements, fetal movements emerge 1–2 weeks later – exceeding even the delay in early growth (Mulder and Visser 1991a, 1991b). The delay is most significant in pregnancies in which the periconceptional quality of glucose is poor (Visser and Prechtl 1988). Initially, total activity also lags behind normal, but it rapidly increases and exceeds normal levels by 12 weeks, due to the higher incidence of breathing movements (Mulder and Visser 1991a).

The development of startles is different (Figure 7.4). Normally, startles show a considerable initial increase in their rate of occurrence, followed by a gradual decrease (see Figure 2.4). In fetuses of mothers with diabetes, the rate of occurrence increases progressively up to 13 weeks, to reach a level similar to normal fetuses (Mulder et al 1991).

General movements have a different quality in fetuses of mothers with diabetes (Kainer et al 1997). From 20 weeks onwards, the complexity of general movements tends to be reduced, and movement components become repetitive, leading to the abnormally 'poor repertoire of general movements' (Einspieler et al 1997, 2004). Interestingly, the degree of abnormality is not related to the White classification of obstetric diabetes but to the Bayley developmental indices, obtained at 10 months of age (Kainer et al 1997).

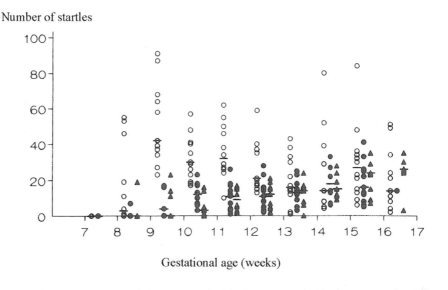

Figure 7.4 Number of startles observed in fetuses of women with diabetes in the preconceptional (●) or postconceptional (▲) continuous subcutaneous insulin infusion therapy subgroups as compared to control values (○). The differences in the rate of occurrence between the control and diabetes groups are statistically significant (*p*<0.01) between weeks 9 and 12. From Mulder EJH, Visser GHA, Morssink LP, de Vries JIP. (1991) Growth and motor development in fetuses of women with type 1 diabetes. III. First trimester quantity of fetal movement patterns. *Early Hum Dev* 25: 117–133, with permission.

In spite of an overall delay in the emergence of the various motor patterns, breathing movements emerge even earlier (Figure 7.5) than in normal fetuses (Mulder and Visser 1991b). From 10–14 weeks onwards, fetuses of mothers with diabetes show more breathing movements than normal fetuses (Roberts et al 1980, Mulder et al 1990, 1991, Devoe et al 1994, Florido et al 2008). Hence, glucose makes breathing movements appear sooner – and continues to affect them thereafter. The underlying mechanism, however, seems to be unrelated to the actual glucose level (Wladimiroff and Roodenburg 1982, Mulder et al 1991). Studies on fetal lambs have revealed that hyperglycaemia resulted in increased cerebral glucose consumption and concomitant carbon dioxide production (Richardson et al 1983). Hypercapnia increases the incidence of fetal breathing movements in both the fetal lamb (Bowes et al 1981) and the human fetus (Ritchie and Lakhani 1980) and is probably mediated by fetal chemoreceptors (see Chapter 2, p 38). As fetal breathing movements consume significant amounts of oxygen and glucose, it has been speculated that the increased incidence of breathing movements in the fetus of a woman with diabetes might be a mechanism to compensate for the excessive delivery of energy substrate. The fact that third-trimester fetuses of women with diabetes spend less time in coincidence/state 1F and have longer activity cycles than control fetuses (Mulder et al 1987, 1990) might serve a similar purpose (Mulder et al 1991). The organisation of behavioural states remains poor even after birth (Mulder et al 1990).

Fetuses of mothers with diabetes exhibit a less mature response to vibroacoustic stimulation (Allen and Kisilevsky 1999); in addition, it takes longer for them to habituate (Doherty and Hepper 2000, Gonzalez-Gonzalez et al 2009).

FETAL BEHAVIOUR REMAINS UNALTERED AFTER INSULIN-INDUCED HYPOGLYCAEMIA
Fetal breathing movements, body movements and fetal heart rate do not alter because of insulin-induced symptomatic maternal hypoglycaemia, although maternal adrenaline and growth hormone levels may increase (Reece et al 1995).

Maternal hypertension
Maternal hypertension is a rather common complication in 6–8% of pregnancies (American College of Obstetricians and Gynecologists 1996). Hypertension is found in women with different medical backgrounds and disparate aetiology and treatments. Maternal complications may include eclampsia and hepatic and/or renal failure, while fetal risks include stillbirth, placental abruption, growth retardation and preterm birth (Warner et al 2002). All of this is due to an impairment of the uteroplacental blood flow (Brown 1995) and thus to a reduction of fetal nutrition and oxygenation.

The Fels study (see Chapter 1, p 2) revealed that, during pre-eclampsia, fetal activity increased to a much higher level than in other, i.e. 'normal', pregnancies. However, after maternal symptoms were brought under control, which at that time took about 10 days, fetal activity decreased and eventually returned to normal (Sontag and Wallace 1934). In

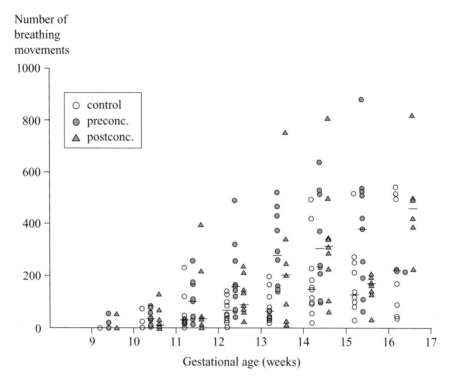

Number of
breathing
movements

Figure 7.5 Number of breathing movements observed in fetuses of women with diabetes in the preconceptional (preconc.) or postconceptional (postconc.) continuous subcutaneous insulin infusion therapy subgroups as compared to control values. The differences in the rate of occurrence between the control and diabetes groups are statistically significant ($p<0.05$) between weeks 10 and 14. From Mulder EJH, Visser GHA, Morssink LP, de Vries JIP. (1991) Growth and motor development in fetuses of women with type 1 diabetes. III. First trimester quantity of fetal movement patterns. *Early Hum Dev* 25: 117–133, with permission.

subsequent studies, no such increase of movements was observed (Warner et al 2002, Lee et al 2007).

Behavioural deviations mainly occur in fetal responsiveness. Normally, the fetus' heart accelerates as a response to the mother's voice, whereas in fetuses of hypertensive mothers, the fetal heart rate does not alter until the offset of the mother's voice, if at all (Lee et al 2007). Furthermore, vibroacoustic stimulation elicits fewer body movements in fetuses of hypertensive mothers: although they exhibit a similar cardiac acceleration response pattern as the normotensive group, they do not peak as high or for as long as the controls (Warner et al 2002). A possible explanation for these rather vague behavioural deviations could be that women with hypertension have, on average, a higher body mass index, and hence the stimulus transmission through the maternal tissue might be less effective (Lee et al 2007).

There is little information available on the possible effects of antihypertensive drugs on fetal behaviour. It is known that methyldopa and isradipine do not alter fetal heart-rate characteristics (Wideswensson et al 1993), but their potential influence on fetal behaviour has never been investigated. The beta-adrenergic-blocking agent labetalol, on the other hand, seems to impede the development of behavioural states, resulting in a higher percentage of non-coincidence, a higher percentage of state 1F at the expense of state 2F, and higher umbilical artery resistance indices (Gazzolo et al 1998).

Maternal epilepsy

Approximately one in 200 pregnant women has epilepsy (Swartjes and van Geijn 1998). This group is at risk of a variety of complications: pregnancy may influence the course of epilepsy by, for example, altering the seizure frequency; on the other hand, epilepsy and antiepileptic drug therapy may have an impact on the course of pregnancy or pregnancy outcome (Koch et al 1992, Kayemba Kay'S et al 1997, Titze et al 2008). Fetal malformation and cerebral dysfunction are associated with epilepsy, depending on the genetic predisposition, the severity of seizure disorder, and the type of anticonvulsant therapy (Lösche et al 1994, Koch et al 1996, Boyle 2002).

Tonic–clonic seizures of either epileptic or eclamptic origin cause fetal heart-rate decelerations and periods of bradycardia, which can be classified as signs of serious fetal hypoxia (Swartjes and van Geijn 1998). Hence, prevention of epileptic attacks throughout pregnancy is in the interest of both the mother and the child; continuation of antiepileptic drugs during pregnancy is advocated. On the other hand, antiepileptic drugs pass the placenta easily, and when in the fetal blood, pass through the immature blood–brain barrier into the fetal central nervous system (Swartjes et al 1992). Although little is known about the susceptibility of fetal brain cells to antiepileptic drugs, there is no antiepileptic drug that has not been a subject of teratology studies.

Regarding the quantity of movements, fetuses exposed to antiepileptic medication follow a similar developmental trend as unaffected fetuses (van Geijn et al 1986, Swartjes et al 1992). However, during state 2F only, fetuses exposed to sodium valproate or carbamazepine move less than they normally would (Kean et al 2001), with reduced eye movements as well (Swartjes et al 1991).

More significant than these subtle quantitative alterations, however, is the fact that movement quality is different in fetuses exposed to antiepileptic drugs: their general movements are classified as abnormal or suspect more often than in control fetuses (Swartjes et al 1992).

Decreased fetal movements as a result of viral infections

In the case of cytomegaly virus infection, fetal breathing movements decrease (Shinozuka et al 1989). Maternal varicella zoster infection during early gestation may result in a reduction of fetal movements throughout gestation (Taylor et al 1993). A parvovirus infection was reported to cause total absence of fetal body movements, including breathing movements and eye movements, and ultimately resulting in intrauterine death (Shinozuka et al 1989).

REFERENCES

Abd-El-Aal DE, Shahin AY, Hamed HO. (2009) Effect of short-term maternal fasting in the third trimester on uterine, umbilical, and fetal middle cerebral artery Doppler indices. *Int J Gynaecol Obstet* 107: 23–25.

Adzick NS, Harrison MR, Glick Pl, Villa RL, Finkbeiner W. (1984) Experimental pulmonary hypoplasia in oligohydramnios: relative contributions of lung fluid and fetal breathing movements. *J Pediatr Surg* 19: 658–665.

Aladjem S, Feria A, Rest J, Gull K, O'Conor M. (1979) Effect of maternal glucose load on fetal activity. *Am J Obstet Gynecol* 134: 276–280.

Allen CL, Kisilevsky BS. (1999) Fetal behaviour in diabetic and non-diabetic women: an exploratory study. *Dev Psychobiol* 35: 69–81.

Allister L, Lester BM, Carr S, Liu J. (2001) The effects of maternal depression on fetal heart rate response to vibroacoustic stimulation. *Dev Neuropsychol* 20: 639–651.

Almli CR, Ball RH, Wheeler ME. (2001) Human fetal and neonatal movement patterns: Gender differences and fetal-to-neonatal continuity. *Dev Psychobiol* 38: 252–273.

American College of Obstetricians and Gynecologists. (1996) Technical bulletin. Hypertension in pregnancy. *Int J Gynaecol Obstet* 53: 175–183.

Andersson JE, Odén A. (2001) The breech presentation and the vertex presentation following an external version represent risk factors for neonatal hip instability. *Acta Paediatr* 90: 895–898.

Archibald SL, Fennema-Notestine C, Gamst A, Riley EP, Mattson SN, Jernigan TL. (2001) Brain dysmorphology in individuals with severe prenatal alcohol exposure. *Dev Med Child Neurol* 43: 148–154.

Archie CL, Lee MI, Sokol RJ, Norman G. (1989) The effects of methadone treatment on the reactivity of the nonstress test. *Obstet Gynecol* 74: 254–255.

Artal R, Platt LD, Sperling M, Kammula RK, Jilek J, Nakamura R. (1981) Exercise in pregnancy. I. Maternal cardiovascular and metabolic responses in normal pregnancy. *Am J Obstet Gynecol* 140: 123–127.

Artal R, Romem Y, Paul RH, Wiswell R. (1984) Fetal bradycardia induced by maternal exercise. *Lancet* 2(8397): 258–260.

Artal R, Rutherford S, Romem Y, Kammula RK, Dorey FJ, Wiswell RA. (1986) Fetal heart rate response to maternal exercise. *Am J Obstet Gynecol* 155: 729–733.

Austin MP, Hadzi-Pavlovic D, Leader L, Saint K, Parker G. (2005) Maternal trait anxiety, depression and life event stress in pregnancy: relationship with infant temperament. *Early Hum Dev* 81: 183–190.

Bartha JL, Martinez-del-Fresno P, Romero-Carmona R, Hunter A, Comino-Delgado R. (2003) Maternal anxiety and fetal behaviour at 15 weeks' gestation. *Ultrasound Obstet Gynecol* 22: 57–62.

Bartlett DJ, Okun NB, Byrne PJ, Watt JM, Piper MC. (2000) Early motor development of breech- and cephalic-presenting infants. *Obstet Gynecol* 95: 425–432.

Benediktsson R, Lindsay RS, Noble J, Seckl JR, Edwards CRW. (1993) Glucocorticoid exposure in utero: new model for adult hypertension. *Lancet* 341: 339–341.

Benveniste H, Fowler JS, Rooney WD, Scharf BA, Backus WW, Izrailtyan I, Knudsen GM, Hasselbalch SG, Volkow ND. (2010) Cocaine is pharmacologically active in the nonhuman primate fetal brain. *Proc Natl Acad Sci U S A* 107: 1582–1587.

Bernardes G, Gonçalves H, Ayres-de-Campos D, Rocha AP. (2008) Linear and complex heart rate dynamics vary with sex in relation to fetal behavioural states. *Early Hum Dev* 84: 433–439.

Blood-Siegfried J, Rende EK. (2010) The long-term effects of prenatal nicotine exposure on neurologic development. *J Midwifery Womens Health* 55: 143–152.

Blott M, Greenough A, Nicolaides KH, Campbell S. (1990) The ultrasonographic assessment of the fetal thorax and fetal breathing movements in the prediction of pulmonary hypoplasia. *Early Hum Dev* 21: 143–151.

Bocking AD, Adamson SL, Cousin A, Campbell K, Carmichael L, Natale R, Patrick J. (1982) Effects of intravenous glucose injections on human fetal breathing movements and gross fetal body movements at 38 to 40 weeks gestational age. *Am J Obstet Gynecol* 142: 606–611.

Bowes G, Wilkinson MH, Dowling M, Ritchie BC, Brodecky V, Maloney JE. (1981) Hypercapnic stimulation of respiratory activity in unanesthetized fetal sheep in utero. *J Appl Physiol* 50: 701–708.

Bowie JD, Clair MR. (1982) Fetal swallowing and regurgitation: observation of normal and abnormal activity. *Radiology* 144: 877–878.

Boyle RJ. (2002) Effects of certain prenatal drugs on the fetus and newborn. *Pediatr Rev* 23: 17–24.

Brien JF, Smith GN. (1991) Effects of alcohol (ethanol) on the fetus. *J Dev Physiol* 15: 21–32.

Brown MA. (1995) The physiology of pre-eclampsia. *Clin Exp Pharmacol Physiol* 22: 781–791.

Buss C, Davis EP, Class QA, Gierczak M, Pattillo C, Glynn LM, Sandman CA. (2009) Maturation of the human fetal startle response: evidence for sex-specific maturation of the human fetus. *Early Hum Dev* 85: 633–638.

Buss C, Davis EP, Muftuler LT, Head K, Sandman CA. (2010) High pregnancy anxiety during mid-gestation is associated with decreased gray matter density in 6–9-year-old children. *Psychoneuroendocrinol* 35: 141–153.

Cardini F, Weixin H. (1998) Moxibustion for correction of breech presentation: A randomized controlled trial. *J Am Med Assoc* 280: 1580–1584.

Castillo RA, Devoe LD, Ruedrich DA, Gardner P. (1989) The effects of acute alcohol intoxication on biophysical activities: a case report. *Am J Obstet Gynecol* 160: 692–693.

Cejtin HE, Mills A, Swift EL. (1996) Effects of methadone on the biophysical profile. *J Reprod Med* 41: 819–822.

Centers for Disease Control and Prevention. (2004) Alcohol consumption among women who are pregnant or who might become pregnant – United States, 2002. *MMWR Morb Mortal Wkly Rep* 24: 1178–1181.

Chasnoff IJ, Landress HJ, Barrett ME. (1990) The prevalence of illicit-drug or alcohol use during pregnancy and discrepancies in mandatory reporting in Pinellas county Florida. *N Engl J Med* 322: 202–206.

Chiriboga CA, Vibbert M, Malouf R, Suarez MS, Abrams EJ, Heagarty MC, Brust JC, Hauser WA. (1995) Neurological correlates of fetal cocaine exposure: transient hypertonia of infancy and early childhood. *Pediatr* 96: 1070–1077.

Clapp JF 3rd. (1991) Exercise and fetal health. *J Dev Physiol* 15: 9–14.

Clarke C, Clarke K, Muneyyirci J, Azmitia E, Whitaker-Azmitia PM. (1996) Prenatal cocaine delays astroglial maturity: immunodensitometry shows proliferation and production of the growth factor S-100. *Brain Res Dev Brain Res* 91: 268–273.

Cohlen BJ, Stigter RH, Derks JB, Mulder EJH, Visser GHA. (1996) Absence of significant haemodynamic changes in the uterus following maternal betamethasone administration. *Ultrasound Obstet Gynecol* 8: 252–255.

Collaer ML, Hines M. (1995) Human behavioural sex differences: a role for gonadal hormones during early development? *Psychol Bull* 118: 55–107.

Collings CA, Curet LB. (1985) Fetal heart rate response to maternal exercise. *Am J Obstet Gynecol* 151: 498–501.

Coppens M, Vindla S, James DK, Sahota DS. (2001) Computerized analysis of acute and chronic changes in fetal heart rate variation and fetal activity in association with maternal smoking. *Am J Obstet Gynecol* 185: 421–426.

Copper RL, Goldenberg RL, Das A, Elder N, Swain M, Norman G, Ramsey R, Cotroneo P, Collins BA, Johnson F, Jones P, Meier A. (1996) The preterm prediction study: Maternal stress is associated with spontaneous preterm birth at less than 35 weeks' gestation. *Am J Obstet Gynecol* 175: 1286–1292.

Cosmi EV, Cosmi E, La Torre R. (2001) The effects of fetal breathing movements on the utero-fetal-placental circulation. *Early Pregn* 5: 51–52.

Cowperthwaite B, Hains SM, Kisilevsky BS. (2007) Fetal behaviour in smoking compared to non-smoking pregnant women. *Infant Behav Dev* 30: 422–430.

Dale E, Mullinax KM, Bryan DH. (1982) Exercise during pregnancy: effects on the fetus. *Can J Appl Sport Sci* 7: 98–103.

Dawes GS, Houghton CW, Redman CW, Visser GH. (1982) Pattern of the normal human fetal heart rate. *Br J Obstet Gynecol* 89: 276–284.

Dawes GS, Serra-Serra V, Moulden M, Redman CWG. (1994) Dexamethasone and fetal heart rate variation. *Br J Obstet Gynaecol* 101: 675–679.

Day NL, Richardson GQ. (1991) Prenatal alcohol exposure: a continuum of effect. *Semin Perinatol* 15: 271–279.

de Heus R, Mulder EJ, Derks JB, Koenen SV, Visser GHA. (2008) Differential effects of betamethasone on the fetus between morning and afternoon recordings. *J Matern Fetal Neonatal Med* 21: 549–554.

de Heus R, Mulder EJ, Derks JB, Visser GHA. (2009) The effects of the tocolytics atosiban and nifedipine on fetal movements, heart rate and blood flow. *J Matern Fetal Neonatal Med* 22: 485–490.

Derks JB, Mulder EJH, Visser GHA. (1995) The effects of maternal betamethasone administration on the fetus. *Br J Obstet Gynaecol* 102: 40–46.

Devoe LD, Murray C, Youssif A, Arnaud M. (1993) Maternal caffeine consumption and fetal behaviour in normal third-trimester pregnancy. *Am J Obstet Gynecol* 168: 1105–1111.

Devoe LD, Youssef AA, Castillo RA, Croom CS. (1994) Fetal biophysical activities in 3rd trimester pregnancies complicated by diabetes mellitus. *Am J Obstet Gynecol* 171: 298–305.

de Vries JIP, Visser GHA, Prechtl HFR. (1985) The emergence of fetal behaviour. II: Quantitative aspects. *Early Hum Dev* 12: 99–120.

de Vries JIP, Visser GHA, Mulder EJH, Prechtl HFR. (1987) Diurnal and other variations in fetal movements and other heart rate patterns. *Early Hum Dev* 15: 99–114.

de Vries JIP, Visser GHA, Prechtl HFR. (1988) The emergence of fetal behaviour. III. Individual differences and consistencies. *Early Hum Dev* 16: 85–103.

de Weerth C, van Hees Y, Buitelaar JK. (2003) Prenatal maternal cortisol levels and infant behaviour during the first 5 months. *Early Hum Dev* 74: 139–151.

Diego MA, Dieter JNI, Field T, Lecanuet JP, Hernandez Reif M, Beutler J, Largie S, Redzepi M, Salman FA. (2002) Fetal activity following stimulation of the mother's abdomen, feet, and hands. *Dev Psychobiol* 41: 396–406.

Dieter JN, Field T, Hernandez-Reif M, Jones NA, Lecanuet JP, Salman FA, Redzepi M. (2001) Maternal depression and increased fetal activity. *J Obstet Gynaecol* 21: 468–473.

DiPietro JA, Hodgson DM, Costigan KA, Hilton SC, Johnson TR. (1996) Fetal neurobehavioural development. *Child Dev* 67: 2553–2567.

DiPietro JA, Costigan KA, Shupe AK, Pressman EK, Johnson TRB. (1998) Fetal neurobehavioural development: associations with socioeconomic class and fetal sex. *Dev Psychobiol* 33: 79–91.

DiPietro JA, Costigan KA, Gurewitsch ED. (2003) Fetal response to induced maternal stress. *Early Hum Dev* 74: 125–138.

DiPietro JA, Caulfield L, Costigan KA, Merialdi M, Nguyen RH, Zavaleta N, Gurewitsch ED. (2004) Fetal neurobehavioural development: a tale of two cities. *Dev Psychol* 40: 445–456.

DiPietro JA, Costigan KA, Nelson P, Gurewitsch ED, Laudenslager ML. (2008a) Fetal responses to induced maternal relaxation during pregnancy. *Biol Psychol* 77: 11–19.

DiPietro JA, Ghera MM, Costigan KA. (2008b) Prenatal origins of temperamental reactivity in early infancy. *Early Hum Dev* 84: 569–575.

Divon MY, Zimmer EZ, Yeh SY, Vilenski A, Sarna Z, Paldi E, Platt LD. (1985) Effect of maternal intravenous glucose administration on fetal heart rate patterns and fetal breathing. *Am J Perinatol* 2: 292–294.

Doherty NN, Hepper PG. (2000) Habituation in fetuses of diabetic mothers. *Early Hum Dev* 59: 85–93.

Edelberg SC, Dierker L, Kalhan S, Rosen MG. (1987) Decreased fetal movements with sustained maternal hyperglycemia using the glucose clamp technique. *Am J Obstet Gynecol* 156: 1101–1105.

Einspieler C, Prechtl HFR, Ferrari F, Cioni G, Bos AF. (1997) The qualitative assessment of general movements in preterm, term and young infants – review of the methodology. *Early Hum Dev* 50: 47–60.

Einspieler C, Prechtl HFR, Bos AF, Ferrari F, Cioni G. (2004) *Prechtl's Method on the Qualitative Assessment of General Movements in Preterm, Term and Young Infants. Clinics in Developmental Medicine No. 167.* London: Mac Keith Press.

Eriksen PS, Gennser G, Löfgren O, Nilsson K. (1983) Acute effects of maternal smoking on fetal breathing and movements. *Obstet Gynecol* 61: 367–372.

Erkkola RU, Pirhonen JP, Kivijärvi AK. (1992) Flow velocity waveforms in uterine and umbilical arteries during submaximal bicycle exercise in normal pregnancy. *Obstet Gynecol* 79: 611–615.

Ernst M, Moolchan ET, Robinson ML. (2001) Behavioural and neural consequences of prenatal exposure to nicotine. *J Am Acad Child Adolesc Psychiatr* 6: 630–641.

Etherton GM, Kochar MS. (1993) Coffee. Facts and controversies. *Arch Fam Med* 2: 317–322.

Faden VB, Graubard BI. (2000) Maternal substance use during pregnancy and developmental outcome at age three. *J Substance Abuse* 12: 329–340.

Ferreira AJ. (1965) Emotional factors in prenatal environment. *J Nerv Ment Dis* 141: 108–118.

Ferriero DM, Dempsey DA. (1999) Impact of addictive and harmful substance on fetal brain development. *Curr Opin Neurol* 12: 161–166.

Field T, Sandberg D, Quetel T, Garcia R, Rosario M. (1985) Effects of ultrasound feedback on pregnancy anxiety, fetal activity, and neonatal outcome. *Obstet Gynecol* 66: 525–528.

Field T, Miguel AD, Dieter J, Hernandez-Reif M, Schanberg S, Kuhn C, Yando R, Bendell D. (2001) Depressed withdrawn and intrusive mothers' effects on their fetuses and neonates. *Infant Behav Dev* 24: 27–39.

Florido J, Padilla MC, Soto V, Camacho A, Moscoso G, Navarrete L. (2008) Photogrammetry of fetal breathing movements during the third trimester of pregnancy: observations in normal and abnormal pregnancies. *Ultrasound Obstet Gynecol* 32: 515–519.

Fong BF, Savelsbergh GJP, van Geijn HP, de Vries JIP. (2005) Does intra-uterine environment influence fetal head-position preference? A comparison between breech and cephalic presentation. *Early Hum Dev* 81: 507–517.

Fong BF, Savelsbergh GJ, de Vries JIP. (2008) Is there an effect of prenatal breech position on locomotion at 2.5 years? *Early Hum Dev* 84: 211–216.

Fong BF, Savelsbergh GJ, de Vries JIP. (2009a) Fetal leg posture in uncomplicated breech and cephalic pregnancies. *Eur J Pediatr* 168: 443–447.

Fong BF, Savelsbergh GJ, Leijsen MR, de Vries JIP. (2009b) The influence of prenatal breech presentation on neonatal leg posture. *Early Hum Dev* 85: 201–206.

Fox HE, Steinbrecher M, Pessel D, Inglis J, Medvid L, Angel E. (1978) Maternal ethanol ingestion and the occurrence of human fetal breathing movements. *Am J Obstet Gynecol* 132: 354–358.

Fox HE, Hohler CW, Steinbrecher M. (1982) Human fetal breathing movements after carbohydrate ingestion in fasting and nonfasting subjects. *Am J Obstet Gynecol* 144: 213–217.

Gabriel K, Hofmann C, Glavas M, Weinberg J. (1998) The hormonal effects of alcohol use on the mother and fetus. *Alcohol Health Res World* 22: 170–177.

Gazzolo D, Visser GHA, Russo A, Scopesi F, Santi F, Bruschettini PL. (1998) Pregnancy-induced hypertension, antihypertensive drugs, and the development of fetal behavioural states. *Early Hum Dev* 50: 149–157.

Gelman S, Spellacy WN, Wood S, Birk SA, Buhi WC. (1980) Effect of maternal intravenous glucose administration. *Am J Obstet Gynecol* 137: 459–461.

Gennser G, Maršál K, Brantmark B. (1975) Maternal smoking and fetal breathing movements. *Am J Obstet Gynecol* 123: 861–867.

Gingras JL, O'Donell KJ. (1998) State control in the substance-exposed fetus. I. The fetal neurobehavioural profile: an assessment of fetal state, arousal, and regulation competency. *Ann N Y Acad Sci* 846: 262–276.

Gingras JL, Weese-Mayer DE, Hume RF Jr, O'Donell KJ. (1992) Cocaine and development: mechanisms of fetal toxicity and neonatal consequences of prenatal cocaine exposure. *Early Hum Dev* 31: 1–24.

Gingras JL, Mitchell EA, Grattan KJ, Stewart AW. (2004) Effects of maternal cigarette smoking and cocaine use in pregnancy on fetal response to vibroacoustic stimulation and habituation. *Acta Paediatr* 93: 1479–1485.

Goldstein A, Warren R. (1962) Passage of caffeine into human gonadal and fetal tissue. *Biochem Pharamacol* 11: 166–168.

Goldstein I, Romero R, Merrill S, Wan M, O'Connor TZ, Mator M, Hobbins JC. (1988) Fetal body and breathing movements as predictors of intraamniotic infection in preterm premature rupture of membranes. *Am J Obstet Gynecol* 159: 363–368.

Goldstein I, Makhoul IR, Nisman D, Tamir A, Escalante G, Itskovitz-Eldor J. (2003) Influence of maternal carbohydrate intake on fetal movements at 14 to 16 weeks of gestation. *Prenat Diagn* 23: 95–97.

Gonzalez-Gonzalez NL, Medina V, Pardon E, Domenech E, Diaz Gomez NM, Armas H, Bartha JL. (2009) Fetal and neonatal habituation in infants of diabetic mothers. *J Pediatr* 154: 492–497.

Goodman JD. (1980) The effect of intravenous glucose on human fetal breathing measured by Doppler ultrasound. *Br J Obstet Gynaecol* 87: 1080–1083.

Goodman JD, Visser FGA, Dawes GS. (1984) Effects of maternal cigarette smoking on fetal trunk movements, fetal breathing movements and fetal heart rate. *Br J Obstet Gynaecol* 91: 657–661.

Gorski J. (1985) Exercise during pregnancy: maternal and fetal responses. A brief review. *Med Sci Sports Exerc* 17: 407–416.

Graça LM, Cardoso CG, Clode N, Calhaz-Jorge C. (1991) Acute effects of maternal cigarette smoking on fetal heart rate and fetal movements felt by the mother. *J Perinat Med* 19: 385–390.

Gutteling BM, de Weerth C, Willemsen-Swinkels SH, Huizink AC, Mulder EJH, Visser GHA, Buitelaar JK. (2005) The effects of prenatal stress on temperament and problem behaviour of 27-month-old toddlers. *Eur Child Adolesc Psychiatr* 14: 41–51.

Habek D. (2007) Effects of smoking and fetal hypokinesia in early pregnancy. *Arch Med Res* 38: 864–867.

Hafström M, Kjellmer I. (2000) Non-nutritive sucking in the healthy preterm infant. *Early Hum Dev* 60: 13–24.

Hallak M, Moise KJ, Lira N, Dorman KF, O'Brian-Smith E, Cotton DB. (1992) The effect of tocolytic agents (indomethacin and terbutaline) on fetal breathing and body movements: a prospective, randomized, double-blind, placebo-controlled clinical trial. *Am J Obstet Gynecol* 167: 1059–1063.

Harper MA, Meis PJ, Rose JC, Swain M, Burns J, Kardon B. (1987) Human fetal breathing response to intravenous glucose is directly related to gestational age. *Am J Obstet Gynceol* 157: 1403–1405.

Hatoum N, Clapp JF 3rd, Newman MR, Dajani N, Amini SB. (1997) Effects of maternal exercise on fetal activity in late gestation. *J Matern Fetal Med* 6: 134–139.

Hellman LM, Johnson HL, Tolles WE, Jones EH. (1961) Some factors affecting the fetal heart rate. *Am J Obstet Gynecol* 82: 1055–1063.

Hellström-Lindahl E, Gorbounova O, Seiger A, Mousavi M, Nordberg A. (1998) Regional distribution of nicotinic receptors during prenatal development of human brain and spinal cord. *Brain Res Dev Brain Res* 108: 147–160.

Hepper PG, Shahidullah S. (1990) Fetal response to maternal shock. *Lancet* 336: 1068.

Hepper PG, Shahidullah S. (1991) Seasonal overeating and fetal movements. *Lancet* 337: 252.

Hepper PG, Shannon EA, Dornan JC. (1997) Sex differences in fetal mouth movements. *Lancet* 350: 1820.

Hepper PG, Dornan JC, Little JF. (2005) Maternal alcohol consumption during pregnancy may delay the development of spontaneous fetal startle behaviour. *Physiol Behav* 83: 711–714.

Hinderaker T, Daltveit AK, Irgens LM, Uden A, Reikeras O. (1994a) The impact of intra-uterine factors on neonatal hip instability. An analysis of 1,059,479 children in Norway. *Acta Orthop Scand* 65: 239–242.

Hinderaker T, Uden A, Reikeras O. (1994b) Direct ultrasonographic measurement of femoral anteversion in newborns. *Skelet Radiol* 23: 133–135.

Hjelmstedt A, Asplund S. (1983) Congenital dislocation of the hip: a biomechanical study in autopsy specimens. *J Pediatr Orthop* 3: 491–497.

Hsieh YY, Tsai FJ, Lin CC, Chang FC, Tsai CH. (2000) Breech deformation complex in neonates. *J Reprod Med* 45: 933–935.

Huisman M, Risseeuw B, van Eyck J, Arabin B. (1997) Nicotine and caffeine. Influence on prenatal hemodynamics and behaviour in early twin pregnancy. *J Reprod Med* 42: 731–734.

Huizink AC, Mulder EJH. (2006) Maternal smoking, drinking or cannabis use during pregnancy and neurobehavioural and cognitive functioning in human offspring. *Neurosci Biobehav Rev* 30: 24–41.

Huizink AC, Robles de Medina PG, Mulder EJH, Visser GHA, Buitelaar JK. (2002) Psychological measures of prenatal stress as predictors of infant temperament. *J Am Acad Child Adolesc Psychiatry* 41: 1078–1085.

Hume RF Jr, O'Donnell KJ, Stanger CL, Killam AP, Gingras JL. (1989) In utero cocaine exposure: observations of fetal behavioural state may predict neonatal outcome. *Am J Obstet Gynecol* 161: 685–690.

Hume RF Jr, Gingras JL, Martin LS, Hertzberg BS, O'Donell K, Killam AP. (1994) Ultrasound diagnosis of fetal anomalies associated with in utero cocaine exposure: further support for cocaine-induced vascular disruption teratogenesis. *Fetal Diagn Ther* 9: 239–245.

Ianniruberto A, Tajani E. (1981) Ultrasonographic study of fetal movements. *Semin Perinatol* 5: 175–181.

Jackson JR, Kleeman S, Doerzbacher M, Lambers DS. (2003) The effect of glucocorticosteroid administration on fetal movements and biophysical scores in normal pregnancies. *J Matern Fetal Neonatal Med* 13: 50–53.

Janke J. (1999) The effect of relaxation therapy on preterm labour outcomes. *J Obstet Gynecol Neonat Nurs* 28: 255–263.

Jansson LM, DiPietro J, Elko A (2005). Fetal response to maternal methadone administration. *Am J Obstet Gynecol* 193: 611–617.

Jansson LM, DiPietro JA, Velez M, Elko A, Knauer H, Kivlighan KT. (2009) Maternal methadone dosing schedule and fetal neurobehaviour. *J Matern Fetal Neonatal Med* 22: 29–35.

Jones KL. (1988) *Smith's Recognizable Pattern of Human Malformation*. Philadelphia, PE: WB Saunders

Jones RL, Botti JJ, Anderson WM, Bennett NL. (1985) Thermoregulation during aerobic exercise in pregnancy. *Obstet Gynecol* 65: 340–345.

Jørgensen NP, Maršal K. (1988) Influence of thiopental anaesthesia on fetal behaviour in early pregnancy. *Early Hum Dev* 17: 71–78.

Kainer F, Prechtl HFR, Engele H, Einspieler C. (1997) Assessment of the quality of general movements in fetuses and infants of women with type-1 diabetes mellitus. *Early Hum Dev* 50: 13–25.

Katz VL, McMurray R, Berry MJ, Cefalo RC. (1988) Fetal and uterine responses to immersion and exercise. *Obstet Gynecol* 72: 225–230.

Kayemba Kay'S S, Beust M, Aboulghit H, Voisin M, Mourtada A. (1997) Carbamazepine and vigabatrin in epileptic pregnant woman and side effects in the newborn infant. *Arch Pediatr* 4: 975–978.

Kean LH, Suwanrath C, Gargari SS, Sahota DS, James DK. (1999) A comparison of fetal behaviour in breech and cephalic presentations at term. *Br J Obstet Gynaecol* 106: 1209–1213.

Kean LH, Gargari SS, Suwanrath C, Sahota DS, James DK. (2001) A comparison of fetal behaviour in term fetuses exposed to anticonvulsant medication with unexposed controls. *Br J Obstet Gynaecol* 108: 1159–1163.

Kelly MK, Schneider EP, Petrikovsky BM, Lesser ML. (2000) Effect of antenatal steroid administration on the fetal biophysical profile. *J Clin Ultrasound* 28: 224–226.

Khoury MJ, Marks JS, McCarthy BJ, Zaro SM. (1985) Factors affecting the sex differential in neonatal mortality: The role of respiratory distress syndrome. *Am J Obstet Gynecol* 151: 777–782.

Kivikovski A, Amon E, Vaalamo PO, Pirhonen J, Kopta MM. (1988) Effect of third-trimester premature rupture of membranes on fetal breathing movements: A prospective case-control study. *Am J Obstet Gynecol* 159: 1474–1477.

Koch S, Lösche G, Jager-Romän E, Jakob S, Rating D, Deichl A, Helge H. (1992) Major and minor birth malformations and antiepileptic drugs. *Neurology* 42 (Suppl 5): 83–88.

Koch S, Jäger-Roman E, Lösche G, Nau H, Rating D, Helge H. (1996) Antiepileptic drug treatment in pregnancy: drug side effects in the neonate and neurological outcome. *Acta Paediatr* 85: 739–746.

Koenen SV, Mulder EJH, Wijnberger LD, Visser GHA. (2005) Transient loss of the diurnal rhythms of fetal movements, heart rate, and its variation after maternal betamethasone administration. *Pediatr Res* 57: 662–666.

Kopecky E, Ryan ML, Barret JFR, Seaward PG, Ryan G, Koren G, Amankwah K. (2000) Fetal response to maternally administered morphine. *Am J Obstet Gynecol* 183: 424–430.

Korner AF. (1969) Neonatal startles, smiles, erections, and reflex sucks as related to state, sex, and individuality. *Child Dev* 40: 1039–1053.

Korner AF. (1973) Sex differences in newborns with special reference to differences in the organization of oral behaviour. *J Child Psychol Psychiatr* 14: 19–29.

Lasegreid LM, Bruaroy S, Reigstad H. (2005) Fetal injury and alcohol drinking during pregnancy. *Tidsskr Not Laegeforen* 125: 445–447.

Leader LR. (1987) The effects of cigarette smoking and maternal hypoxia on fetal habituation. In: Maeda K, editor. *The Fetus as a Patient.* Amsterdam: Elsevier. p 83–88.

Leader LR. (1995) The potential value of habituation in the prenate. In: Lecanuet JP, Krasnegor N, Fifer WP, Smotherman WP, editors. *Fetal Development: A Psychobiological Perspective.* Hillsdale, NJ: Lawrence Erlbaum Associates. p 383–404.

Leader LR, Baille P, Martin B, Vermeulen E. (1982) The assessment and significance of habituation to a repeated stimulus by the human fetus. *Early Hum Dev* 7: 211–219.

Lee CT, Brown CA, Hains SMJ, Kisilevsky BS. (2007) Fetal development: voice processing in normotensive and hypertensive pregnancies. *Biol Res Nurs* 8: 272–282.

Levine A, Rebarber A. (1995) Methadone maintenance treatment and the nonstress test. *J Perinatol* 15: 229–231.

Lewis PJ, Trudinger BJ, Mangez J. (1978) Effect of maternal glucose ingestion on fetal breathing and body movements in late pregnancy. *Br J Obstet Gynaecol* 85: 86–89.

Li Y, Wang H. (2004) In utero exposure to tobacco and alcohol modifies neurobehavioural development in mice offspring: Consideration of a role of oxidative stress. *Pharmacol Res* 49: 467–473.

Little JF, Hepper PG, Dornan JC. (2002) Maternal alcohol consumption during pregnancy and fetal startle behaviour. *Physiol Behav* 76: 691–694.

Lotgering FK, Gilbert RD, Longo LD. (1984) The interactions of exercise and pregnancy: a review. *Am J Obstet Gynecol* 149: 560–568.

Lösche G, Steinhausen HC, Koch S, Helge H. (1994) the psychological development of children of epileptic parents. II. The differential impact of intrauterine exposure to anticonvulsant drugs and further influential factors. *Acta Paediatr* 83: 961–966.

Lou HC, Hansen D, Nordentoft M, Pryds O, Jensen F, Nim J, Hemmingsen R. (1994) Prenatal stressors of human life affect fetal brain development. *Dev Med Child Neurol* 36: 826–832.

Lundqvist C, Hafström M. (1999) Non-nutritive sucking in full-term and preterm infants studied at term conceptional age. *Acta Paediatr* 88: 1287–1289.

Lunshof MS, Boer K, Wolf H, Koppen S, Velderman JK, Mulder EJ. (2005) Short-term (0–48 h) effects of maternal betamethasone administration on fetal heart rate and its variability. *Pediatr Res* 57: 545–549.

Luterkort M, Maršál K. (1985) Fetal motor activity in breech presentation. *Early Hum Dev* 10: 193–200.

Magee LA, Dawes GS, Moulden M, Redman CWG. (1997) A randomized controlled comparison of betamethasone with dexamethasone: effects on the antenatal fetal heart rate. *Br J Obstet Gynaecol* 104: 1233–1238.

Manders MAM, Sonder GJB, Mulder EJH, Visser GHA. (1997) The effects of maternal exercise on fetal heart rate and movement patterns. *Early Hum Dev* 48: 237–247.

Manning FA, Feyerabend C. (1976) Cigarette smoking and fetal breathing movements. *Br J Obstet Gynaecol* 83: 262–270.

Manning FA, Wyn Pugh E, Boddy K. (1975) Effect of cigarette smoking on fetal breathing movements in normal pregnancies. *Br J Obstet Gynaecol* 82: 552–553.

Maršál K, Löfgren O, Gennser G. (1979) Fetal breathing movements and maternal exercise. *Acta Obstet Gynecol Scand* 58: 197–201.

May LE, Glaros A, Yeh HW, Clapp JF 3rd, Gustafson KM. (2010) Aerobic exercise during pregnancy influences fetal cardiac autonomic control of heart rate and heart rate variability. *Early Hum Dev* 86: 213–217.

McDonald RL. (1968) The role of emotional factors in obstetric complications: a review. *Psychosom Med* 30: 222–237.

McGowan J, Devoe LD, Searle N, Altman R. (1987) The effects of long- and short-term maternal caffeine ingestion on human fetal breathing and body movements in term gestations. *Am J Obstet Gynecol* 157: 726–729.

McLeod W, Brien J, Loomis C, Carmichael L, Probert C, Patrick J. (1983) Effect of maternal ethanol ingestion on fetal breathing movements, gross body movements and heart rate at 37 to 40 weeks gestational age. *Am J Obstet Gynecol* 145: 251–257.

McLeod W, Brien J, Carmichael L, Probert C, Steenaart N, Patrick J. (1984) Maternal glucose injection do not alter the suppression of fetal breathing following maternal ethanol ingestion. *Am J Obstet Gynecol* 148: 634–639.

Meis PM, Rose JC, Swain M, Nelson LH. (1985) Gestational age alters fetal breathing response to intravenous insulin and intravenous glucose administration. *Am J Obstet Gynecol* 151: 438–440.

Mennes M, Stiers P, Lagae L, van den Berg BRH. (2006) Long-term cognitive sequelae of antenatal maternal anxiety: involvement of the orbitofrontal cortex. *Neurosci Biobehav Rev* 30: 1078–1086.

Miller FC, Skiba H, Klapholz H. (1978) The effect of maternal blood sugar levels on fetal activity. *Obstet Gynecol* 52: 662–665.

Miller JL, Macedonia C, Sonies BC. (2006) Sex differences in prenatal oral-motor function and development. *Dev Med Child Neurol* 48: 465–470.

Mirghani HM, Weerasinghe DS, Ezimokhai M, Smith JR. (2003) The effect of maternal fasting on the biophysical profile. *Int J Gynaecol Obstet* 81: 17–21.

Monk C, Fifer WP, Myers MM, Sloan RP, Trien L, Hurtado A. (2000) Maternal stress responses and anxiety during pregnancy: effects on fetal heart rate. *Dev Psychobiol* 36: 67–77.

Monk C, Sloan RP, Myers MM, Ellman L, Werner E, Jeon J, Tager F, Fifer WP. (2004) Fetal heart rate reactivity differs by women's psychiatric status: an early marker for developmental risk? *J Am Acad Child Adolesc Psychiatr* 43: 283–290.

Morrow CE, Bandstra ES, Anthony JC, Ofir AY, Xue L, Reyes ML. (2001) Influence of prenatal cocaine exposure on full-term infant neurobehavioural functioning. *Neurotoxicol Teratol* 23: 533–544.

Mulder EJH, Visser GHA. (1987) Braxton Hicks' contractions and motor behaviour in the near-term human fetus. *Am J Obstet Gynecol* 156: 543–549.

Mulder EJH, Visser GHA. (1991a) Growth and motor development in fetuses of women with type 1 diabetes. I. Early growth patterns. *Early Hum Dev* 25: 91–106.

Mulder EJH, Visser GHA. (1991b) Growth and motor development in fetuses of women with type 1 diabetes. II. Emergence of specific motor pattern. *Early Hum Dev* 25: 107–115.

Mulder EJ, Kamstra A, O'Brien MJ, Visser GHA, Prechtl HFR. (1986) Abnormal fetal behavioural state regulation in a case of high maternal alcohol intake during pregnancy. *Early Hum Dev* 14: 321–326.

Mulder EJH, Visser GHA, Bekedam DJ, Prechtl HFR. (1987) Emergence of behavioural states in fetuses of type I diabetic mothers. *Early Hum Dev* 15: 231–252.

Mulder EJH, O'Brien MJ, Lems YL, Visser GHA, Prechtl HFR. (1990) Body and breathing movements in fetuses and infants of women with type-1 diabetes. *Early Hum Dev* 24: 131–152.

Mulder EJH, Visser GHA, Morssink LP, de Vries JIP. (1991) Growth and motor development in fetuses of women with type 1 diabetes. III. First trimester quantity of fetal movement patterns. *Early Hum Dev* 25: 117–133.

Mulder EJH, Derks JB, Zonneveld MF, Bruinse HW, Visser GHA. (1994) Transient reduction in fetal activity and heart rate variation after maternal betamethasone administration. *Early Hum Dev* 36: 49–60.

Mulder EJH, Leiblum DM, Visser GHA. (1995) Fetal breathing movements in late diabetic pregnancy: relationship to fetal heart rate patterns and Braxton Hicks' contractions. *Early Hum Dev* 43: 225–232.

Mulder EJH, Derks JB, Visser GHA. (1997) Antenatal corticosteroid therapy and fetal behaviour: a randomised study of the effects of betamethasone and dexamethasone. *Br J Obstet Gynaecol* 104: 1239–1247.

Mulder EJH, Morssink LP, van der Schee T, Visser GHA. (1998) Acute maternal alcohol consumption disrupts behavioural state organization in the near-term fetus. *Pediatr Res* 44: 774–779.

Mulder EJH, Robles de Medina PG, Huizink AC, van den Bergh BRH, Buitelaar JK, Visser GHA. (2002) Prenatal maternal stress: effects on pregnancy and the (unborn) child. *Early Hum Dev* 70: 3–14.

Mulder EJH, Koenen SV, Blom I, Visser GHA. (2004a) The effects of antenatal betamethasone administration on fetal heart rate and behaviour depend on gestational age. *Early Hum Dev* 76: 65–77.

Mulder EJH, Derks JB, Visser GHA. (2004b) Effects of antenatal betamethasone administration on fetal heart rate and behavior in twin pregnancy. *Pediatr Res* 56: 35–39.

Mulder EJH, de Heus R, Visser GH. (2009) Antenatal corticosteroid therapy: short-term effects on fetal behaviour and haemodynamics. *Semin Fetal Neonatal Med* 14: 151–156.

Mulder EJH, Tegaldo L, Bruschettini P, Visser GH. (2010) Foetal response to maternal coffee intake: role of habitual versus non-habitual caffeine consumption. *J Psychopharmacol* 24: 1641–1648.

Mushkat Y, Ascher-Landsberg J, Keidar R, Carmon E, Panzner D, David MP. (2001) The effect of betamethasone versus dexamethasone on fetal biophysical parameters. *Eur J Obstet Gynecol Reprod Biol* 97: 50–52.

Nagy E, Loveland KA, Orvos H, Molnár P. (2001) Gender-related physiological differences in human neonates and the greater vulnerability of males to developmental brain disorders. *J Gend Specif Med* 4: 41–49.

Narendran S, Nagarathna R, Narendran C, Gunasheela S, Nagendra HRR. (2005) Efficacy of yoga on pregnancy outcome. *J Altern Complement Med* 11: 237–244.

Natale R, Richardson B, Patrick J. (1983) The effect of maternal hyperglycemia on gross body movements in human fetuses at 32–34 weeks' gestation. *Early Hum Dev* 8: 13–20.

Natale R, Nasello-Paterson C, Connors G. (1988) Patterns of fetal breathing activity in the human fetus at 24 to 28 weeks of gestation. *Am J Obstet Gynecol* 158: 317–321.

Newnham JP. (1991) Smoking in pregnancy. *Fetal Med Rev* 3: 115–132.

Niederhofer H. (2004) A longitudinal study: some preliminary results of association of prenatal maternal stress and fetal movements, temperament factors in early childhood and behaviour at age 2 years. *Psychol Rep* 95: 767–770.

Nijhuis JG, Jongsma HW, Crijns IJMJ, de Valk IMGM, van der Velden JWHJ. (1986) Effects of maternal glucose ingestion on human fetal breathing movements at weeks 24 and 28 of gestation. *Early Hum Dev* 13: 183–188.

Nijhuis JG, van de Pas M, Jongsma HW. (1998) State transitions in uncomplicated pregnancies after term. *Early Hum Dev* 52: 125–132.

Nimrod C, Varela-Gittings F, Machin G, Campbell D. (1984) The effect of very prolonged membrane rupture on fetal development. *Am J Obstet Gynecol* 148: 540–543.

Nordstrom L, Ingemarsson I. (1998) Transient fetal cerebral dysfunction after road traffic accident. A case report. *Eur J Obstet Gynecol Reprod Biol* 80: 29–32.

Oguch O, Steer P. (1998) Gender does not affect fetal heart rate variation. *Br J Obstet Gynaecol* 105: 1312–1314.

Omeroglu H, Koparal S. (2001) The role of clinical examination and risk factors in the diagnosis of developmental dysplasia of the hip: a prospective study in 188 referred young infants. *Arch Orthop Trauma Surg* 121: 7–11.

Pagliaro AM, Pagliaro L. (1997) Teratogenic effects of in utero exposure to alcohol and other abusable psychotropics. In: Haak MR, editor. *Drug Dependent Mothers and Their Children: Issues in Public Policy and Public Health*. New York: Springer. p 31–63.

Patrick J, Fetherston W, Vick H, Voegelin R. (1978) Human fetal breathing movements and gross fetal body movements at weeks 34 to 35 gestation. *Am J Obstet Gynecol* 130: 693–699.

Patrick J, Campbell K, Carmichael L, Natale R, Richardson B. (1980) Patterns of human fetal breathing during the last 10 days of pregnancy. *Obstet Gynecol* 56: 24–30.

Patrick J, Campbell K, Carmichael L, Natale R, Richardson B. (1982) Patterns of gross fetal body movements over 24-hour observation intervals during the last 10 weeks of pregnancy. *Am J Obstet Gynecol* 146: 363–371.

Petrie B, Segalowitz SJ. (1980) Use of fetal heart rate, other perinatal and maternal factors as predictors of sex. *Percept Mot Skills* 50: 871–874.

Pillai M, James D. (1990) Are the behavioural states of the newborn comparable to those of the fetus? *Early Hum Dev* 22: 39–49.

Pillai M, James D, Parker M. (1992) The development of ultradian rhythms in the human fetus. *Am J Obstet Gynecol* 167: 172–177.

Platt LD, Artal R, Semel J, Sipos L, Kammula RK. (1983) Exercise in pregnancy. II. Fetal responses. *Am J Obstet Gynecol* 147: 487–491.

Pratt O. (1981) Alcohol and the women of childbearing age – a public health problem. *Br J Addict* 76: 383–390.

Prechtl HFR. (1977) *The Neurological Examination of the Fullterm Newborn Infant. Second revised and enlarged edition. Clinics in Developmental Medicine No. 63.* London: Heinemann.

Prechtl HFR, Knol AR. (1958) The influence of the basin end position on the sole reflexes with the newborn child . Der Einfluß der Beckenendlage auf die Fußsohlenreflexe beim neugeborenen Kind. *Arch Psychiatr Ztsch Gesell Neurol* 196: 542–553.

Pressman EK, DiPietro JA, Costigan KA, Shupe AK, Johnson TRB. (1998) Fetal neurobehavioural development: associations with socioeconomic class and fetal sex. *Dev Psychobiol* 33: 79–91.

Previc FH. (1991) A general theory concerning the prenatal origins of cerebral lateralisation in humans. *Psychol Rev* 98: 299–334.

Preyer W. (1885) [*Special Physiology of the Embryo*]. Leipzig: Grieben. (In German)

Rauramo I. (1987) Effect of short-term physical exercise on fetal heart rate and uterine activity in normal and abnormal pregnancies. *Ann Chir Gynaecol* 76: 1–6.

Rayburn WF. (1982) Antepartum fetal assessment. Monitoring fetal activity. *Clin Perinatol* 9: 231–252.

Rayburn WF. (1990) Fetal body movement monitoring. *Obstet Gynecol Clin North Am* 17: 899–911.

Reddy UM, Paine LL, Gegor CL, Johnson MJ, Johnson TRB. (1991) Fetal movement during labor. *Am J Obstet Gynecol* 165: 1073–1076.

Reece EA, Hagay Z, Roberts AB, DeGennaro N, Homko CJ, Conolly-Diamond M, Sherwin R, Tamborlane WV, Diamond MP. (1995) Fetal Doppler and behavioural responses during hypoglycaemia induced with the insulin clamp technique in pregnant diabetic women. *Am J Obstet Gynecol* 172: 151–155.

Reinhard J, Hüsken-Janssen H, Hatzmann H, Schiermeier S. (2009) Changes in resistance of the umbilical artery, foetal movements and short time variation through clinical hypnosis – preliminary results. *Z Geburtshilfe Neonatol* 213: 23–26.

Reynolds SRM. (1962) Nature of fetal adaptation to the uterine environment: A problem of sensory deprivation. *Am J Obstet Gynecol* 83: 800–808.

Rhainds M, Levallois P. (1997) Effects of maternal cigarette smoking and alcohol consumption on blood lead levels of newborns. *Am J Epidemiol* 145: 250–257.

Richardson BS, Hohimer AR, Bissonette JM, Machida CM. (1983) Cerebral metabolism in hypoglycaemic and hyperglycaemic fetal lambs. *Am J Physiol* 245: R730–R736.

Riikonen R, Salonen I, Partanen K, Verho S. (1999) Brain perfusion SPECT and MRI in foetal alcohol syndrome. *Dev Med Child Neurol* 41: 652–659.

Ritchie K. (1980) The response to changes in the composition of maternal inspired air in human pregnancy. *Semin Perinatol* 4: 295–299.

Ritchie JWK, Lakhani K. (1980) Fetal breathing movements in response to maternal inhalation of 5% carbon dioxide. *Am J Obstet Gynecol* 136: 386–388.

Roberts AB, Mitchell J. (1995) Pulmonary hypoplasia and fetal breathing in preterm premature rupture of membranes. *Early Hum Dev* 41: 27–37.

Roberts AB, Stubbs SM, Mooney R, Cooper D, Brudenell JM, Campbell S. (1980) Fetal activity in pregnancies complicated by maternal diabetes mellitus. *Br J Obstet Gynaecol* 87: 485–489.

153

Roberts AB, Goldstein I, Romero R, Hobbins JC. (1991) Fetal breathing movements after preterm rupture of membranes. *Am J Obstet Gynecol* 164: 821–825.

Roberts D, Dalziel S. (2006) Antenatal corticosteroids for accelerating fetal lung maturation for women at risk of preterm birth. *Cochrane Database Syst Rev* 3: CD004454.

Robles de Medina PG, Visser GH, Huizink AC, Buitelaar JK, Mulder EJ. (2003) Fetal behaviour does not differ between boys and girls. *Early Hum Dev* 73: 17–26.

Romanini C, Rizzo G. (1995) Fetal behaviour in normal and compromised fetuses. An overview. *Early Hum Dev* 43: 117–131.

Ronnekliev OK, Naylor BR. (1995) Chronic cocaine exposure in fetal rhesus monkey: consequences for early development of dopamine neurons. *J Neurosci* 15: 7330–7343.

Roodenburg PJ, Wladimiroff JW, van Es A, Prechtl HFR. (1991) Classification and quantitative aspects of fetal movements during the second half of normal pregnancy. *Early Hum Dev* 25: 19–35.

Rosett HL, Snyder PA, Sander LW, Lee A, Cook P, Weiner L, Gould JB. (1979) Effects of maternal drinking on neonate state regulation. *Dev Med Child Neurol* 21: 464–473.

Rosier-van Dunné FMF, van Wezel-Meijler G, Bakker MPS, Odendaal HJ, de Vries JIP. (2010) Fetal general movements and brain sonography in a population at risk for preterm birth. *Early Hum Dev* 86: 107–111.

Rothberg AD, Lits B. (1991) Psychosocial support for maternal stress during pregnancy: effect on birthweight. *Am J Obstet Gynecol* 165: 403–407.

Rotschild A, Ling EW, Puterman ML, Farquharson D. (1990) Neonatal outcome after prolonged preterm rupture of the membranes. *Am J Obstet Gynecol* 162: 46–50.

Rougemont M, Do KQ, Catagne V. (2002) New model of glutathione deficit during development: effect on lipid peroxidation in the rat brain. *J Neurosci Res* 70: 774–783.

Ruhmann O, Lazovic D, Bouklas P, Gosse F, Franke J. (1999) Ultrasound hip joint screening in newborn infants. Correlation of amnestic risk factors and hip dysplasia. *Klin Pädiatr* 211: 141–148.

Sadovsky E, Perlman M. (1978) Decreased fetal movements and polyhydramnios. *Acta Obstet Gynecol Scand* 57: 177–178.

Sadovsky E, Polishuk WZ. (1977) Fetal movements in utero. Nature, assessment, prognostic value, timing of delivery. *Obstet Gynecol* 50: 49–55.

Sadovsky E, Rabinowitz R, Freeman A, Yarkoni S. (1984) The relationship between fetal heart rate accelerations, fetal movements and uterine contractions. *Am J Obstet Gynecol* 149: 187–189.

Salvador HS, Koos BJ. (1989) Effects of regular and decaffeinated coffee on fetal breathing and heart rate. *Am J Obstet Gynecol* 160: 1043–1047.

Samueloff A, Evron S, Sadovsky E. (1984) Fetal movements in isoxsuprine-treated patients. *Am J Obstet Gynecol* 148: 335–356.

Sander LW, Snyder PA, Rosett HL, Lee A, Gould JB, Ouellette EM. (1977) Effects of alcohol intake during pregnancy on newborn state regulation: a progress report. *Alcoholism: Clin Exp Res* 1: 233–241.

Sapolsky RM, Uno H, Rebert CS, Finch CE. (1990) Hippocampal damage associated with prolonged glucocorticoid exposure in primates. *J Neurosci* 10: 2897–2902.

Seckl JR. (2001) Glucocorticoid programming of the fetus; adult phenotypes and molecular mechanism. *Mol Cell Endocrinol* 185: 61–71.

Sekulić S, Zarkov M, Slankamenac P, Bozić K, Vejnović T, Novakov-Mikić A. (2009) Decreased expression of the righting reflex and locomotor movements in breech-presenting newborns in the first days of life. *Early Hum Dev* 85: 263–266.

Senecal PE, Osterloh JD. (1991) Normal fetal outcome after maternal ciguateric toxin exposure in the 2nd trimester. *J Toxicol Clin Toxicol* 29: 473–478.

Shinozuka N, Masuda H, Okai T, Kuwabara Y, Mizuno M. (1989) Computer-assisted analysis of fetal behaviour in fetal abnormalities. *Fetal Ther* 4: 97–109

Sival DA, Visser GHA, Prechtl HFR. (1992) Fetal breathing movements are not a good indicator of lung development after premature rupture of membranes and oligohydramnios – a preliminary study. *Early Hum Dev* 28: 133–143.

Sival DA, Prechtl HFR, Sonder GHA, Touwen BCL. (1993) The effect of intra-uterine breech position on postnatal motor functions of the lower limbs. *Early Hum Dev* 32: 161–176.

Sjöström K, Valentin L, Thelin T, Maršal K. (1997) Maternal anxiety in late pregnancy and fetal hemodynamics. *Eur J Obstet Gynaecol Reprod Biol* 74: 149–155.

Sjöström K, Valentin L, Thelin T, Maršal K. (2002) Maternal anxiety in late pregnancy: effect on fetal movements and fetal heart rate. *Early Hum Dev* 67: 87–100.

Slotkin TA. (1998) Fetal nicotine or cocaine exposure: which one is worse? *J Pharmacol Exp Ther* 285: 931–945.

Sontag LW. (1941) The significance of fetal environmental differences. *Am J Obstet Gynecol* 42: 86–103.

Sontag LW, Wallace RF. (1934) Preliminary report of the Fels Fund study of fetal activity. *Am J Dis Child* 48: 1050–1057.

Sørensen KE, Børlum KG. (1987) Acute effects of maternal smoking on human fetal heart function. *Acta Obstet Gynaecol Scand* 66: 217–220.

Sowell ER, Jernigan TL, Mattson SN, Riley EP, Sobel DF, Jones KL. (1996) Abnormal development of the cerebellar vermis in children prenatally exposed to alcohol: size reduction in lobules I-V. *Alcohol Clin Exp Res* 20: 31–34.

Sowell ER, Mattson SN, Thompson PM, Jernigan TL, Riley EP, Toga AW. (2001) Mapping callosal morphology and cognitive correlates: effects of heavy prenatal alcohol exposure. *Neurology* 57: 235–244.

Spencer JAD, Ryan G, Ronderosdumit D, Nicolini U, Rodeck CH. (1994) The effect of neuromuscular blockade on human fetal heart rate and its variation. *Br J Obstet Gynaecol* 101: 121–124.

Spinillo A, Capuzzo E, Nicola S, Colonna L, Iasci A, Zara C. (1994) Interaction between fetal gender and risk factors for fetal growth retardation. *Am J Obstet Gynecol* 171: 1273–1277.

Swartjes JM, van Geijn HP. (1998) Pregnancy and epilepsy. *Eur J Obstet Gynaecol Reprod Biol* 79: 3–11.

Swartjes JM, van Geijn HP, Meinardi H, van Alphen M, Schoemaker HC. (1991) Fetal rest-activity cycles and chronic exposure to antiepileptic drugs. *Epilepsia* 32: 722–728.

Swartjes JM, van Geijn HP, Meinardi H, van Woerden EE, Mantel R. (1992) Fetal motility and chronic exposure to antiepileptic drugs. *Eur J Obstet Gynecol Reprod Biol* 16: 37–45.

Takashima T, Koyanagi T, Horimoto N, Satoh S, Nakano H. (1995) Breech presentation: is there a difference in eye movement patterns compared with cephalic presentation in the human fetus at term? *Am J Obstet Gynecol* 172: 851–855.

Taylor WG, Walkinshaw SA, Thomson MA. (1993) Antenatal assessment of neurological impairment. *Arch Dis Child* 68: 604–605.

Teixeira JMA, Fisk NM, Glover V. (1999) Association between maternal anxiety in pregnancy and increased uterine artery resistance index: cohort based study. *BMJ* 318: 153–157.

Teixeira J, Martin D, Prendiville O, Glover V. (2005) The effects of acute relaxation on indices of anxiety during pregnancy. *J Psychosom Obstet Gynaecol* 26: 271–276.

Thaler I, Goodman JDS, Dawes GS. (1980) Effects of maternal cigarette smoking on fetal breathing and fetal movements. *Am J Obstet Gynecol* 138: 282–287.

Thompson PJ, Greenough A, Nicolaides KH. (1992) Fetal breathing movements and prostaglandin levels in pregnancies complicated by premature rupture of the membranes. *J Perinat Med* 20: 209–213.

Titze K, Koch S, Helge H, Lehmkuhl U, Rauh H, Steinhausen HC. (2008) Prenatal and family risks of children born to mothers with epilepsy: effects on cognitive development. *Dev Med Child Neurol* 50: 117–122.

Ullian ME. (1999) The role of corticosteroids in the regulation of vascular tone. *Cardiovasc Res* 41: 55–64.

Valentin L, Lofgren O, Maršál K, Gullberg B. (1984) Subjective recording of fetal movements. I. Limits and acceptability in normal pregnancies. *Acta Obstet Gynecol Scand* 63: 223–228.

van den Bergh BR, Marcoen A. (2004) High antenatal anxiety is related to ADHD symptoms, externalizing problems, and anxiety in 8- and 9-year-olds. *Child Dev* 75: 1085–1097.

van den Bergh BRH, Mulder EJH, Visser GHA, Poelmann-Weesjes G, Bekedam DJ, Prechtl HFR. (1989) The effect of (induced) maternal emotions on fetal behaviour: a controlled study. *Early Hum Dev* 19: 9–19.

155

van den Bergh BR, Mennes M, Oosterlaan J, Stevens V, Stiers P, Marcoen A, Lagae L. (2005) High antenatal maternal anxiety is related to impulsivity during performance on cognitive tasks in 14- and 15-year-olds. *Neurosci Biobehav Rev* 29: 259–269.

van den Bergh BRH, Mennes M, Stevens V, van der Meere J, Börger N, Stiers P, Marcoen A, Lagae L. (2006) ADHD deficit as measured in adolescent boys with a continuous performance task is related to antenatal maternal anxiety. *Pediatr Res* 59: 78–82.

van den Bergh BRH, van Calster B, Smits T, van Huffel S, Lagae L. (2008) Antenatal maternal anxiety is related to HPA-axis dysregulation and self-reported depressive symptoms in adolescence: a prospective study on the fetal origins of depressed mood. *Neuropsychopharmacology* 33: 536–545.

van der Meulen JA, Davies GA, Kisilevsky BS. (2008) Fetal sensory-elicited body movements differ in breech compared to cephalic position. *Dev Psychobiol* 50: 530–534.

van Geijn HP, Swartjes JM, van Woerden EE, Caron FJM, Brons JTJ, Arts NTF. (1986) Fetal behavioural states in epileptic pregnancies. *Eur J Obstet Gynec Reprod Biol* 21: 309–314.

Ververs IAP, de Vries JIP, van Geijn HP, Hopkins B. (1994) Prenatal head position from 12 to 38 weeks. I. Developmental aspects. *Early Hum Dev* 39: 83–91.

Ville Y, Vincent Y, Tordjman N, Hue MV, Fernandez H, Frydman R. (1995) Effect of betamethasone on the fetal heart rate pattern assessed by computerized cardiotocography in normal twin pregnancies. *Fetal Diagn Ther* 10: 301–306.

Vindla S, Sahota DS, Coppens M, James DK. (1997) Computerized analysis of behaviour in fetuses with congenital abnormalities. *Ultrasound Obstet Gynecol* 9: 302–309.

Visser GHA, Anceschi MM. (2001) Guidelines on antepartum corticosteroids. *Prenat Neonat Med* 6 (Suppl 2): 78–81.

Visser GHA, Prechtl HFR. (1988) Movements and behavioural states in the human fetus. In: Jones CT, editor. *Fetal and Neonatal Development*. Ithaca, New York: Perinatology Press. p 581–590.

Visser GHA, Csermely T, Cosmi EV. (2001) Side-effects of prenatal corticosteroids. *Prenat Neonat Med* 6 (Suppl 2): 42–49.

Walker A, Rosenberg M, Balaban-Gil K. (1999) Neurodevelopmental and neurobehavioural sequelae of selected substances of abuse and psychiatric medications in utero. *Child Adolesc Psychiatr Clin North Am* 8: 845–867.

Ward SL, Schuetz S, Wachsman L, Bean XD, Bautista D, Buckley S, Sehgal S, Warburton D. (1991) Elevated plasma norepinephrine levels in infants of substance-abusing mothers. *Am J Dis Child* 145: 44–48.

Warner J, Hains SM, Kisilevsky BS. (2002) An exploratory study of fetal behaviour at 33 and 36 weeks gestational age in hypertensive women. *Dev Psychobiol* 41: 156–168.

Weinberg MK, Tronick EZ, Cohn JF, Olson KL. (1999) Gender differences in emotional expressivity and self-regulation during early infancy. *Dev Psychol* 35: 175–188.

Whitehead J. (1867) Convulsions in utero. *BMJ* 2: 59–61.

Wideswensson D, Montan S, Arulkumaran S, Ingemarsson I, Ratnam SS. (1993) Effect of methyldopa and isradipine on fetal heart rate pattern assessed by computerized cardiotocography in human pregnancy. *Am J Obstet Gynecol* 169: 1581–1585.

Wigglesworth JS, Desai R. (1982) Is fetal respiratory function a major determinant of perinatal survival? *Lancet* 1(8266): 264–267.

Wilkinson C, Robinson J. (1982) Braxton Hicks' contractions and fetal breathing movements. *Aust N Z J Obstet Gynecol* 22: 212–214.

Windle WF. (1940) *Physiology of the Fetus. Origin and Extent of Function in Fetal Life*. Philadelphia: WB Saunders.

Winn HN, Hess O, Goldstein I, Wackers F, Hobbins JC. (1994) Fetal responses to maternal exercise: effect on fetal breathing and body movements. *Am J Perinatol* 11: 263–266.

Wittman B, Segal S. (1991) A comparison of the effects of the single- and split-dose methadone administration on the fetus: ultrasound evaluation. *Int J Addict* 26: 213–218.

Wittmann BK, Lyons E, Frohlich J, Towell ME. (1979) Real-time ultrasound observation of fetal activity in labour. *Br J Obstet Gynaecol* 86: 278–281.

Wladimiroff JW, Roodenburg PJ. (1982) Human fetal breathing and gross body activity relative to maternal meals during insulin-dependent pregnancy. *Acta Obstet Gynecol Scand* 61: 65–68.

Wolkind S. (1981) Prenatal emotional stress-effects on the fetus. In: Wolkind S, Zajiceck E, editors. *Pregnancy. A Psychological and Social Study*. London: Academic Press. p 177–183.

Wood C, Gilbert M, O'Connor A, Walters WA. (1979) Subjective recording of fetal movements. *Br J Obstet Gynaecol* 86: 836–842.

Wouldes TA, Roberts AB, Pryor JE, Bagnall C, Gunn TR. (2004) The effect of methadone treatment on the quantity and quality of human fetal movement. *Neurotoxicol Teratol* 26: 23–34.

Yoles I, Hod M, Kaplan B, Ovadia J. (1993) Fetal 'fright-bradycardia' brought on by air-raid alarm in Israel. *Int J Gynaecol Obstet* 40: 157–160.

Zeskind PS, Gingras JL. (2006). Maternal cigarette smoking during pregnancy disrupts rhythms in fetal heart rate. *J Pediatr Psychol* 31: 5–14.

Zimmer EZ, Goldstein I, Alglay S. (1988a) Simultaneous recording of fetal breathing movements and body movements in twin pregnancy. *J Perinat Med* 16: 109–112.

Zimmer EZ, Divon MY, Vadasz A. (1988b) The relationship between fetal movements and uterine contractions in the active phase of labour. *J Reprod Med* 33: 289–291.

Zimmer E, Peretz B, Eyal E, Fuchs K. (1988c) The influence of maternal hypnosis on fetal movements in anxious pregnant women. *Eur J Obstet Gynecol Reprod Biol* 27: 133–137.

Zuckerman B, Frank DA, Hingson R, Amaro H, Levenson SM, Kayne H, Parker S, Vinci R, Aboagye K, Fried LE. (1989) Effects of marijuana and cocaine on fetal growth. *N Engl J Med* 320: 762–768.

8
FUNCTIONAL ASSESSMENT OF THE FETAL NERVOUS SYSTEM

An ability to assess the functional condition of the fetal nervous system is very important to the clinician, since a considerable percentage of early brain damage is of prenatal origin (Scher et al 1991, Sherer et al 1998, Rezaie and Dean 2002, Ghi et al 2003, Yoon et al 2003, Rosier-van Dunné et al 2007, Gávai et al 2008).

This chapter reviews the research conducted so far on the behavioural effects of various neurological conditions of the fetus. Clearly, some results – especially those related to the behaviour of fetuses with genetic disorders – are based on a small number of case studies and were published when ultrasonographic observation was still in its infancy. Nonetheless, we feel obliged to give a brief overview of former related work, as its results may stimulate future research.

Assessments based on the observation of fetal behaviour
THE NON-STRESS TEST (DETERMINATION OF FETAL ACTIVITY ACCELERATION)
Fetal movements are usually associated with heart-rate accelerations. At term, there are, on average, 35 accelerations per hour, with a mean amplitude of 25 beats per minute and a mean duration of 40 seconds. Movement-related accelerations of this type occur in 85% of fetuses (Patrick et al 1984).

The following criteria are considered to constitute a reassuring non-stress test result in the term fetus: two to five heart-rate accelerations of a least 15 beats per minute, lasting for at least 15 seconds, coupled with fetal body movements within a 40-minute recording. A non-reactive test indicates a high likelihood of fetal hypoxaemia (Rochard et al 1976, Kisilevsky and Low 1998). However, it is important to take the behavioural state of the fetus into account: during state 1F it is very rare that a fetus shows heart-rate accelerations! To claim that every second fetus fails to achieve a 'normal' result is to disregard the typical developmental characteristics of fetal behaviour.

THE FETAL BIOPHYSICAL PROFILE

The criteria for a normal fetal biophysical profile are as follows: (1) fetal heart-rate reactivity; (2) at least 30 seconds of continuous fetal breathing movements; (3) at least three body movements consisting of a brisk flexion or extension of the limb, head or trunk; (4) an adequate fetal tone that manifests itself in the posture as well as in flexor and extensor movements; and (5) an age-adequate amniotic fluid volume (Manning et al 1980). Most frequently, a 10-point scale is applied, with two points given for each of the five variables. A total score of 0–2 raises a strong suspicion of chronic fetal asphyxia and indicates the need for urgent delivery; a score of 3–7 still raises suspicion of chronic asphyxia. The test should be repeated within 24 hours; a score of 8–10 is regarded as normal (Kisilevsky and Low 1998).

A diagnostically conclusive interpretation must also take into account the respective behavioural state. If the fetus is in state 2F or 4F, satisfactory results are obtained in a matter of 5 minutes. However, if the fetus is in state 1F, it may take half an hour or more for the clinician to obtain a biophysical profile. Pillai and James (1990a) found that 44 out of 100 fetuses were assessed as 'abnormal', while in fact they showed a perfectly normal profile, typical of state 1F.

THE FETAL NEUROBEHAVIOURAL PROFILE

The fetal neurobehavioural profile comprises the following variables: (1) fetal responsiveness and arousal after perturbation with a vibroacoustic stimulus; (2) habituation to vibroacoustic stimulation; (3) state recovery; and (4) the so-called self-regulation after stimulation (Gingras and O'Donell 1998). As discussed in Chapter 5 (p 99), we consider that vibroacoustic stimulation is an invasive method that is ultimately harmful to the fetus, especially during state 1F.

THE ZAGREB SCORING SYSTEM

Kurjak and colleagues (2008) proposed a special scoring system, which was to be applied during three-dimensional (3D)/4D ultrasonography. Their assessment includes measurement of the cranial sutures and the head circumference, observation of isolated head anteflexion, isolated eye blinking, facial alterations, mouth opening, isolated arm and leg movements, hand-to-face contacts, finger movements and thumb position, as well as general movements.

There are a number of serious shortcomings to the proposed scoring system. The quality of general movements cannot be assessed by means of 3D/4D sonography, as the current time resolution does not allow the recognition of fluent and smooth movements (see also Chapter 1, p 7). Furthermore, no age range or statistics are available for the reference group. Last but not least, the authors consider a score of 14–20 low risk, although each of the 10 parameters is supposed to score between 1 and 3, which means there is a maximum score of 30.

ASSESSMENT BY THE KYUSHU UNIVERSITY, JAPAN

Horimoto and colleagues (1993) suggested application of the following criteria as markers of a normal, functioning nervous system: (1) there has to be at least one episode of limb motion per hour (extension, flexion, external and internal rotation, or abduction and adduction of any extremity); (2) breathing movements must reoccur at intervals of 120 minutes at most; (3) there must be an episode of eye movements lasting 2–30 minutes, and an episode of no eye movements lasting 2–25 minutes; (4) rapid eye movements co-exist with slow eye movements; (5) repetitive mouth movements occur at an interval of 300–600 milliseconds during a no-eye-movement episode; and (6) over a period of 120–180 minutes, the fetal heart rate alternates several times between active and quiet.

Based on this rather lengthy assessment, Morokuma and colleagues (2007) developed a less time-consuming screening system that is based on two steps: (1) fetuses are considered to have an impairment of brain function if at least one of the following three indicators is observed: (a) a decrease or lack of fetal movements, whereby the mother experiences fewer than three fetal movements per 12 hours or even a complete cessation of fetal movements over 24 hours; (b) a persistently non-reactive fetal heart-rate pattern, which implies that there are no accelerations over a period of 2 hours; (c) a central nervous system malformation. (2) As a second screening step in the assessment of brain function, the examiner should look out for five specific behavioural patterns adapted from Horimoto and colleagues (1993) by means of a short ultrasound evaluation: (a) movements of the extremities (normal = one or more episodes of motion including extension, flexion, external and internal rotation or abduction and adduction of all four extremities); (b) breathing movements (normal = at least one incidence of 30-second-long breathing movements); (c) alternating episodes of eye movements and no eye movements (normal = each episode lasts longer than 5 minutes); (d) rapid and slow eye movements (normal = coexistence of rapid and slow eye movements); (e) concurrence of regular mouthing movements and episodes of no eye movement (normal = one burst of regular mouthing during a no-eye-movement episode).

ASSESSING THE QUALITY OF FETAL GENERAL MOVEMENTS

An integral part of any neurological examination is to evaluate the quality of movements. This is also true for functional assessment of the fetal nervous system. As early as 1971, Reinold described a correlation between the quality of fetal movements and the pregnancy outcome, even though, for him, the only indicator of movement quality was speed (Reinold 1971, 1973).

In 1985, Prechtl introduced a more comprehensive assessment technique. With general movements being the most complex fetal motor pattern, they are most suitable for a qualitative assessment. Moreover, they are frequently present and of long duration. Provided that the examiner holds the probe still and is trained in this assessment technique, a few minutes of recording during bouts of activity should suffice. A lot of experience in Gestalt perception is required to decode the complex picture of a normal or abnormal pattern by assessing the sequence, speed, amplitude and intensity of movements and establishing the presence – or absence – of rotations (Prechtl 1985, Prechtl and Einspieler 1997). In the case of brain dysfunction, general movements lose their complexity (Prechtl 1990, Einspieler et al 2004, Einspieler and Prechtl 2005): their pace tends to be slow and their amplitude too small, but the most striking feature is the overall monotony of the movement sequence (Table 8.1). Such a pattern of abnormal fetal general movements can be observed in growth-retarded fetuses (Bekedam et al 1985) and in fetuses exposed to oligohydramnios (Sival et al 1992a, Rosier-van Dunné et al 2010), antiepileptic drugs (Swartjes et al 1992) or maternal diabetes (Kainer et al 1997). Abnormally abrupt, brusque and jerky fetal general movements in a repetitive sequence can be seen during the early stages of Pena–Shokeir syndrome (Mulder et al 2001a), in restrictive dermopathy (Mulder et al 2001b), myotonic dystrophy (Hsu et al 1993) or anencephalic fetuses (Visser et al 1985, Visser and Prechtl 1988, Shahidullah and Hepper 1992).

TABLE 8.1
TABLE 8.1 Quality of fetal general movements

	Sequence	Character	Amplitude	Speed
Normal	Variable	Smooth	Variable	Variable
Intrauterine growth retardation	Monotonous	Smooth	Small	Slow
Oligohydramnios	Monotonous	Smooth or jerky	Small	Slow
Exposure to antiepileptic drugs	Monotonous	Jerky	Small	Fast or slow
Maternal diabetes	Monotonous	Jerky, abrupt	Invariable	Invariable
Prader–Willi syndrome	Monotonous	Abnormal	Small	Slow
Trisomy 21	Variable or monotonous	Smooth or jerky, brisk	Not reported	Fast
Fanconi anaemia	Monotonous	Abrupt	Large	Fast
Anencephaly	Monotonous	Abrupt and jerky, forceful	Large	Fast

Adapted from Boué et al (1982), Bekedam et al (1985), Visser et al (1985), Shahidulla and Hepper (1992), Sival et al (992a), Swartjes et al 1992, de Vries et al (1994), Kainer et al (1997), Fong and de Vries (2003), Rosier-van Dunné et al (2010).

Since the same criteria can be applied in assessment of the fetus, neonate and young infant, it is possible to determine a certain consistency in the movement quality. If, for example, the general movements in offspring of mothers with diabetes are consistently normal pre- and postnatally, their neural development will be normal as well. General movements that are consistently abnormal pre- and postnatally, by contrast, are associated with a developmental delay (Kainer et al 1997). In the case of normal fetal but abnormal postnatal general movements, difficulties during labour, or postnatal complications, may be responsible for neurological dysfunction (Kainer et al 1997, Prechtl and Einspieler 1997).

While Prechtl's assessment of general movements has long been an established standard for the preterm and young infant (Ferrari et al 1990, Prechtl 1997a, Prechtl et al 1997, Einspieler et al 2004, Einspieler and Prechtl 2005), it still awaits a breakthrough in fetal neurology, although many researchers agree that qualitative evaluation is the only option when it comes to the assessment of fetal neurofunctions (e.g. Boué et al 1982, Maršál 1983, Hill 1989, Pillai and James 1990b, Amiel-Tison et al 2006, de Vries and Fong 2007, Rosier-van Dunné et al 2010).

Behaviour of fetuses with structural malformations
THE ANENCEPHALIC FETUS

The abnormal behaviour of anencephalic fetuses is in striking contrast to the almost normal posture and muscle tone and to some neonatal reflexes found in the anencephalic neonate (Lou 1982, Prechtl 1985). As early as 1885, Preyer noted that anencephalic fetuses moved excessively and forcefully, which is not only noticed by the mothers concerned (Rayburn et al 1983, Visser et al 1985), but is also confirmed by ultrasound studies: the forceful and abrupt general movements of anencephalic fetuses are clearly distinguishable from the fluency and the waxing and waning of normal fetal general movements (Table 8.1; Visser et al 1985, Visser and Prechtl 1988, Kurauchi et al 1995a, Andonotopo et al 2005). By a mere 10 weeks, a fetus with structural abnormalities consistent with anencephaly shows fast, powerful and explosive general movements (Shahidullah and Hepper 1992). Observational studies suggest that, while a few motoneurones may suffice for movements to emerge at such an early stage, an intact nervous system is necessary for them to be executed normally (Visser and Prechtl 1988).

Movement patterns and rest–activity cycles

The most striking abnormality in the anencephalic fetus is the quality of the various movement patterns, especially of the general movements. This is due to the reduced supraspinal ability to induce variance and complexity of movement (Visser et al 1985, Visser and Prechtl 1988, Shahidulla and Hepper 1992).

General movements appear abruptly, maintaining the force and (usually large) amplitude until the movement suddenly ceases (Table 8.1; Visser et al 1985, Kurauchi et al 1995a). There are large interfetal differences, but each fetus executes his/her general movements highly consistently. The temporal patterning of general movements is also abnormal: they either come in the form of excessive activity, scattered throughout the observation time (Figure 8.1a), or occur in bursts and pauses (Figure 8.1b). In the latter case, the rate of occurrence can be normal (Rayburn and Barr 1982, Visser et al 1985).

If startles are present (Table 8.2), their rate of occurrence exceeds the values of normal fetuses, even at late gestation (Visser et al 1985, Kurauchi et al 1995a).

Isolated arm movements are scarce and jerky (Visser et al 1985, Andonotopo et al 2005). Hand-to-face contact can sometimes be observed (Table 8.2). It is impressive that even in the histologically proven absence of a cervical cord, isolated arm and hand movements can be observed (Cases 4, 6, and 7 in Table 8.2), which suggests that, in spite of missing supraspinal connections, parts of the body can move by the mere means of ectopic motoneurones inside or outside the central nervous system (Visser et al 1985).

Isolated leg movements are scarce but also jerky and abrupt (Visser et al 1985, Warsof et al 1988, Andonotopo et al 2005).

Hiccups can occasionally be observed (Kurauchi et al 1995a). If present, they appear excessive (Visser et al 1985).

Breathing movements are limited (or missing entirely) if the medulla oblongata is dysplastic and a nucleus ambiguous-like structure can be found in the region of the medulla (Kurauchi et al 1995a). If the medulla is absent and only part of the spinal cord is present, albeit aplastic in the cervical region, there are usually no breathing movements or

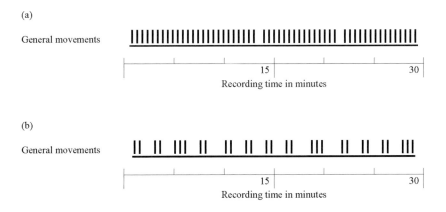

Figure 8.1 Actograms (30-minute recordings) of fetal general movements in two anencephalic fetuses: (a) excessive activity in a fetus with spinal cord, medulla oblongata and pons, dysplasia of the cerebellum, 16 weeks old; (b) burst–pause pattern of general movements in a fetus with a thoracic and lumbosacral spinal cord, 19 weeks old. Adapted from Visser GHA, Laurini RN, de Vries JIP, Bekedam DJ, Prechtl HFR. (1985) Abnormal motor behaviour in anencephalic fetuses. *Early Hum Dev* 12: 173–182, with permission.

TABLE 8.2
Presence of movement patterns in seven anencephalic fetuses

	Case 1	Case 2	Case 3	Case 4	Case 5	Case 6	Case 7
Recording age	**16 weeks**	**16 weeks**	**16 weeks**	**17 weeks**	**17 weeks**	**19 weeks**	**33 weeks**
Hindbrain[a]	Dysplasia of the medulla	Normal pons and medulla; dysplasia of the cerebellum	Normal pons and medulla; dysplasia of the cerebellum	Aplasia	Aplasia	Aplasia	Aplasia
Spinal cord[a]	Normal	Normal	Normal	Dysplasia of the thoracic and lumbosacral spinal cord	Dysplasia of the cervical spinal cord; normal thoracic and lumbosacral spinal cord	Normal thoracic and lumbosacral spinal cord	Dysplasia of the thoracic and lumbosacral spinal cord
General movements	+	+	+	+	+	+	+
Startle	−	+	+	+	+	−	+
Isolated arm movements	+	+	+	+	−	+	+
Isolated leg movements	−	+	+	+	−	+	+
Breathing movements	+	−	−	+	−	−	−
Hiccup	−	−	−	+	−	−	−
Hand-to-face contact	−	+	−	+	−	+	−
Head rotation	+	−	−	−	−	−	−

[a]Normal is defined by the presence of white and grey matter structures corresponding to those found in normal fetuses with comparable gestational age. Dysplasia indicates anomalies in the arrangement and the amount of white and/or grey matter. Aplasia indicates that no white and/or gray matter structures corresponding to the brain or spinal cord can be identified; only fetal leptomeninges and glial tissue are sometimes present, together with dorsal ganglions. + = present; − = absent. From Visser GHA, Laurini RN, de Vries JIP, Bekedam DJ, Prechtl HFR. (1985) Abnormal motor behaviour in anencephalic fetuses. *Early Hum Dev* 12: 173–182, with permission.

hiccups (Kurauchi et al 1996), although Visser and associates (1985) did observe a few breathing movements and hiccups in a fetus with only a hypoplastic and dysplastic spinal cord at the lower thoracic level and groups of motoneurones in the lumbosacral segments (Case 4 in Table 8.2). In the cervical region, only fetal meninges, scarce glial tissue and dorsal ganglia were present, but there was no spinal cord at all, which shows how little structure of the central nervous system is required to generate movements, albeit abnormal ones. The absence of breathing movements is typically associated with lung hypoplasia (Chapter 2, p 35), which is also common in anencephalic fetuses (Dornan et al 1984a, Kurauchi et al 1996). If an anencephalic fetus does show fetal breathing movements, the lungs are appropriately grown and surfactant-active material is released into the alveolar and amniotic fluids (Table 8.3).

TABLE 8.3
Fetal breathing movements and lung growth in five anencephalic fetuses

	Case 1	Case 2	Case 3	Case 4	Case 5
Recording age	**40 weeks**	**34 weeks**	**36 weeks**	**35 weeks**	**40 weeks**
Brain tissue	Absent, and spina bifida	Neural tissue in a sac of meninges, but no spinal cord	Absent, lumbar myelocele	Grossly disorganised brain in a meningeal sac and spina bifida	Absent
Diaphragm	Intact	Intact	Intact	Intact	Intact
Lungs	Hypoplasia	Hypoplasia	Hypoplasia	Appropriately grown	Hypoplasia
Breathing movements	–	–	–	+	–
Production (and storage) of surface-active material in type II cells	+	+	+	+ but no storage	+
Release of surface-active material into the alveolar and amniotic fluids	–	–	–	+	–

+ = present; – = absent. Created using data from Dornan et al (1984a).

Swallowing movements can also occur in anencephalic fetuses (Pritchard 1965, Peleg and Goldman 1978).

Rest–activity cycles may occur when a rudiment of the midbrain is present, but they do not increase with progressing gestational age, and rarely exceed 6 minutes (Kurauchi et al 1995a, Belich et al 1996).

Sometimes the motor activity of anencephalic fetuses shows so little resemblance to the patterns observed in normal fetuses that it is hard to classify movements at all (Visser and Prechtl 1988).

Fetal heart rate and its diurnal rhythm
The biological clock in the brain, which regulates diurnal rhythms, is located in the suprachiasmatic nuclei of the anterior hypothalamus. It would seem obvious, therefore, that an anencephalic fetus whose respective cerebral regions are missing does not have diurnal rhythms (Lunshof et al 1997). In fact, some fetuses demonstrate diurnal rhythms in spite of an aplasia rostral to the medulla (Muro et al 1998). It has therefore been speculated that maternal factors might influence these oscillations (Lunshof et al 1997, Muro et al 1998).

If the anencephalic fetus is younger than 30 weeks and has an intact medulla oblongata, his/her heart-rate pattern is similar to that of a normally developing fetus (Yoshizato et al 1994). Only then does the heart-rate pattern alter: severe V-shaped, W-shaped or prolonged decelerations (but no accelerations) occur (Terao et al 1984, Kurauchi et al 1995b, Belich et al 1996), which suggests that more rostral parts of the brain are now involved in the regulation of the fetal heart rate (Yoshizato et al 1994). If the brainstem is missing altogether, either the heart rate is persistently flat (de Haan and Stolte 1971, Belich et al 1996), or continuous V-shaped decelerations occur, which indicates an intrinsic cardiac rhythmicity (Terao et al 1984).

Fetal responsiveness
Anencephalic fetuses do not show any alteration in their heart rate or movements in response to acoustic or vibroacoustic stimulation (Leader et al 1982, Park and Kim 1989, van Heteren et al 2000).

SPINA BIFIDA APERTA
Spina bifida aperta is characterised by a defective fusion of the neural tube, resulting in exposure of the myelomeningocele to the amniotic fluid. Despite this defect, leg movements are present prenatally, and sometimes even normal in quality (Korenromp et al 1986, Warsof et al 1988, Chervanek and Isaacson 1989, Sival et al 1997, 2008, Prayer and Brugger 2007, Verbeek et al 2009). If leg movements are abnormal, they are abrupt, or hardly discernible at all (Sival et al 2008).

Fetal bladder function is normal (Warsof et al 1988). Responsiveness to vibroacoustic stimulation is within the normal range (Vindla et al 1999a), although the leg does not withdraw if directly contacted with an amniocentesis needle (Petrikovsky and Kaplan 1995). The quantity of fetal movements is reduced during behavioural states 2F and 4F, whereas state 1F sometimes lasts longer than in normal fetuses (Vindla et al 1997a).

During the first 2 days of life, general movements are still normal if the myelomeningocele is located caudally from L3 (Sival et al 2004). After this, leg movements become increasingly abnormal and eventually disappear altogether (Sival et al 2006).

OTHER BRAIN MALFORMATIONS

Some brain malformations, such as cerebral cortical dysgenesis (du Plessis et al 1993), olivopontocerebellar hypoplasia (Mitra et al 1999), hydranencephaly (Conover et al 1986), or microcephaly (Landy et al 1989), are associated with seizure-like activity.

A fetus with multiple congenital anomalies shows either a bizarre behaviour with no rest–activity cycles (Pillai and James 1990b) or reduced body movements (Vindla et al 1997a), but interestingly enough achieves normal results in the non-stress test or the biophysical profile (Pillai and James 1990b, Vindla et al 1997a, 1999a).

Microcephaly

Microcephalic fetuses show abnormally fast body movements (Shinozuka et al 1989); a severe reduction of breathing movements (Shinozuka et al 1989) or abnormal, staccato-like excursions of the chest wall, not accompanied by abdominal movements (Dornan et al 1984a); an abnormal pattern of habituation to vibroacoustic stimulation (Leader et al 1982); and seizure-like movements (Landy et al 1989).

Corpus callosum agenesis

Reduced fetal activity with a normal heart-rate variation was reported in a fetus with corpus callosum agenesis and mild ventriculomegaly (Vindla et al 1997a). Vibroacoustic stimulation revealed normal results (Vindla et al 1999a).

Holoprosencephaly and porencephaly

In the case of holoprosencephaly and porencephaly, body movements can be excessive (Vindla et al 1997a); breathing movements are sometimes normal (Morokuma et al 2007); eye movements only occur sporadically (Shinozuka et al 1989, Horimoto et al 1993); regular mouthing is absent during state 1F (Morokuma et al 2007); and fetal activity decreases in response to vibroacoustic stimulation (Vindla et al 1999a).

167

Owing to some form of dysgenesis, fetuses with porencephaly or ventriculomegaly have an increased rate of fetal activity – even during state 1F (Vindla et al 1997a). Their responsiveness to vibroacoustic stimulation is within the normal range (Vindla et al 1999a).

Lissencephaly
Nothing is known about general movements of term fetuses with lissencephaly; breathing movements can be normal, abnormal or missing altogether, and there is regular mouthing during state 1F (Morokuma et al 2007). The duration of both eye-movement and no-eye-movement episodes is abnormal (Horimoto et al 1993).

Hydrocephalus
In hydrocephalus, general movements are reduced and jerky in appearance (Ianniruberto and Tajani 1981, Rayburn and Barr 1982, Visser and Prechtl 1988); breathing movements are reduced (Shinozuka et al 1989); and cogwheel-like tremor sometimes occurs (Ianniruberto and Tajani 1981). After 36 weeks, eye movements occur less often, which suggests a delay in the control of eye movement (Awoust and Lewi 1984, Arduini et al 1987).

The appearance of behavioural states is also delayed, so that the degree of discordance of the state variables is related to the severity of the neonatal outcome (Arduini et al 1987, Romanini and Rizzo 1995). The rate of occurrence of fetal heart-rate patterns A and B can be normal, but the clustering of heart-rate patterns with body and eye movements is very low, resulting in a high percentage of non-coincidence (see Chapter 4, Figure 4.8).

Arnold–Chiari malformation
In Arnold–Chiari malformation, motor activity is reduced during states 2F and 4F but it is normal during behavioural state 1F (Vindla et al 1997a).

Moebius syndrome
A case report on Moebius syndrome with linear calcifications in the periependymal areas of the anterior aspect of the fourth ventricle from the pons to the medulla described a fetus with abnormal eye movements: they occurred sporadically; neither their presence nor their absence lasted for more than 1 minute. No breathing movements were reported, but irregular mouthing was observed (Horimoto et al 1993, Koyanagi et al 1993, Morokuma et al 2007).

Cardiac abnormalities

Body movements are normal in fetuses with a tricuspid atresia or Fallot's tetralogy (Vindla et al 1997a, 1999a). However, heart-rate variation is low (Vindla et al 1997a). Fetuses with hydrops due to severe heart anomalies display fewer breathing and trunk movements (Shinozuka et al 1989).

Gastrointestinal abnormalities

A fetus with tracheal atresia can have jerky, vigorous breathing movements of high speed and large amplitude (Baarsma et al 1993). Fetuses with oesophageal atresia appear to be vomiting: mouth opening, neck extension and tongue protrusion can be observed (Bowie and Clair 1982, de Vries and Fong 2007). Fetal vomiting is shown in Video 26, although not in a fetus with gastrointenstinal abnormalities but one with brainstem hypoplasia. Fetuses with gastroschisis move normally (Ianniruberto and Tajani 1981), although mothers may experience a decrease of fetal movements (Rayburn and Barr 1982).

Genetic disorders and fetal behaviour

Obviously, behavioural observation provides no evidence of a particular genetic disorder, since behavioural abnormalities are too unspecific and often very subtle. They can, nevertheless, indicate an underlying neurological disorder that needs further detailed assessment.

TRISOMY 1Q

The fetal movements in trisomy 1q are abrupt and jerky and show no modulation. The trunk does not rotate but shows hyperextension and flexion. Rest–activity cycles are absent (Boué et al 1982).

TRISOMY 4P

In trisomy 4p, the fetus is very active. Fetal movements are rough, jerky and sometimes synchronised. Hyperextensions of the trunk are frequent (Boué et al 1982).

MONOSOMY 5P, CRI-DU-CHAT SYNDROME

In this syndrome, the fetus is very active, displaying abrupt movements. Twitches occur frequently, and the trunk is sometimes hyperextended (Boué et al 1982).

TRISOMY 5P

Fetal movements are continuously present in trisomy 5p. They are brisk, with sudden jerks of the whole body and hyperextension of the head. There are no rest–activity cycles (Boué et al 1982). Interestingly, some fetuses with trisomy 5p display normal and fluent body movements (Boué et al 1982).

TRISOMY 8

Fetal breathing movements are reduced in trisomy 8 (Shinozuka et al 1989).

TRISOMY 13

In trisomy 13, fetal body, breathing and eye movements are inconspicuous (Shinozuka et al 1989).

PRADER–WILLI SYNDROME

In the majority of patients with Prader–Willi syndrome, genes on chromosome 15 (bands 15q11–q13) are deleted. This affects the central nervous system, predominantly the hypothalamus. Due to hypokinesia and hypotonia, Prader–Willi syndrome can cause complications during labour. Therefore, prenatal diagnosis can help to optimise perinatal care.

A prominent feature of Prader–Willi syndrome is polyhydramnios, presumably caused by diminished fetal swallowing, in analogy with the sucking problems encountered in neonatal life. General movements are reduced and of short duration. They are abnormal in that they hardly vary in amplitude (mostly small) and speed (mostly slow); their complexity is reduced (Table 8.1; Fong and de Vries 2003). Isolated arm, finger and leg movements can be normal (Fong and de Vries 2003), although their posture is sometimes peculiar: the hands can be clenched, with the thumbs adducted over the index and middle fingers; the toes are often flexed in spite of extended legs and feet (Bigi et al 2008). The duration of fetal heart-rate pattern A (state 1F) is prolonged, whereas active states are short (Hiroi et al 2000, Fong and de Vries 2003).

TRISOMY 18, EDWARDS SYNDROME

Apart from a severe symmetrical growth retardation in trisomy 18, with a deformity of the skull and craniofacial abnormalities, the mouth is persistently open, with the tongue protruding. The fingers are flexed, the index finger is clasped over the middle finger and the small finger clutches the ring finger. Rocker bottom feet and a ventricular septum defect of the heart are further features (Hepper et Shahidullah 1992a). The behaviour is bizarre: fetal body movements, monotonous in appearance, are continuously present, with a fine tremor superimposed (Boué et al 1982, Shinozuka et al 1989, Hepper and

Shahidulla 1992a). The legs of the fetus are mainly extended, as though the fetus lies outstretched. This conspicuous posture is accompanied by an unusual side-to-side movement of the trunk. A fetus with trisomy 18 shows a predominance of vertical eye movements (Hepper and Shahidulla 1992a), while normally developing fetuses mainly move their eyes horizontally (see Figure 2.14). Since the fetus is continuously active, no rest–activity cycles or behavioural states occur (Hepper and Shahidulla 1992a).

TRISOMY 21, DOWN SYNDROME

The appearance of fetal body movements is inconclusive in Down syndrome: sometimes they appear normal and harmonious, sometimes scarce and jerky. The majority of fetuses with trisomy 21 move continuously and quickly, in a brisk and abrupt manner (Table 8.1; Boué et al 1982). Cogwheel-like movements of the limbs may occur (Boué et al 1982). The basal fetal heart rate is low during early pregnancy (Schats et al 1990). Behavioural states are disorganised (Vindla et al 1997a). The response to vibroacoustic stimulation is normal (Vindla et al 1999a), but habituation is slower or missing altogether (Hepper and Shahidullah 1992b).

SMITH–LEMLI–OPITZ SYNDROME

Smith–Lemli–Opitz syndrome is caused by mutations in the *DHCR7* gene, which generates an enzyme responsible for the final step in the production of cholesterol. Cholesterol, a structural component of cell membranes and myelin, is a nutrient that is essential for normal embryonic development. Infants with Smith–Lemli–Opitz syndrome have a reduced muscle tone, they experience feeding difficulties and tend to grow more slowly than normal infants. Their fetal behaviour is bizarre and inappropriate: fetal movements occur sporadically; breathing movements are intermittent; and mouthing is absent. The behavioural states are dissociated; none of the behavioural-state patterns that are normally present can be recognised around term. And yet the conventional non-stress test yields normal results, with several accelerations during fetal movements (Pillai et al 1991).

FANCONI ANAEMIA

Fanconi anaemia is an autosomal recessive disease characterised by the association of aplastic anaemia, a variety of congenital anomalies and an increased risk of malignancy (Auerbach et al 1985). There are at least 13 genes where mutations are known to cause Fanconi's anaemia. De Vries and colleagues (1994) reported a case of prenatal diagnosis presenting with abnormal fetal behaviour along with brain damage, such as spongiform degeneration of the white matter in multiple areas and a small subarachnoid haemorrhage in the cerebellum.

At 22 weeks' gestation, only four specific motor patterns were observed: general movements, isolated arm movements, isolated leg movements and side-to-side movement of the head. Breathing movements, hiccups, and jaw movements were missing, which is unusual at that age. The rate of occurrence of each of the four patterns observed was low, though within the normal range. Total activity, however, was well below normal.

The most striking abnormality was found in the general movements (Table 8.1), which occurred in burst and pauses; their onset was abrupt and flexions and extensions were only performed to the highest possible extent. Isolated arm and leg movements were performed abruptly and with large amplitudes. The fetus frequently shifted from the dorsal to a lateral position. Overall motor activity was monotonous in character, since all movements were performed at a high speed and large amplitude (de Vries et al 1994).

SCHWARTZ–JAMPEL SYNDROME

Schwartz–Jampel syndrome is a rare autosomal recessive disorder characterised by myotonia, a mask-like face with narrow palpebral fissures and microstomia, short stature and osteochondrodysplasia (Schwartz and Jampel 1962). Fetal activity is distinctly decreased. Movements of the head and trunk are more or less absent; arm and leg movements are scarce. When moving the arms, the fetus flexes the fingers of both hands, with intermittent extension of the second digit, and sometimes also the fifth digit (Hunziker et al 1989).

SPINAL MUSCULAR ATROPHY, ESPECIALLY WERDNIG–HOFFMANN DISEASE

Werdnig–Hoffmann disease is an autosomal recessive disorder linked to a mutation in the survival motor neurone gene. It results in a fatal progressive degeneration of motor neurones. The degree of profound hypotonia and paresis often present at birth – and progressively deteriorating from then – is such that the condition must have existed for weeks or months prior to delivery. Although the first maternal notion of quickening is not delayed, mothers describe the intensity of fetal movements as reduced compared to that of normal siblings (Kirkinen et al 1994, Rayburn 1995, Kobayashi et al 1996). One pregnant woman gave an account of rapid, jerky, fluttering movements during the last few weeks of pregnancy. At birth, her infant was severely affected with obvious muscle fasciculations (Pearn 1973).

In one case documented by means of sonographic examination, fetal movements were normal at 17 weeks. Leg movements were so frequent that femoral length measurement was difficult (Kirkinen et al 1994). At 36 weeks, however, no limb movements were observed. The elbows and knees were flexed and the hands open. By contrast, the rate of occurrence of breathing and swallowing movements was normal. The examination was repeated on four consecutive days, with similar findings. Fetal cardiotocograms revealed normal fetal heart-rate accelerations. Labour was induced at 37 weeks' gestation. The only muscular activity in the newborn was in the form of faint movements in the eyelids and tongue. Otherwise, the boy was severely hypotonic and could not suck or swallow. Spinal muscular atrophy type I was diagnosed (Kirkinen et al 1994).

WALKER–WARBURG SYNDROME AND OTHER MYOPATHIES

Walker–Warburg syndrome is a rare form of autosomal recessive congenital muscular dystrophy associated with cerebral and occular abnormalities such as lissencephaly, hydrocephalus, cerebellar malformations and retina dysplasia. It presents at birth with generalised hypotonia, muscle weakness, and occasional seizures. Several mutations are found in the protein-*O*-mannosyltransferase *POMT1* and *POMT2* genes, as well as in the fukutin-related protein genes (Vajsar and Schachter 2006).

Nothing is known about the quality of fetal movements. However, their quantity is reduced, especially during the last 10 weeks of pregnancy (Vindla et al 1997a). Despite a low activity rate, the number of episodes with high fetal heart-rate variability (patterns B and D) increases with advancing gestation, reaching the 90th centile at 36 weeks (Vindla et al 1997a). This discrepancy results in a disorganisation of behavioural states. Vibroacoustic stimulation does not elicit a fetal response (Vindla et al 1999a).

Fetuses of mothers with myotonic dystrophy or X-linked myotubular myopathy show decreased fetal movements of a poor quality (Stoll et al 1991, Tyson et al 1992, Hageman et al 1993, Hsu et al 1993).

A fetus with generalised amyoplasia presenting at mid-gestation shows no fetal movements, which results in severe multiple congenital contractures and polyhydramnios (Sepulveda et al 1995).

Fetal akinesia deformation sequence

Normal fetal growth – and brain development in particular – is highly dependent on adequate fetal movements (see Chapter 2, p 19). Limitation of movements results in a particular pattern of abnormal fetal morphogenesis, regardless of the underlying cause. This phenotype was termed 'fetal akinesia deformation sequence' (FADS) (Moessinger 1983). Whereas the term 'arthrogryposis multiplex congenital' describes contractures alone, FADS includes the entire spectrum of anomalies that originate in a decrease of fetal movements: diffuse joint contractures, hypertelorism, micrognathia, small nose and mouth, intrauterine growth restriction, polyhydramnios, pulmonary hypoplasia and a short umbilical cord. The term was proposed by Moessinger (1983), who showed in curarised rats that such anomalies were the consequence of decreased embryonic movement. It is now assumed that Pena–Shokeir sequence (Pena and Shokeir 1974) is just another name for the same constellation of findings. The FADS is seen in a number of syndromes: Neu–Laxova syndrome, dermal disorders such as restrictive dermopathy and multiple pterygium syndrome, acquired intrauterine brain damage, Marden–Walker syndrome (decreased number of anterior horn cells), pancreatic cell hyperplasia or proliferative vasculopathy (Hall 1986).

This heterogeneous aetiopathology may start its destructive effects on the various systems at different gestational ages (de Vries and Fong 2007). In addition, there must be a variable expression of the FADS, since the onset of the disease differs by weeks among the offspring of the same parents (Bacino et al 1993, Paladini et al 2001). The majority of cases are diagnosed before 24 weeks' gestation, although the abnormal behaviour emerges between 12 and 29 weeks (de Vries and Fong 2007, Donker et al 2009, Senocak et al 2009).

Postural anomalies tend to be the initial behavioural signs. The upper limbs are flexed, whereas the lower limbs are extended and crossed (Ajayi et al 1995, Paluda et al 1996, Paladini et al 2001). There can also be a chronological discrepancy: sometimes the leg posture precedes the arm posture in becoming abnormal by 3–8 weeks (Mulder et al 2001a, Paladini et al 2001). In the case of 'focal akinesia', only one extremity is involved (Tongsong et al 2000).

Fetal movements are normal until the end of the first trimester (Kirkinen et al 1987, Bacino et al 1993). After this time, the quantity of movement decreases substantially (Paladini et al 2001). By this time, normal general movements are interspersed with jerky movements until eventually, a few weeks later, all general movements become abnormal and monotonous, with an abrupt and jerky onset (Hill et al 1983, Mulder et al 2001a, Donker et al 2009). Some fetuses show seizure-like movements (Skupski et al 1996); others are totally inactive (Kirkinen et al 1987, Yfantis et al 2002, Romero et al 2003).

Breathing movements are of small amplitude (Dornan et al 1984a). As gestation progresses, they are barely visible (Mulder et al 2001a).

Fetal heart rate is sometimes within the limits of normal, as is fetal heart-rate variation (Kirkinen et al 1987, Mulder et al 2001a). Fetal heart-rate patterns A and B may even develop. However, as fetal quiescence increases rapidly, the temporal association between fetal movements and heart-rate patterns loosens (Mulder et al 2001a).

Interestingly, the heart-rate response to vibroacoustic stimulation can be normal, in spite of a significantly reduced fetal activity (Vindla et al 1999a).

FOCAL AKINESIA

Tongsong and colleagues (2000) reported a fetus whose postmortem examination revealed a reduction of motor cells in the anterior horn of both the cervical and thoracic spinal cords, with clear evidence that the body parts with no movements showed contractures or hypoplasia, while body parts with active movements developed normally.

Although the mother perceived a normal fetal motion, a sonographic examination at 28 weeks' gestation revealed polyhydramnios and contractures of the upper limbs. Both upper limbs were in fixed flexion at the wrist, elbow and shoulder. There were no breathing movements for a full 2 hours. The lower extremities, however, were normal, in both morphology and activity. Fetal head movements and blinking were occasionally noted, but the mouth was fixed open.

When vibroacoustic stimulation was applied, an unusual partial fetal response was noted: the lower limbs moved normally, and normal heart-rate accelerations could be elicited, but the upper limbs remained motionless and fetal breathing movements could not be triggered; the mouth remained opened (Tongsong et al 2000).

Neu–Laxova syndrome is an autosomal recessive disorder with a poor prognosis. The syndrome comprises malformations of the central nervous system, limb deformities, lung hypoplasia, ichthyosis, growth retardation and polyhydramnios. Fetal movements can be normal until 16 weeks (Bacino et al 1993). Thereafter, activity is reduced, and the remaining movements occur in bursts and pauses (Kirkinen et al 1987). Episodes of complete quiescence can be interrupted by adductor cloni of all the limbs or abrupt arm or leg movements (Kainer et al 1996).

RESTRICTIVE DERMOPATHY

Restrictive dermopathy is a rare lethal autosomal recessive disorder characterised by a thin, shiny and rigid skin, facial dysmorphism, and multiple joint contractures. Clinically, preterm birth is usually preceded by polyhydramnios, preterm rupture of membranes, and growth retardation (Hoffmann et al 1993).

Fetal general movements are abnormally monotonous, abrupt and short lived; they usually start in the legs, hips and lower trunk. With advancing gestation, these brief bursts of movement increase, resulting in an abnormal temporal organisation of activity (Mulder et al 2001b).

Isolated limb or head movements sometimes occur; an abnormal posture of the feet and a rigid head–thorax junction can only be observed shortly before term. Unexpectedly, fetal breathing movements and hiccups occur episodically, with normal amplitude and a normal rate of occurrence. Mouth movements can also be normal, although from time to time they are exaggerated and repetitive. The fetal heart rate may be high, though within normal range (Mulder et al 2001b).

Sudden changes in the quantity of fetal movements

Both a sudden increase and a sudden decrease of fetal movements can be a serious – albeit unspecific – sign of fetal compromise (Table 8.4), but can also occur during physiological conditions (see Chapter 2, p 52, and Chapter 4, p 81).

A sudden reduction or cessation of fetal movements causes concern and anxiety in the pregnant woman, as such a change of state can obviously be associated with an adverse pregnancy outcome (Olesen and Svare 2004, Heazell and Frøen 2008). Indeed, fetal death is preceded by a sudden reduction of fetal movements (Hill et al 1983); a cessation of activity is also associated with cerebellar haemorrhage (Hadi et al 1994), massive feto-

TABLE 8.4
TABLE 8.4 Sudden quantitative changes in fetal motility

Sudden increase	Sudden decrease
Acute fetal stress	Cerebellar haemorrhage
Cord complications	Feto-maternal haemorrhage
Placental abruption	Nuchal cord

Sadovsky and Polishuk (1977), Steinfeld et al (1992), Kosasa et al (1993), Hadi et al (1994).

maternal haemorrhage (Kosasa et al 1993, Mahendru et al 2007), or a nuchal cord (Steinfeld et al 1992). More often, however, a pathological decrease of fetal movements is associated with chronic rather than acute complications. Approximately half of inactive fetuses tolerate labour poorly or need resuscitation at birth (Mathews 1973, Birnholz et al 1978, Rayburn 1995); in addition, they are at high risk for neuromuscular disorders (Hill 1989, Christensen and Rayburn 1999, Vasta et al 2005) or sudden infant death (Einspieler et al 1988). The aetiological factor that is usually associated with diminished fetal movements is hypoxia. As the fetus responds to chronic hypoxia by conserving energy, the subsequent reduction in fetal movements is an adaptive mechanism to reduce oxygen consumption (Velazquez and Rayburn 2002, Olesen and Svare 2004). This goes hand in hand with a loss of fetal heart-rate variability, followed by heart-rate decelerations (Kirkinen et al 1994).

A sudden increase of fetal movements can also be a sign of acute fetal distress; it occurs in cases of cord complications or placental abruption (Sadovsky and Polishuk 1977).

Fetal seizures

Mothers occasionally give an account of their babies having fits (Whitehead 1867, Badr El-Din 1960, Isler 1964, Bejšovec et al 1967, Conover et al 1986, Landy et al 1989, Osiovich and Barrington 1996, Mitra et al 1999, Amiel-Tison et al 2006). Sonographic examination reveals episodes of rapid, sometimes explosive, jerking motion of the head and all four extremities (Conover et al 1986, Landy et al 1989, Shimizu et al 1991, du Plessis et al 1993, Skupski et al 1996, Osiovich and Barrington 1996, Usta et al 2007, Jung et al 2008). They may last 5–10 seconds and recur every 20–30 seconds for a period of 3–5 minutes, followed by an interval of 5–10 minutes during which no fetal movements are observed (Conover et al 1986, Skupski et al 1996). The entire sequence then repeats itself. Seizure activity can also be subtle in the case of multiple ankylosis or joint contractures (Skupski et al 1996).

Underlying causes are brain malformations (Conover et al 1986, Abrams and Balducci 1996, Patane and Ghidini 2001, Usta et al 2007), including neural migration disorder (du Plessis et al 1993) and olivopontocerebellar hypoplasia (Mitra et al 1999); fetal akinesia deformations sequence (Skupski et al 1996, de Vries 2008); brain lesion (Landy et al 1989, Ingemarsson and Spencer 1998); congenital arthrogryposis due to congenital muscular dystrophy (Skupski et al 1996); pyrodixine deficiency (Isler 1964, Bejšovec et al 1967, Gospe and Hecht 1998); or severe growth restriction with oligohydramnios (Landy et al 1989, Shimizu et al 1991).

FETAL BRAIN DEATH

James (1998) reported a case of fetal brain death that presented itself as abnormal, seizure-like fetal movements. At 36 weeks, polyhydramnios rapidly developed, without obvious cause. Sonography revealed normal fetal movements. A day later, the mother felt the fetus was shaking regularly and repetitively. Cardiotocography showed a baseline tachycardia of 165 beats per minute, with no variation. At this point, the ultrasound examination revealed a morphologically normal fetus, although with convulsive movements of all limbs, lasting for about 2 seconds and recurring in a sequence of approximately 10 seconds. A Caesarean section was performed. The convulsive movements of the limbs continued during and after delivery. The infant was clinically brain dead; the abnormal movements were found to be decerebrate spinal reflexes. The underlying cause of the decerebration remained unknown.

Prenatal brain lesions

The most frequent patterns of prenatal brain lesions are periventricular white-matter damage and germinal matrix haemorrhage (Sherer et al 1998, van Gelder-Hasker et al 2001, Volpe 2001, Ghi et al 2003, Scher 2003, Rosier-van Dunné et al 2007). Cystic lesions can have multiple causes, both congenital and acquired. A congenital cystic lesion is believed to occur at an earlier stage of the first half of pregnancy (encephaloclastic lesions such as schizencephaly or arachnoid cysts), while acquired lesions due to intravascular occlusive events generally occur at a later point, during the second half of pregnancy (encephalomalacia from stroke syndromes associated with maternal pre-eclampsia or thrombotic vasculopathy of the placenta).

Unfortunately, little is known about the behaviour of fetuses with brain lesions. It is very likely that fetal movements, and in particular fetal general movements, lack variation in sequencing, amplitude and speed (Prechtl 1989, 1997b, Pillai and James 1992, Prechtl and Einspieler 1997). Rest–activity cycles can also be disturbed (Pillai and James 1992, Horimoto et al 1993). An absence of regular mouthing during state 1F has been described in fetuses with white-matter lesions (Horimoto et al 1993, Koyanagi et al 1993).

Intrauterine growth retardation, an exposure to chronic nutritional deprivation

Fetal growth ranging below the 5th percentile is defined by the term 'intrauterine growth retardation' (Kloosterman 1973). Its aetiology is varied. There can be both physiological (i.e. constitutional) and pathological causes. The latter are numerous, including, for example, uteroplacental insufficiency, which can itself be secondary to a number of pathologies, chromosomal abnormalities and congenital infections. The result is a diminished fetal supply of oxygen and/or nutrients (van Vliet et al 1985a, Sival 1993, Romanini and Rizzo 1995, Vindla et al 1997b). Under these circumstances, a shift of blood flow to the fetus's central nervous system occurs (Wladimiroff et al 1986, 1987). This relative redistribution of fetal blood flow is a 'brain-sparing' mechanism, but the neurological outcome may still be adverse (Blair and Stanley 1990). In this respect, it is not clear whether hypoxia or the deprivation of other nutrients such as glucose and amino acids is the major cause of damage to the central nervous system. Deteriorating growth-retarded fetuses show behavioural abnormalities before they become hypoxic, which indicates that nutritional deprivation is the primary cause (Visser et al 1990).

In the course of intrauterine growth retardation, the quantity and quality of general movements alter. Movements decrease and are generally monotonous, as opposed to the variable motor repertoire of a normal fetus (Table 8.1; Ianniruberto and Tajani 1981, Bekedam et al 1985, van Vliet et al 1985a, Sival et al 1992a, Ribbert et al 1993, Vindla et al 1997b, 1999b). The movements alter in four stages (Figure 8.2): (1) general movements are normal during uncomplicated and mild intrauterine growth retardation; (2) as the amniotic fluid volume decreases, general movements become slower and decrease in amplitude; (3) after the fetal heart-rate pattern deteriorates – this comprises reduced heart-rate variability or heart rate decelerations – the complexity of general movements decreases and the movement sequence becomes monotonous; (4) with further deterioration of the fetal clinical condition (e.g. reduction in the amount of amniotic fluid along with repetitive fetal heart-rate decelerations), general movements become ever harder to discern (Sival et al 1992a, Sival 1993). It seems to be the case that the stepwise decrease of general movements marks a continuous adaptation to a limited oxygen delivery, whereby the fetal organism struggles to keep the oxygen level high by reducing physical movements (Ribbert et al 1993).

Startles, twitches, isolated arm movements and side-to-side movements of the head occur less often; head movements in particular are performed at a slow pace and with small amplitude (Bekedam et al 1985). Breathing movements are also reduced, especially if the fetal heart rate becomes abnormal. Unlike in the normal fetus, breathing movements do not increase when the growth-retarded fetus reaches term age (Bots et al 1978, Trudinger et al 1979, Dornan et al 1984b, Shinozuka et al 1989, Bekedam et al 1991, Sival et al 1992b, Ribbert et al 1993).

Positional changes occur less often than in the normal fetus. The posture of the growth-retarded fetus is slightly more crouched, as the vertebral column tends to be more flexed, especially at the cervical level (Bekedam et al 1985).

The fetal heart rate is generally higher in the growth-retarded fetus, whereas heart-rate variation is initially within or below the norm – falling further as the deterioration of the fetal condition progresses (Bekedam et al 1987, Ribbert et al 1993, Gagnon 1995, Nijhuis et al 2000). Consequently, there is no diurnal pattern of fetal heart rate (Koenen et al

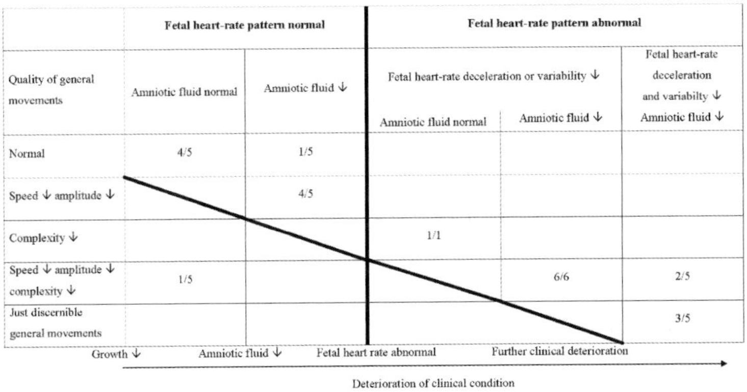

Quality of general movements	Fetal heart-rate pattern normal		Fetal heart-rate pattern abnormal		
	Amniotic fluid normal	Amniotic fluid ↓	Fetal heart-rate deceleration or variability ↓		Fetal heart-rate deceleration and variabilty ↓ Amniotic fluid ↓
			Amniotic fluid normal	Amniotic fluid ↓	
Normal	4/5	1/5			
Speed ↓ amplitude ↓		4/5			
Complexity ↓			1/1		
Speed ↓ amplitude ↓ complexity ↓	1/5			6/6	2/5
Just discernible general movements					3/5

Growth ↓   Amniotic fluid ↓   Fetal heart rate abnormal   Further clinical deterioration →

Deterioration of clinical condition

Figure 8.2 Relationship between the quality of general movements and indices of fetal clinical condition in 17 growth-retarded fetuses. All fetuses entered the study at a certain point on the horizontal axis indicating the fetal clinical condition, and were followed longitudinally upon deterioration (indicated by the horizontal arrow from left to right). The quality of general movements is indicated on the vertical axis. The boxes show how many fetuses out of a total number of examined fetuses showed a certain quality of general movements, given a particular clinical condition. Adapted from Sival DA, Visser GHA, Prechtl HFR. (1992a) The effect of intra-uterine growth retardation on the quality of general movements in the human fetus. *Early Hum Dev* 28: 119–132, with permission.

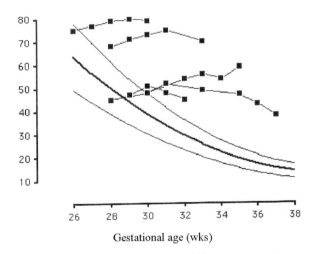

Percentage of non-coincidence

Gestational age (wks)

Figure 8.3 Individual values of percentage of non-coincidence in five intrauterine growth-retarded fetuses (– ■ –) who were diagnosed in early pregnancy by means of Doppler ultrasonography and later developed abnormal (late decelerations) heart-rate tracings within 48 hours from the last recording. Reference values are shown as mean ±2 standard deviations. From Romanini C, Rizzo G. (1995) Fetal behaviour in normal and compromised fetuses. An overview. *Early Hum Dev* 43: 117–131, with permission.

2002). A rapid decrease in heart-rate variation and reversed end-diastolic velocities indicate a poor outcome (Ribbert et al 1993).

Correlating with the degree of peripheral vascular resistance – and hence with the diastolic peak flow – the appearance of behavioural states is delayed (van Vliet et al 1985b, Rizzo et al 1987, Shinozuka et al 1989, Prechtl 1992, Gazzolo et al 1994, Romanini and Rizzo 1995). Consequently, transitions between coincidences are longer and the sequence of change of state variables is disorganised (Arduini et al 1989, Nijhuis et al 1999). The incidence of periods of non-coincidence is significantly elevated, relative to the reference limits for gestation (Figure 8.3).

Responsiveness to acoustic or vibroacoustic stimulation is also diminished (Trudinger and Boylan 1980, Ianniruberto and Tajani 1981, Vindla et al 1999b).

REFERENCES

Abrams LA, Balducci J. (1996) Fetal seizures: a case study. *Obstet Gynecol* 88: 661–663.
Ajayi RA, Keen CE, Knott PD. (1995) Ultrasound diagnosis of the Pena Shokeir phenotype at 14 weeks of pregnancy. *Prenat Diagn* 15: 762–764.
Amiel-Tison C, Gosselin J, Kurjak A. (2006) Neurosonography in the second half of fetal life: a neonatologist's point of view. *J Perinat Med* 34: 437–446.
Andonotopo W, Kurjak A, Ivancic Kosuta M. (2005) Behavior of an anencephalic fetus studied by 4D sonography. *J Matern Fetal Neonat Med* 17: 165–168.
Arduini D, Rizzo G, Caforio L, Mancuso S. (1987) Development of behavioural states in hydrocephalic fetuses. *Fetal Ther* 2: 135–143.
Arduini D, Rizzo G, Caforio L, Boccolini MR, Romanini C, Mancuso S. (1989) Behavioural state transitions in healthy and growth retarded fetuses. *Early Hum Dev* 19: 155–165.
Auerbach AD, Sagi M, Adler B. (1985) Fanconi anemia: prenatal diagnosis in 30 fetuses at risk. *Pediatr* 76: 794–800.
Awoust J, Lewi S. (1984) New aspects of fetal dynamics with a special emphasis on eye movements. *Ultrasound Med Biol* 10: 107–116.
Baarsma R, Bekedam DJ, Visser GHA. (1993) Qualitative abnormal fetal breathing movements, associated with tracheal atresia. *Early Hum Dev* 32: 63–69.
Bacino CA, Platt LD, Garber A, Carlson D, Pepkowitz S, Lachman RS, Sharony R, Rimoin DL, Graham JM Jr. (1993) Fetal akinesia/hypokinesia sequence: prenatal diagnosis and intra-familial variability. *Prenat Diagn* 13: 1001–1019.
Badr El-Din MK. (1960) A familial convulsive disorder with an unusual onset during intrauterine life: a case report. *J Pediatr* 56: 655–657.
Bejšovec M, Kulenda Z, Ponča E. (1967) Familial intrauterine convulsions in pyridoxine dependency. *Arch Dis Child* 42: 201–207.
Bekedam DJ, Visser GHA, de Vries JIP, Prechtl HFR. (1985) Motor behaviour of the growth retarded fetus. *Early Hum Dev* 12: 155–165.
Bekedam DJ, Visser GHA, Mulder EJH, Poelmann-Weesjes G. (1987) Heart rate variation and movement incidence in growth-retarded fetuses: the significance of antenatal late heart rate decelerations. *Am J Obstet Gynecol* 157: 126–133.
Bekedam DJ, Mulder EJH, Snijders RJM, Visser GHA. (1991) The effects of maternal hypoxia on fetal breathing movements, body movements and heart rate variation in growth retarded fetuses. *Early Hum Dev* 27: 223–232.
Belich AI, Konstantinova NN, Natsvlishvili VV, Pavlova NG, Popova NI. (1996) Morphophysiological analysis of the formation of mechanisms of the activity–rest cycle in human ontogensis. *Vestn Ross Akad Med Nauk* 3: 55–61.

Bigi N, Faure JM, Coubes C, Puechberty J, Lefort G, Sarda P, Blanchet P. (2008) Prader-Willi syndrome: is there a recognizable fetal phenotype? *Prenat Diagn* 28: 796–799.

Birnholz JC, Stephens JC, Faria M. (1978) Fetal movement patterns: a possible means of defining neurological developmental milestones in utero. *Am J Roentgenol* 130: 537–540.

Blair E, Stanley F. (1990) Intrauterine growth and spastic cerebral palsy. I. Association with birth weight for gestational age. *Am J Obstet Gynecol* 162: 229–237.

Bots RSGM, Broeders GHB, Farman DJ, Haverkorn MJ, Stolte LAM. (1978) Fetal breathing movements in the growth retarded human fetus: a multiscan M-mode echofetographic study. *Eur J Obstet Gynecol Reprod Biol* 8: 21–29.

Boué J, Vignal P, Aubry JP, Aubry MC, Mac Aleese J. (1982) Ultrasound movement patterns of fetuses with chromosome anomalies. *Prenat Diagn* 2: 61–65.

Bowie JD, Clair MR. (1982) Fetal swallowing and regurgitation: observation of normal and abnormal activity. *Radiology* 144: 877–878.

Chervenak FA, Isaacson G. (1989) Current perspectives on the diagnosis, prognosis and management of fetal spina bifida. In: Hill A, Volpe JJ, editors. *Fetal Neurology.* New York: Raven Press. p 257–264.

Christensen FC, Rayburn WF. (1999) Fetal movement counts. *Obstet Gynecol Clin North Am* 26: 607–621.

Conover WB, Yarwood RL, Peacock MD, Thomas BA. (1986) Antenatal diagnosis of fetal seizure activity with use of real-time ultrasound. *Am J Obstet Gynecol* 155: 846–847.

de Haan J, Stolte LAM. (1971) Drugs and the fetal heart rate. *BMJ* 4(5780): 171.

de Vries JIP. (2008) Ultrasonographic diagnosis of fetal seizures: a case report and review of the literature. *Br J Obstet Gynaecol* 115: 129–130.

de Vries JIP, Fong BF. (2007) Changes in fetal motility as a result of congenital disorders: an overview. *Ultrasound Obstet Gynecol* 29: 590–599.

de Vries JIP, Laurini RN, Visser GHA. (1994) Abnormal motor behaviour and developmental post-mortem findings in a fetus with Fanconi anaemia. *Early Hum Dev* 36: 137–142.

Donker ME, Eijckelhof BHW, Tan GMB, de Vries JIP. (2009) Serial postural and motor assessment of Fetal Akinesia Deformation Sequence (FADS). *Early Hum Dev* 85: 785–790.

Dornan JC, Ritchie JWK, Meban C. (1984a) Fetal breathing movements and lung maturation in the congenitally abnormal human fetus. *J Dev Physiol* 6: 367–374.

Dornan JC, Ritchie JW, Ruff SS. (1984b) The rate and regularity of breathing movements in the normal and growth-retarded fetus. *Br J Obstet Gynaecol* 91: 31–36.

du Plessis AJ, Kaufmann WE, Kupsky WJ. (1993) Intrauterine-onset myoclonic encephalopathy associated with cerebral cortical dysgenesis. *J Child Neurol* 8: 164–170.

Einspieler C, Prechtl HFR. (2005) Prechtl's assessment of general movements: a diagnostic tool for the functional assessment of the young nervous system. *Ment Retard Dev Disabil Res Rev* 11: 61–67.

Einspieler C, Widder J, Holzer A, Kenner T. (1988) The predictive value of behavioural risk factors for sudden infant death. *Early Hum Dev* 18: 101–109.

Einspieler C, Prechtl HFR, Bos AF, Ferrari F, Cioni G. (2004) *Prechtl's Method on the Qualitative Assessment of General Movements in Preterm, Term and Young Infants. Clinics in Developmental Medicine No. 167.* Cambridge: Cambridge University Press.

Ferrari F, Cioni G, Prechtl HFR. (1990) Qualitative changes of general movements in preterm infants with brain lesions. *Early Hum Dev* 23: 193–231.

Fong BF, de Vries JIP. (2003) Obstetric aspects of the Prader-Willi syndrome. *Ultrasound Obstet Gynaecol* 21: 389–392.

Gagnon R. (1995) Developmental aspects of alterations in fetal behavioural states. In: Lecanuet JP, Fifer WP, Krasnegor NA, Smotherman WP, editors. *Fetal Development. A Psychobiological Perspective.* Hillsdale, Hove: Lawrence Erlbaum Associates. p 129–148.

Gávai M , Hargitai B , Váradi V , Belics Z , Csapó Z , Hajdú J , Hauzman E , Berkes E , Papp Z . (2008) Prenatally diagnosed fetal brain injuries with known antenatal etiologies. *Fetal Diagn Ther* 23: 18–22.

Gazzolo D, Scopesi FA, Bruschettini PL, Marasini M, Esposito V, Di Renzo GC, De Toni E. (1994) Predictors of perinatal outcome in intrauterine growth retardation: a long term study. *J Perinat Med* 22: 71–77.

Ghi T, Pilu G, Savelli L, Segata M, Bovicelli L. (2003) Sonographic diagnosis of congenital anomalies during the first trimester. *Placenta* 24: S84-S87.

Gingras JL, O'Donell KJ. (1998) State control in the substance-exposed fetus. I. The fetal neurobehavioural profile: an assessment of fetal state, arousal, and regulation competency. *Ann N Y Acad Sci* 846: 262–276.

Gospe SM Jr, Hecht ST. (1998) Longitudinal MRI findings in pyridoxine-dependent seizures. *Neurology* 51: 74–78.

Hadi HA, Finley J, Mallette JQ, Strickland D. (1994) Prenatal diagnosis of cerebellar hemorrhage: medicolegal implications. *Am J Obstet Gynecol* 170: 1392–1395.

Hageman ATM, Gabreels FJM, Liem KD, Renkawek K, Boon JM. (1993) Congenital myotonic dystrophy – a report on 13 cases and a review of the literature. *J Neurol Sci* 115: 95–101.

Hall JG. (1986) Analysis of Pena-Shokeir phenotype. *Am J Med Genet* 25: 99–117.

Heazell AE, Frøen JF. (2008) Methods of fetal movement counting and the detection of fetal compromise. *J Obstet Gynaecol* 28: 147–154.

Hepper PG, Shahidullah S. (1992a) Trisomy 18: behavioural and structural abnormalities. A ultrasonographic case study. *Ultrasound Obstet Gynecol* 2: 48–50.

Hepper PG, Shahidullah S. (1992b) Habituation in normal and Down's syndrome fetuses. *Q J Exp Psychol B* 44: 305–317.

Hill A. (1989) Assessment of the fetus: relevance to brain injury. *Clin Perinatol* 16: 413–434.

Hill LM, Breckle R, Wolfgram KR. (1983) An ultrasonic view of the developing fetus. *Obstet Gynecol Surv* 38: 375–398.

Hiroi H, Kozuma S, Hayashi N, Unno N, Fujii T, Tsutsumi O, Okai T, Taketani Y. (2000) A fetus with Prader-Willi syndrome showing normal diurnal rhythm and abnormal ultradian rhythm on heart rate monitoring. *Fetal Diagn Ther* 15: 304–307.

Hoffmann R, Lohner M, Bohm N, Leititis J, Helwig H. (1993) Restrictive dermopathy – a letal congenital skin disorder. *Eur J Pediatr* 152: 95–98.

Horimoto N, Koyanagi T, Maeda H, Satoh S, Takashima T, Minami T, Nakano H. (1993) Can brain impairment be detected by in utero behavioural patterns? *Arch Dis Child* 69: 3–8.

Hsu CD, Feng TI, Crawford TO, Johnson TRB. (1993) Unusual fetal movement in congenital myotonic dystrophy. *Fetal Diagn Ther* 8: 200–202.

Hunziker UA, Savoldelli G, Boltshauser E, Giedion A, Schinzel A. (1989) Prenatal diagnosis of Schwartz-Jampel syndrome with early manifestation. *Prenat Diagn* 9: 127–131.

Ianniruberto A, Tajani E. (1981) Ultrasonographic study of fetal movements. *Semin Perinatol* 5: 175–181.

Ingemarsson I, Spencer JA. (1998) Fetal seizure activity associated with lethal cerebral damage at birth: two cases. *Acta Obstet Gynecol Scand* 77: 127–129.

Isler W. (1964) [Fetal epileptic seizures. Case Report]. *Helv Paediatr Acta* 19: 318–325. (In German)

James SJ. (1998) Fetal brain death syndrome. A case report and literature review. *Aust N Z J Obstet Gynaecol* 38: 217–220.

Jung E, Lee BY, Huh CY. (2008) Prenatal diagnosis of fetal seizure: a case report. *J Korean Med Sci* 23: 906–908.

Kainer F, Prechtl HFR, Dudenhausen JW, Unger M. (1996) Qualitative analysis of fetal movement patterns in the Neu–Laxova syndrome. *Prenat Diagn* 16: 667–669.

Kainer F, Prechtl HFR, Engele H, Einspieler C. (1997) Assessment of the quality of general movements in fetuses and infants of women with type-1 diabetes mellitus. *Early Hum Dev* 50: 13–25.

Kirkinen P, Herva R, Leisti J. (1987) Early prenatal diagnosis of a lethal syndrome of multiple congenital contractures. *Prenat Diagn* 7: 189–196.

Kirkinen P, Ryynänen M, Haring P, Torkkeli H, Pääkkönen L, Martikainen A. (1994) Prenatal activity of a fetus with early onset, severe spinal muscular atrophy. *Prenat Diagn* 14: 1074–1076.

Kisilevsky BS, Low JA. (1998) Human fetal behaviour: 100 years of study. *Dev Rev* 18: 1–29.

Kloosterman GJ. (1973) On intra-uterine growth. *Int J Gynecol Obstet* 8: 895–921.

Kobayashi O, Hayashi Y, Arahata K, Ozawa E, Nonaka I. (1996) Congenital muscular dystrophy: clinical and pathological study of 50 patients with the classical (Occidental) merosin-positive form. *Neurology* 46: 815–818.

Koenen SV, Franx A, Mulder EJH, Bruinse HW, Visser GHA. (2002) Fetal and maternal cardiovascular diurnal rhythms in pregnancies complicated by pre-eclampsia and intrauterine growth restriction. *J Matern Fetal Neonatal Med* 11: 313–320.

Korenromp MJ, van Gool JD, Bruinese HW, Kriek R. (1986) Early fetal leg movements in myelomeningocele. *Lancet* 1(8486): 917–918.

Kosasa TS, Ebesugawa I, Nakayama RT, Hale RW. (1993) Massive fetomaternal hemorrhage preceded by decreased fetal movement and a nonreactive fetal heart pattern. *Obstet Gynecol* 82: 711–714.

Koyanagi T, Horimoto N, Maeda H, Kukita J, Minami T, Ueda K, Nakano H. (1993) Abnormal behavioural patterns in the human fetus at term: correlation with lesion sites in the central nervous system after birth. *J Child Neurol* 8: 19–26.

Kurauchi O, Ohno Y, Mizutani S, Tomoda Y. (1995a) Longitudinal monitoring of fetal behaviour in twins when one is anencephalic. *Obstet Gynecol* 86: 672–674.

Kurauchi O, Ishida T, Ohno Y, Ando H, Nomura S, Mizutani S, Tomoda Y. (1995b) Serial fetal heart rate monitoring in monozygotic twin, one of which was anencephalic. *Arch Gynecol Obstet* 256: 53–56.

Kurauchi O, Ohno Y, Furugori K, Kuno N, Morikawa S, Itakura A, Mizutani S, Tomoda Y. (1996) Comparative study of fetal behaviour in a case of monozygotic twins, one being anencephalic. *Gynecol Obstet Invest* 42: 209–210.

Kurjak A, Miskovic B, Stanojevic M, Amiel-Tison C, Ahmed B, Azumendi G, Vasilj O, Andonotopo W, Turudic T, Salihagic-Kadic A. (2008) New scoring system for fetal neurobehaviour assessed by three- and four-dimensional sonography. *J Perinat Med* 36: 73–81.

Landy HJ, Khoury AN, Heyl PS. (1989) Antenatal ultrasonographic diagnosis of fetal seizure activity. *Am J Obstet Gynecol* 161: 308.

Leader LR, Baille P, Martin B, Vermeulen E. (1982) Fetal habituation in high-risk pregnancies. *Br J Obstet Gynaecol* 89: 441–446.

Lou HC. (1982) *Developmental Neurology*. New York: Raven Press.

Lunshof S, Boer K, van Hoffen G, Wolf H, Mirmiran M. (1997) The diurnal rhythm in fetal heart rate in a twin pregnancy with discordant anencephaly: comparison with three normal twin pregnancies. *Early Hum Dev* 48: 47–57.

Mahendru A, Gajjar K, Bashir T. (2007) Idiopathic chronic fetomaternal haemorrhage presenting with reduced fetal movements. *J Obstet Gynaecol* 27: 848–849.

Manning FA, Platt LD, Sipos L. (1980) Antepartum fetal evaluation: development of fetal biophysical profile. *Am J Obstet Gynecol* 136: 787–793.

Maršál K. (1983) Ultrasonic assessment of fetal activity. Clin Obstet Gynaecol 10: 541–563.

Mathews DD. (1973) Fetal movements and fetal wellbeing. *Lancet* 7815: 1315.

Mitra AG, Salvino AR, Spence JE. (1999) Prenatal diagnosis of fatal infantile olivopontocerebellar hypoplasia syndrome. *Prenat Diagn* 19: 375–378.

Moessinger AC. (1983) Fetal akinesia deformation sequence: an animal model. *Pediatr* 72: 857–863.

Morokuma S, Fukushima K, Yumoto Y, Uchimura M, Fujiwara A, Matsumoto M, Satoh S, Nakano H. (2007) Simplified ultrasound screening for fetal brain function based on behavioural pattern. *Early Hum Dev* 83: 177–181.

Mulder EJ, Nikkels PG, Visser GHA. (2001a) Fetal akinesia deformation sequence: behavioral development in a case of congenital myopathy. *Ultrasound Obstet Gynecol* 18: 253–257.

Mulder EJ, Beemer FA, Stoutenbeek P. (2001b) Restrictive dermopathy and fetal behaviour. *Prenatal Diagn* 21: 581–585.

Muro M, Shono H, Ito Y, Sugimori H. (1998) Diurnal variation in baseline heart rate of anencephalic fetuses. *Psychiatry Clin Neurosci* 52: 173–174.

Nijhuis IJM, ten Hof J, Nijhuis JG, Mulder EJH, Narayan H, Taylor D, Visser GHA. (1999) Temporal organization of fetal behaviour from 24-weeks gestation onwards in normal and complicated pregnancies. *Dev Psychobiol* 34: 257–268.

Nijhuis IJM, ten Hof J, Mulder EJ, Nijhuis JG, Narayan H, Taylor DJ, Visser GHA. (2000) Fetal heart rate in relation to its variation in normal and growth retarded fetuses. *Eur J Obstet Gynecol Reprod Biol* 89: 27–33.

Olesen AG, Svare JA. (2004) Decreased fetal movements: background, assessment, and clinical management. *Acta Obstet Gynecol Scand* 83: 818–826.

Osiovich H, Barrington K. (1996) Prenatal ultrasound diagnosis of seizures. *Am J Perinatol* 13: 499–501.

Paladini D, Tartaglione A, Agangi A, Foglia S, Martinelli P, Nappi C. (2001) Pena-Shokeir phenotype with variable onset in three consecutive pregnancies. *Ultrasound Obstet Gynecol* 17: 163–165.

Paluda SM, Comstock CH, Kirk JS, Lee W, Smith RS. (1996) The significance of ultrasonographically diagnosed fetal wrist position anomalies. *Am J Obstet Gynecol* 174: 1834–1839.

Park M, Kim DS. (1989) The acoustic stimulation test in the anencephalus: preliminary results. *J Perinat Med* 17: 329–331.

Patane L, Ghidini A. (2001) Fetal seizures: case report and literature review. *J Matern Fetal Med* 10: 287–289.

Patrick J, Carmichael L, Chess L, Staples C. (1984) Accelerations of the human fetal heart rate at 38–40 weeks' gestational age. *Am J Obstet Gynecol* 148: 35–41.

Pearn JH. (1973) Fetal movements and Werdnig-Hoffmann Disease. *J Neurol Sci* 18: 373–379.

Peleg D, Goldman JA. (1978) Fetal deglutition: a study of the anencephalic fetus. *Eur J Obstet Gynecol Reprod Biol* 8: 133–136.

Pena SDJ, Shokeir MHK. (1974) Syndrome of camptodactyly, multiple ankyloses, facial anomalies and pulmonary hypoplasia: a lethal condition. *J Pediatr* 85: 373–375.

Petrikovsky BM, Kaplan GP. (1995) Fetal responses to inadvertent contact with the needle during amniocentesis. *Fetal Diagn Ther* 10: 83–85.

Pillai M, James D. (1990a) The importance of the behavioural state in biophysical assessment of the term human fetus. *Br J Obstet Gynaecol* 97: 1130–1134.

Pillai M, James D. (1990b) Development of human fetal behaviour: a review. *Fetal Diagn Ther* 5: 15–32.

Pillai M, James D. (1992) Absence of fetal breathing and abnormal fetal behaviour in prolonged preterm ruptured membranes: case report. *Ultrasound Obstet Gynecol* 2: 44–47.

Pillai M, Garrett C, James D. (1991) Bizarre fetal behaviour associated with lethal congenital anomalies: a case report. *Eur J Obstet Gynecol Reprod Biol* 39: 215–218.

Prayer D, Brugger PC. (2007) Investigation of normal organ development with fetal MRI. *Eur Radiol* 17: 2458–2471.

Prechtl HFR. (1985) Ultrasound studies of human fetal behaviour. *Early Hum Dev* 12: 91–98.

Prechtl HFR. (1989) Fetal behaviour. In: Hill A, Volpe JJ, editors. *Fetal Neurology*. New York: Raven Press. p 1–16.

Prechtl HFR. (1990) Qualitative changes of spontaneous movements in fetus and preterm infants are a marker of neurological dysfunction. *Early Hum Dev* 23: 151–159.

Prechtl HFR. (1992) The organization of behavioral states and their dysfunction. *Semin Perinatol* 16: 258–263.

Prechtl HFR. (1997a) State of the art of a new functional assessment of the young nervous system. An early predictor of cerebral palsy. *Early Hum Dev* 50: 1–11.

Prechtl HFR. (1997b) The importance of fetal movements. In: Connolly KJ, Forssberg H, editors. *Neurophysiology and Psychology of Motor Development. Clinics in Developmental Medicine No. 143/144.* Cambridge: Cambridge University Press. p 42–53.

Prechtl HFR, Einspieler C. (1997) Is neurological assessment of the fetus possible? *Eur J Obstet Gynecol Reprod Biol* 75: 81–84.

Prechtl HFR, Einspieler C, Cioni G, Bos AF, Ferrari F, Sontheimer D. (1997) An early marker for neurological deficits after perinatal brain lesions. *Lancet* 349: 1361–1363.

Preyer W. (1885) [*Special Physiology of the Embryo*]. Leipzig: Grieben. (In German)

Pritchard JA. (1965) Deglutition by normal and anencephalic fetuses. *Obstet Gynecol* 25: 289–297.

Rayburn WF. (1995) Fetal movement monitoring. *Clin Obstet Gynecol* 38: 59–67.

Rayburn WF, Barr M. (1982) Activity patterns in malformed fetuses. *Am J Obstet Gynecol* 142: 1045–1048.

Rayburn WF, Rayburn PR, Gabel LL. (1983) Excess fetal activity: another worrisome sign? *South Med J* 76: 163–165.

Reinold E. (1971) [Observations of fetal activity during the first half of pegnancy by means ultrasonography]. *Pädiat Pädol* 6: 274–279. (In German)

Reinold E. (1973) Clinical value of fetal spontaneous movements in early pregnancy. *J Perinat Med* 1: 65–69.

Rezaie P, Dean A. (2002) Periventricular leukomalacia, inflammation and white matter lesions within the developing nervous system. *Neuropathol* 22: 106–132.

Ribbert LSM, Visser GHA, Mulder EJH, Zonneveld MF, Morssink LP. (1993) Changes with time in fetal heart rate variation, movement incidences and haemodynamics in intrauterine growth retarded fetuses: a longitudinal approach to the assessment of fetal wellbeing. *Early Hum Dev* 31: 195–208.

Rizzo G, Arduini D, Pennestri F, Romanini C, Mancuso S. (1987) Fetal behaviour in growth retardation: its relationship to fetal blood flow. *Prenatal Diagn* 7: 229–238.

Rochard F, Schifrin BS, Goupil F, Legrand H, Blottiere J, Sureau C. (1976) Nonstressed fetal heart rate monitoring in the antepartum period. *Am J Obstet Gynecol* 126: 699–706.

Romanini C, Rizzo G. (1995) Fetal behaviour in normal and compromised fetuses. An overview. *Early Hum Dev* 43: 117–131.

Romero NB, Monnier N, Viollet L, Cortey A, Chevallay M, Leroy JP, Lunardi J, Fardeau M. (2003) Dominant and recessive central core disease associated with RYR1 mutations and fetal akinesia. *Brain* 126: 2341–2349.

Rosier-van Dunné FM, van Wezel-Meijler G, Odendaal HJ, van Geijn HP, de Vries JIP. (2007) Changes in echogenicity in the fetal brain: a prevalence study in fetuses at risk for preterm delivery. *Ultrasound Obstet Gynecol* 29: 644–650.

Rosier-van Dunné FMF, van Wezel-Meijler G, Bakker MPS, Odendaal HJ, de Vries JIP. (2010) Fetal general movements and brain sonography in a population at risk for preterm birth. *Early Hum Dev* 86: 107–111.

Sadovsky E, Polishuk WZ. (1977) Fetal movements in utero. Nature, assessment, prognostic value, timing of delivery. *Obstet Gynecol* 50: 49–55.

Schats R, Jansen CAM, Wladimiroff JW. (1990) Abnormal fetal heart rate pattern in early Rosierpregnancy associated with Down's syndrome. *Hum Reprod* 5: 877–879.

Scher MS. (2003) Fetal neurologic consultations. *Pediatr Neurol* 29: 193–202.

Scher MS, Belfar H, Martin J, Painter MJ. (1991) Destructive brain lesion of presumed fetal onset: antepartum causes of cerebral palsy. *Pediatr* 88: 898–906.

Schwartz O, Jampel RS. (1962) Congenital blepharophimosis associated with a unique generalized myopathy. *Arch Ophthalmol* 68: 52–57.

Senocak EU, Oguz KK, Haliloglu G, Karcaaltincaba D, Akata D, Kandemir O. (2009) Prenatal diagnosis of Pena-Shokeir syndrome phenotype by ultrasonography and MR imaging. *Pediatr Radiology* 39: 377–380.

Sepulveda W, Stagiannis KD, Cox PM, Wigglesworth JS, Fisk NM. (1995) Prenatal findings in generalized amyoplasia. *Prenat Diagn* 15: 660–664.

Shahidullah S, Hepper PG. (1992) Abnormal fetal behaviour in first trimester spontaneous abortion. *Eur J Obstet Gynecol Reprod Biol* 45: 181–184.

Sherer DM, Anyaegbunam A, Onyeije C. (1998) Antepartum fetal intracranial hemorrhage, predisposing factors and prenatal sonography: a review. *Am J Perinatol* 15: 431–441.

Shimizu T, Nagai T, Nishimura R, Amano H, Ihara Y, Yomura W, Shimizu S. (1991) Does fetal seizure activity mean a poor outcome? A case report. *J Reprod Med* 36: 453–454.

Shinozuka N, Masuda H, Okai T, Kuwabara Y, Mizuno M. (1989) Computer-assisted analysis of fetal behaviour in fetal abnormalities. *Fetal Ther* 4: 97–109.

Sival DA. (1993) Studies on fetal motor behaviour in normal and complicated pregnancies. *Early Hum Dev* 34: 13–20.

Sival DA, Visser GHA, Prechtl HFR. (1992a) The effect of intra-uterine growth retardation on the quality of general movements in the human fetus. *Early Hum Dev* 28: 119–132.

Sival DA, Visser GHA, Prechtl HFR. (1992b) The relationship between the quantity and quality of prenatal movements in pregnancies complicated by intrauterine growth retardation and premature rupture of membranes. *Early Hum Dev* 30: 193–209.

Sival DA, Begeer JH, Staal-Schreinemachers AL, Vos-Niel JM, Beekhuis JR, Prechtl HFR. (1997) Perinatal motor behaviour and neurological outcome in spina bifida aperta. *Early Hum Dev* 50: 27–37.

Sival DA, van Weerden TW, Vles JH, Timmer A, den Dunnen WFA, Staal-Schreinemachers AL, Hoving EW, Sollie KM, Kranen-Mastenbroek VJ, Sauer PJ, Brouwer OF. (2004) Neonatal loss of motor function in human spina bifida aperta. *Pediatr* 114: 427–434.

Sival DA, Brouwer OF, Bruggink JLM, Vles JSH, Staal-Schreinemachers AL, Sollie KM, Sauer PJ, Bos AF. (2006) Movement analysis in neonates with spina bifida aperta. *Early Hum Dev* 82: 227–234.

Sival DA, Verbeek RJ, Brouwer OF, Sollie KM, Bos AF, den Dunnen WFA. (2008) Spinal hemorrhages are associated with early neonatal motor function loss in human spina bifida aperta. *Early Hum Dev* 84: 423–431.

Skupski DW, Sepulveda W, Udom-Rice I, Leo MV, Lescale KB, Chervenak FA. (1996) Fetal seizures: further observations. *Obstet Gynecol* 88: 663–665.

Steinfeld JD, Ludmir J, Eife S, Robbins D, Samuels P. (1992) Prenatal detection and management of quadruple nuchal cord. A case report. *J Reprod Med* 37: 989–991.

Stoll C, Ehretmentre MC, Treisser A, Tranchant C. (1991) Prenatal diagnosis of congenital myasthenia with arthrogryposis in a myasthenic mother. *Prenat Diagn* 11: 17–22.

Swartjes JM, van Geijn HP, Meinardi H, van Woerden EE, Mantel R. (1992) Fetal motility and chronic exposure to antiepileptic drugs. *Eur J Obstet Gynecol Reprod Biol* 16: 37–45.

Terao T, Kawashima Y, Noto H, Inamoto Y, Lin TY, Sumimoto K, Maeda M. (1984) Neurological control of fetal heart rate in 20 cases of anencephalic fetuses. *Am J Obstet Gynecol* 149: 201–208.

Tongsong T, Chanprapaph P, Khunamornpong S. (2000) Prenatal ultrasound of regional akinesia with Pena-Shokier phenotype. *Prenat Diagn* 20: 422–425.

Trudinger BJ, Boylan P. (1980) Antepartum fetal heart rate monitoring: Value of sound stimulation. *Obstet Gynecol* 55: 265–268.

Trudinger BJ, Lewis PJ, Petit B. (1979) Fetal breathing patterns in intrauterine growth retardation. *Br J Obstet Gynaecol* 86: 432–436.

Tyson RW, Ringel SP, Manchester DK, Shikes RH, Goodman SI. (1992) X-linked myotubular myopathy – a case report of prenatal and perinatal aspects. *Pediatr Pathol* 12: 535–543.

Usta IM, Adra AM, Nassar AH. (2007) Ultrasonographic diagnosis of fetal seizures: a case report and review of the literature. *Br J Obstet Gynaecol* 114: 1031–1033.

Vajsar J, Schachter H. (2006) Walker-Warburg syndrome. *Orphanet J Rare Dis* 3: 29.

van Gelder-Hasker MR, van Wezel-Meijler G, van Geijn HP, de Vries JIP. (2001) Ultrasonography of the peri- and intraventricular areas of the fetal brain between 26 and 36 weeks' gestational age; a comparison with neonatal ultrasound. *Ultrasound Obstet Gynecol* 17: 34–41.

van Heteren CF, Boekkooi PF, Jongsma HW, Nijhuis JG. (2000) Responses to vibroacoustic stimulation in a fetus with an encephalocele compared to responses of normal fetuses. *J Perinat Med* 28: 306–308.

van Vliet MAT, Martin CB Jr, Nijhuis JG, Prechtl HFR. (1985a) Behavioural states in growth retarded human fetuses. *Early Hum Dev* 12: 183–197.

van Vliet MAT, Martin CB Jr, Nijhuis JG, Prechtl HFR. (1985b) The relationship between fetal activity, and behavioral states and fetal breathing movements in normal and growth retarded fetuses. *Am J Obstet Gynecol* 153: 582–588.

Vasta I, Kinali M, Messina S, Guzzetta A, Kapellou O, Manzur A, Cowan F, Muntoni F, Mercuri E. (2005) Can clinical signs identify newborns with neuromuscular disorders? *J Pediatr* 146: 73–79.

Velazquez M, Rayburn W. (2002) Antenatal evaluation of the fetus using fetal movement monitoring. *Clin Obset Gynecol* 45: 993–1004.

Verbeek RJ, van der Hoeven JH, Sollie KM, Maurits NM, Bos AF, den Dunnen WF, Brouwer OF, Sival DA. (2009) Muscle ultrasound density in human fetuses with spina bifida aperta. *Early Hum Dev* 85: 519–523.

Vindla S, Sahota DS, Coppens M, James DK. (1997a) Computerized analysis of behaviour in fetuses with congenital abnormalities. *Ultrasound Obstet Gynecol* 9: 302–309.

Vindla S, James DK, Sahota DS, Coppens M. (1997b) Computerised analysis of behaviour in normal and growth retarded fetuses. *Eur J Obstet Gynecol Reprod Biol* 75: 169–175.

Vindla S, James DK, Sahota DS. (1999a) Comparison of unstimulated and stimulated behaviour in human fetuses with congenital abnormalities. *Fetal Diagn Ther* 14: 156–165.

Vindla S, James D, Sahota D. (1999b) Computerised analysis of unstimulated and stimulated behaviour in fetuses with intrauterine growth restriction. *Eur J Obstet Gynecol Reprod Biol* 83: 37–45.

Visser GHA, Prechtl HFR. (1988) Movements and behavioural states in the human fetus. In: Jones CT, editor. *Fetal and Neonatal Development*. Ithaca, New York: Perinatology Press.

Visser GHA, Laurini RN, de Vries JIP, Bekedam DJ, Prechtl HFR. (1985) Abnormal motor behaviour in anencephalic fetuses. *Early Hum Dev* 12: 173–182.

Visser GHA, Bekedam Dj, Ribbert LSM. (1990) Changes in antepartum heart rate patterns with progressive deterioration of the fetal condition. *Int J Biomed Comp* 25: 239–246.

Volpe JJ. (2001) *Neurology of the Newborn*, 4th edition. Philadelphia, PA: WB Saunders.

Warsof SL, Abramowicz JS, Sayegh SK, Levy DL. (1988) Lower limb movements and urologic function in fetuses with neural tube and other central nervous system defects. *Fetal Ther* 3: 129–134.

Whitehead J. (1867) Convulsions in utero. *BMJ* 2: 59–61.

Wladimiroff JW, Tonge HM, Steward PA. (1986) Doppler ultrasound assessment of cerebral blood flow in the human fetus. *Br J Obstet Gynaecol* 93: 471–475.

Wladimiroff JW, van den Wijngaard JAGW, Degani S, Noordam MI, van Eyck J, Tonge HM. (1987) Cerebral and umbilical arterial blood flow velocity waveforms in normal and growth retarded pregnancies. *Obstet Gynecol* 69: 705–709.

Yfantis H, Nonaka D, Castellani R, Harman C, Sun CC. (2002) Heterogeneity in fetal akinesia deformation sequence (FADS): autopsy confirmation in three 20–21 week fetuses. *Prenat Diagn* 22: 42–47.

Yoon BH, Park CW, Chaiworapongsa T. (2003) Intrauterine infection and the development of cerebral palsy. *Br J Obstet Gynaecol* 110 (Suppl 20): 124–127.

Yoshizato T, Koyanagi T, Takashima T, Satoh S, Akazawa K, Nakano H. (1994) The relationship between age-related heart rate changes and developing brain function: a model of anencephalic human fetuses in utero. *Early Hum Dev* 36: 101–112.

EPILOGUE

During the last 30 or 40 years, ultrasonography and, more recently, magnetic resonance imaging, have gradually revealed what had hitherto been concealed from our eyes. We thus have a better idea of the complex and surprisingly coordinated motor patterns of fetuses. By visualising the onset of human behaviour, we have come to realise that these early movements are not merely reflexes but are in fact spontaneously generated, and that there is a close relationship between the generation of motor activity and the development of structure.

This book aims to contribute to a standardised description of fetal behavioural patterns, since observers throughout the world still display a great methodological variety in their individual assessments. In a way, fetal movements continue to be diagnosed from an 'adult' perspective, in that the fetus's behaviour is regarded as intentional. But just because a fetus exhibits movements that are similar to those of adults, this does not mean that these movements are directly comparable to adult behaviour.

Apart from the fundamental question of when, how, and why human behaviour evolves, the majority of studies on fetal behaviour deal with the issue of responsiveness. One of their shortcomings is that, in many cases, only heart rate alterations are focused on as a sign of fetal reaction to sensory (usually vibroacoustic) stimulation. Another insufficiency is that study designs often do not take into account just how closely fetal responses are linked to the current behavioural state of the fetus. In fact, the continuous change of states influences not only fetal haemodynamics and metabolism, but also – and most significantly – fetal motility and heart rate. We have frequently pointed out that, although a silent fetal heart rate pattern can indeed indicate fetal stress, it may also signify that the fetus is in quiet sleep, i.e. in behavioural state 1F.

A dysfunction of behavioural states can be caused by a number of fetal and maternal maldevelopments, such as fetal growth retardation, hydrocephaly or various congenital abnormalities, as well as by maternal intake of caffeine, alcohol or corticosteroids. It is therefore extremely difficult to interpret alterations of fetal activity or heart rate in fetuses with disorganised behavioural states.

According to its proponents, one of the rationales for testing fetal responsiveness is the prospect that such a procedure might provide a more comprehensive insight into the neural performance, as it embraces both the sensory and the motor domains. However, apart from the fact that observers tend to disregard the state dependency of fetal responsiveness (which may even result in inappropriate patient management), there are a number of neurological conditions, such as porencephaly, corpus callosum agenesis, trisomy 21 or early fetal akinesia deformation sequence, in which fetal responsiveness appears normal, especially if only the heart rate response is measured. Even a fetus with multiple congenital anomalies may react properly to vibroacoustic stimulation. In other words, to focus on fetal responsiveness alone is to be misled by the assumption that normal behaviour reflects neural integrity – particularly if 'behaviour' is assessed in the reductionist approach of strictly recording the heart rate.

A number of studies – especially those on preterm infants – have shown that the quality of spontaneous activity changes if the nervous system is impaired. The complex general movements have proven most suitable for a functional assessment of the nervous system at this early stage. Some 10 years ago, we were rather optimistic that this assessment method – well established in preterm, full-term and young infants – would also make its breakthrough in fetal neurology. Today, we have to concede that we are nowhere near that objective. First of all, there are only a handful of obstetricians trained in the assessment of fetal general movements. It may only take a few minutes during bouts of fetal activity to decode the complex picture of normal or abnormal general movements, yet the observer needs a lot of experience in the Gestalt perception of general movements. Secondly, there are hardly any longitudinal studies on the predictive value of abnormal fetal general movements, especially in fetuses with acquired brain lesions. We know, for instance, that the general movements are grossly impaired in many growth-retarded fetuses, but we still do not know if and how the quality of fetal movements predicts the further development. The same holds true for fetuses with periventricular white matter damage or germinal matrix haemorrhage. Interdisciplinary longitudinal studies are urgently needed in order to assess whether fetal general movements and their degree of abnormality reflect, for example, the degree of white matter injuries. Only such studies can provide clarity, if neurological assessment of the fetuses is possible at all.

LIST OF VIDEOS

1. First movements at 7.5 weeks' gestation
2. Startle at 10 weeks' gestation
3. Startles at 16.5 weeks' gestation
4. General movements in a preterm infant at 29 weeks' postmenstrual age
5. General movements at 10 weeks' gestation
6. General movements at 14 weeks' gestation
7. General movements at 27 weeks' gestation
8. Isolated arm movements at 14 weeks' gestation
9. Pointing index finger at 27 weeks' gestation
10. Hand-to-face contact (thumb approaching mouth) at 14 weeks' gestation
11. Isolated leg movements including a clonus at 19 weeks' gestation
12. Alternating leg movements (the so-called "newborn stepping") in an infant at term
13. Hiccup at 14 weeks' gestation
14. Breathing movements at 12 weeks' gestation
15. Irregular and regular breathing movements at 14 weeks' gestation
16. Side-to-side movements of the head at 36 weeks' gestation
17. Rooting in a newborn infant
18. Anteflexion of the head at 14 weeks' gestation
19. Conjugate eye movements at 30 weeks' gestation
20. Opening and closing of the eyelids at 36 weeks' gestation
21. Fetal stretch at 14 weeks' gestation
22. Yawn at 14 weeks' gestation
23. Sucking and swallowing at 14 weeks' gestation
24. Neonatal sucking
25. General movements in twins at 22 weeks' gestation
26. Vomiting due to brainstem hypoplasia at 23.5 weeks' gestation videos

Acknowledgements

The transvaginal (videos 1, 2, and 5) and abdominal (videos 6, 8, 10, 11, 13-16, 18, 20-23) ultrasound recordings were made by Heinz Prechtl, JIP (Hanneke) de Vries, and Gerard Visser. The dynamic MRI sequences (videos 3, 7, 9, 19, 25 and 26) were provided by Daniela Prayer. Movie 4 is from the CD that accompanies Prechtl's Method on the Qualitative Assessment of General Movements in Preterm, Term and Young Infants by

190

Einspieler C, Prechtl HFR, Bos AF, Ferrari F and Cioni G (Clinics in Developmental Medicine No. 167, London: Mac Keith Press, 2004). Videos 12, 17, 24 were taken from the film on the Development of the Newborn Infant by Heinz Prechtl, Institute for Scientific Films, Göttingen 1952 (with permission).

INDEX

acoustic stimulation 96–8
    habituation and 110
    see also auditory system; noise; sound;
    vibroacoustic stimulation
activity/rest cycles 53
    anencephaly 162–6
    see also movements
actocardiotocography 9
acupuncture 130
afferent control, postnatal change of endogenously
    generated motility to 56–7
Ahlfeld, Johann F 1, 35
akinesia deformation sequence 20, 173–5, 189
alcohol 133, 135
amniocentesis 80, 105, 167
amniotic fluid 49–50
    chemical compounds and their sensation 107
    swallowing 48, 49, 50
    volume
        abnormalities 127–9
        regulation 49, 49–50
amyoplasia 173
anencephaly 161, 162–6
anteflexion of head 39
    postnatal 55
antiepileptic drugs 143–4, 161
antigravity movements 56
antihypertensive drugs 143
anxiety, maternal 130–1
arm
    movements 28
        anencephaly 163
    posture, age-related 52
    see also limb movements

Arnold–Chiari malformation 168
auditory system 92–9
    development 92
    see also acoustic stimulation; noise; sound;
    vibroacoustic stimulation
axodendritic synapses 21, 27

B-mode linear scanners 4–5
behaviour, our (book's) definition xi
benzodiazepines, maternal 137
betamethasone 85, 138
biophysical profile 159
Birnholz JC 5
blinking 45–6
blood gases and fetal movements 38
blood pressure (maternal), high (hypertension)
    141–3
body movements 24
    in behavioural states
        recording 73, 74
        state 1F 75
        state 2F 77
    first 20–1
    maternal glucose intake and 139
    see also specific parts
bone conduction, sound 93
brain
    death 177
    hemispheric dominance 69
    lesions 177
    malformations 162–8, 176–7
Braxton Hicks contractions 36, 75, 125
breathing (respiratory) movements 34–8
    akinesia deformation sequence and 173

anencephaly and 163–5
in behavioural states 73
  state 1F 77
  state 2F 77, 78
growth-retarded fetus 178
historical studies 35
maternal factors affecting
  fasting 36, 139
  glucose intake 37, 139
  type 1 diabetes 139–40
oligohydramnios and 127
breech position 125–7
  arm posture 52
  head in 70, 126

caffeine and coffee 134
callosal agenesis 167
carbon dioxide levels (maternal) affecting
  movements 37
carbon monoxide (from smoking) 133
  and haemoglobin (carboxyhaemoglobin) 133,
  134
cardiotocography in behavioural state recording 74
  see also actocardiotocography
central pattern generators 18
  sucking 48–9
cephalic fetuses 70, 125–6
  arm posture 52
chemosensation 105–8
Christmas, overeating at 139
cigarette smoking in pregnancy 133–4
classical conditioning 110–11
cocaine 133, 135–6
coffee and caffeine 134
Coghill GE 3
coincidence (of state variables) 81
  growth-retarded fetus 179
conditioning, classical 110–11
congenital malformations see structural
  malformations
corpus callosum agenesis 167
corticospinal tract 27

corticosteroids 85, 138
cri-du-chat syndrome 169
crying, fetal homologue 80
cutaneous... see skin
cystic brain lesions 177

da Vinci, Leonardo 1, 50
depression, maternal 132–3
dermopathy, restrictive 161, 175
developmental malformations see structural
  malformations
dexamethasone 85, 138
diabetes, maternal 139-40, 161–2
diaphragmatic movements 30
diet see nutrition and diet
diurnal variations in activities 53
  heart rate 53
  anencephaly 166
dopamine and yawning 48
Doppler actocardiotocography 9
Down syndrome (trisomy 21) 161, 171
drugs (maternal)
  abuse 133–7
  therapeutic 137–8, 143–4
dynamic MRI 10–11

ear, sound reaching see sound
eating, maternal see mother
Edwards syndrome (trisomy 18) 170–1
EEG 9
elbow flexion 52
electroencephalogram 9
embryonic motility
  evidence 17–18
  functions of 19–20
emotions, maternal 130
epileptic seizures see seizures
epiphenomenal concept of embryonic/fetal
  movements 19
exercise (physical), mother's 129–30
expressions, facial 43
extension

legs, postnatal 55
    spinal 26–7
exteriorised (miscarried) fetuses, studies 3–4
exteroception see sensory stimuli
eye development and light sensation 108–9
eye movements 43–6
    in behavioural states
        recording 73, 74
        state 1F 75
        state 2F 75, 77
        state 3F 75, 79
        state 4F 75, 79

face
    expressions 43
    touching with hand 28–9
Fanconi anaemia 161, 171–2
Fels Research Institute study 2–3
    maternal stress 132
    pre-eclampsia 141
    vibroacoustic stimulation 99
female and male fetuses, behavioural comparisons
    124–5
finger movements 28, 52
flexion
    arm/wrist/fingers 52
    neck/head 21, 39, 47
        postnatal 55
focal akinesia 174–5
food intake, maternal see mother
four-dimensional ultrasonography 6
    in Zagreb neurological scoring system 159
functional hypothesis of embryonic/fetal
    movements 19
functional MRI 11
    light stimulation 109

gastrointestinal abnormalities 169
gastroschisis 169
genetic disorders 169–73
genitourinary function 50–1
gestational age

breathing movements and 36
definition xii
first movements and 21
    reported by mother 5
heart rate from 32-42 weeks 78
parity and behavioural state appearance
related to 82
posture and 51
    arm 52
glucocorticoids 138–9
glucose, maternal
    blood levels and fetal consumption 141
    intake 37, 139
    see also hyperglycaemia; hypoglycaemia
glycaemic load 139
gravity, movements against 55
Greeks, ancient 1
Groningen fetal ultrasound studies 6–7
growth, intrauterine
    retardation effects 161, 177–8
        behavioural states 85
    ultrasound effects 8
gustation (taste sensation) 105–8

habituation 110
    maternal smoking and 134
haemodynamic changes
    invasive procedures causing 105
    in state 2F 78, 84
haemoglobin and carbon monoxide (from
    smoking) 133, 134
hand
    movements 28
    touching face 28–9
handedness 69, 70
head
    movements 38–45, 46
        postnatal 55
        sideward 22, 38–9, 126
    position
        in breech position 70, 126
        lateralisation 70, 126

presentation see cephalic fetuses
    see also microcephaly
health assessment and behavioural states 84–5
hearing see acoustic stimulation; auditory system;
    sound; vibroacoustic stimulation
heart
    motion/beating, start of 20–1
    abnormalities 169
heart rate
    acceleration, determination 158
    akinesia deformation sequence 174
    anencephaly 166
    in behavioural states
        recording 73, 74, 75, 76
        silent heart rate pattern 84
        state 1F 73, 75, 84
        state 2F 74, 77–8
        state 3F 74, 79
        state 4F 74, 79
    diurnal variations see diurnal variations
    gestational age (32-42 weeks) and 78
    growth-retarded fetus 178–80
    historical studies 3, 9
    maternal physical activity and 129–30
    twins, synchronicity 121–2
hemispheric dominance 69
hereditary (genetic) disorders 169–73
hiccups 33–4
    anencephaly 163
historical studies 1–11
    breathing movements 2, 35
    reflexes 3, 17, 28, 29
    ultrasound 4–9
holoprosencephaly 167–8
Hooker, Davenport 3
hunger and swallowing 49
hydrocephalus 168
hyperglycaemia 141
hyperoxia (maternal) affecting movements 38
hypertension (high blood pressure), maternal
    141–3
hypocapnia (maternal) affecting movements 37

hypoglycaemia, insulin-induced 141
hypoxia (maternal) affecting movements 38

inactivity see rest
index finger pointing 29
infections, viral 144
inherited (genetic) disorders 169–73
insulin-induced hypoglycaemia 141
invasive procedures, responses 105

jaw movements 40

Kyushu University (Japan) neurological
    assessment system 160

labour
    breathing movements in 36
    uterine contractions 76, 125
laryngeal movements 49
laterality 69–71
    head position 70, 126
learning, prenatal 109
left vs right handedness 69, 70
leg movements 28, 30
    alternating 30
    anencephaly 163
    postnatal 55
    see also limb movements
Leonardo da Vinci 1, 50
light stimuli 108–9
limb movements 28–30
    akinesia deformation sequence 174
    anencephaly 163
    brain death 177
    focal akinesia 174, 175
    Neu–Laxova syndrome 175
    startles 23–4
    see also arm; leg
lingual movements see tongue movements
lissencephaly 168
lungs
    development and breathing movements 35–6
    hypoplasia 127

magnetic resonance imaging (MRI) 10–11
functional see functional MRI
magnetocardiography 10
magnetoencephalography 10
male and female fetuses, behavioural comparisons 124–5
maternal... see mother
Mayor F 20–1
medications, maternal 137–8, 143–4
memory (remembering) 109–10
neonatal, of prenatal experiences 98
methadone 134, 137
microcephaly 167
micturition (urination; voiding) 50, 78, 84
inhibition in 1F 77, 84
miscarried (exteriorised) fetuses, studies 3–4
Moebius syndrome 168
monosomy 5p 169
monozygotic twins 120, 121–2
mother
blood gases affecting movements 37
diabetes 138–41, 161
drugs see drugs
eating/food/diet 108, 139–40
amniotic food odour and 107
movements affected by 37
epilepsy 143–4
hypertension (high blood pressure) 141–3
physical exercise 129–30
poisoning 137
psychological status 130–3
reporting of movements, vs ultrasound recording 5–6
viral infections 144
voice, as stimulant from prenatal to postnatal life 96–7
motor behaviour see movements
mouthing, rhythmical/regular 40
state 1F 77
movements/motions/activity (motor behaviour), spontaneous 17–56
amniotic fluid volume abnormalities and 127

endogenous generation
evidence for 17–19
postnatal change to afferent (sensory) control 55
Fels study see Fels Research Institute study
first 20–3
functions of 19–20
generalised 22–8
assessing quality of 160–2
historical perspectives 3, 4, 5–6, 10–11
maternal factors affecting
diabetes type 1 139–41
fasting 139
glucose intake 37, 139–141
stress 131–2
substance abuse 134, 135, 136–7
therapeutic drugs 137–8, 143–4
viral infections 144
maternal reports, vs ultrasound 5–6
in neurological assessment (incl. neurological disorders) 159–62
akinesia deformation sequence 173–5
genetic disorders 169–73
growth-retarded fetus 178
structural malformations 162–9
sudden changes in quantity 175–6
pathological suppression 38
qualitatively abnormal 38
quantitative aspects 52–3
sensory stimuli evoking 91
specific 28–52
ultrasound effects on 8–9
see also activity/rest cycles; body movements and specific parts
multiple fetuses (incl. twins) 120–2
sensation and contact between 101–2, 120–1
muscle relaxants see neuromuscular blocking agents
muscular atrophy, spinal 172–3
music 97–8
myelomeningocele 166, 167
myopathies 173–4

myotonic dystrophy 161, 173
myotubular myopathy, X-linked 173

nasal chemoreceptors 105, 106, 107
neck flexion see flexion
neonate see postnatal life
nervous system 158–80
    disorders of (and their assessment) 158–80,
    188–9
        habituation testing 110
    minimal neural structures for generating well-
    organised movements 27–8
    pain sensation and 103
    yawning and the 48
    see also brain
nervus terminalis 106
Neu–Laxova syndrome 175
neural tube defects 166–7
neurobehavioural profile 159
neuroendocrine responses to invasive procedures
    105
neurological disorders see nervous system
neuromuscular blocking agents (muscle relaxants)
    experimental studies 19–20
    maternal 137
neurones
    migration, ultrasound effects 8
    nociception and pain perception and 103
neurotransmitters and yawning 48
newborns see postnatal life
nicotine chewing gum 134
nociception 103
noise
    external 94
        intense, adverse effects 98–9
        in magnetic resonance imaging 10
    habituation to 110
    intrauterine 94
non-stress test 158
nutrition and diet
    fetal, chronic deprivation 177–8
    maternal see mother

nystagmoid eye movements 44

ocular development and movements see eye
odour (smell) sensation 106–8
oesophageal atresia 169
olfaction (smell sensation) 106–8
oligohydramnios 127, 161
oral chemoreceptors 105–6
overeating at Christmas 139
oxygen levels (maternal) affecting movements 37

pain sensation 102–5
Pajot, Charles 1
parents, ultrasound examination and its effects on
    8–9
Pena–Shokeir syndrome 161
penile tumescence 51, 78
pharmaceuticals, maternal 137–8, 143–4
physical exercise, mother's 129–30
physiological conditions affecting breathing
    movements 36–7
poisoning, maternal 137
polyhydramnios 127–8
porencephaly 167–8
position 51–2
    changes in 51
        growth-retarded fetus 178
        movements causing 20
    head, lateralisation 70, 126
postnatal life (incl. neonate)
    behavioural states 72–3, 83
    breech position and 126–7
    continuity from prenatal to
        of mother's voice (as salient stimulus)
        96–7
        of motor patterns 54–6
    memory of prenatal experiences 98
    odour preferences 107–8
    sex differences in behaviour 124
posture 51–2
    deformities 52
    growth-retarded fetus 178

Prader–Willi syndrome 161, 170
Prechtl's assessment of quality of movement 162
pre-eclampsia 3, 38, 141
pregnant mother see mother
premature rupture of the membranes, prolonged 127
preparatory hypothesis of embryonic/fetal movements 19
Preyer, William T 2, 17, 55, 162
prolonged premature rupture of the membranes 127
proprioception 102
psychological status, maternal 130–3
pulmonary... see lungs
pulsatility index 78

quickening 5
quiescence see rest

rapid eye movements (REMs) 43, 44, 77
reactions to sensory stimuli see sensory stimuli
real-time ultrasound, advent 4–5
reflexes 17, 19, 21
    historical studies 3, 28, 29
    postnatal, breech position and 126
Reinold, Emil 4
relaxation, maternal 130
respiration see breathing movements
responsiveness see sensory stimuli
rest (inactivity; quiescence) 81
    cycles of activity and see activity/rest cycles
restrictive dermopathy 161, 175
retroflexion of head 39, 47
rhythmical mouthing see mouthing
rhythmical sounds (environmental) 97–8
right vs left handedness 69, 70
rooting 55–6
Rösslin, Eucharius 1
rotations 24, 27

Schwartz–Jampel syndrome 172
sedatives, maternal 137

seizures (epileptic)
    fetal 176–7
    maternal 143
sensory (afferent) control, postnatal change of endogenously generated motility to 56
sensory stimuli, responses to 91–112, 188
    anencephaly 166
    substance abuse and 134
    twins fetuses 101–2, 120–1
sex differences 124–5
side-to-side head movements 38–39, 56, 126
skin
    restrictive dermopathy 161, 175
    tactile sensation see touch
sleep states 75, 77–8
smell sensation (olfaction) 106–8
smiling, endogenous, superseded by social smiling 56
Smith–Lemli–Opitz syndrome 171
smoking in pregnancy 133–4
sonography see ultrasound
Soranus of Ephesus 1
sound reaching fetal ear 92–3
    discrimination 95–6
    pressure levels 95
    see also acoustic stimulation; noise; vibroacoustic stimulation
spina bifida aperta 166–7
spinal cord, nociception and pain perception and 103
spinal extension 26–7
spinal muscular atrophy 172–3
startles 22–3
    anencephaly 163
    maternal type 1 diabetes and 139
state(s) (behavioural), fetal 72–85
    1F 73, 74, 75, 82
        heart rate 73, 74, 84
        transition to 2F from 81–2
        voiding inhibition 77, 85
    2F 73, 74, 75, 82
        haemodynamic changes 78, 84–5

transition from 1F to 81–2
3F 73, 74, 75
4F 73, 74, 75
5F 73
in biophysical profiling 159
developmental course 81–3
dysfunctions 85–6
recording 73–5
substance abuse and 134
state(s) (behavioural), neonatal 72–3, 83
state concomitants 72
1F 77
2F 78
stepping movements 30
steroid therapy, prenatal 138–9
Strassmann P 2
stress
physical (fetus), maternal exercise causing 129–30
psychological (maternal) 130–3
stretching 46
postnatal 55
structural (congenital) malformations 162–9
brain 162–8, 176–7
subplate (developing nervous system) 27
substance abuse, maternal 133–7
sucking 48–9, 79
postnatal 55–6
swallowing 48, 49, 50
acoustic stimulation and 96
anencephaly 166
synapses, axodendritic 21, 27

tactile sensation see touch
taste sensation 105–8
temperature sensation 102
terminal nerve (nervus terminalis) 106
three-dimensional ultrasonography 6–7
in Zagreb neurological scoring system 159
tobacco smoking in pregnancy 133–4
tongue (lingual) movements 40–3
swallowing and 49

touch
face with hand 28–9
sensation of 100–2
twin fetuses 101–2, 120–1
tracheal atresia 169
transitions between behavioural states 81–2
transvaginal ultrasound, first body movements 21
trigeminal system 106
trisomy 1q 169
trisomy 4p 169
trisomy 5p 170
trisomy 8 170
trisomy 13 170
trisomy 18 170–1
trisomy 21 161, 171
twins see multiple fetuses

ultrasound (sonography) 4–9
in behavioural state recording 74
effects on parents and fetus 8–9
eye movements 43
first body movements 21
historical studies 4–9, 45
in Zagreb neurological scoring system 159
umbilical cord
grasping 31
sucking 49
urine production see micturition
urogenital function 50–1
uterine contractions 125
Braxton Hicks contractions 36, 75, 125
in labour 75, 125

vagitus uterinus 80
vasoconstriction with smoking 133
vernix caseosa 49
vibroacoustic stimulation 30, 45, 50, 80, 84, 99–100, 125, 159, 167
in focal akinesia 175
habituation and 110
harmful effects 99–100
in hypertensive mothers 142

in neurobehavioural profile 159
see also auditory system; noise; sound
viral infections 144
visual stimuli 108–9
vocalisation
fetal, in state 5F 73, 80
maternal, as stimulant from prenatal to
postnatal life 96–7
voiding see micturition
vomeronasal system 106

wakefulness 79, 82, 130

Walker–Warburg syndrome 173
well-being, historical assessment 1–2
Werdnig–Hoffmann disease 172–3
Whitehead, James 2
withdrawal reflex and breech position 126

Yanase J 2
yawning 39, 46, 47–8
postnatal 55
state 1F 77

Zagreb scoring system 159

Other titles from Mac Keith Press www.mackeith.co.uk

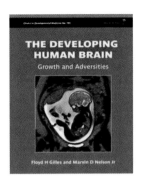

The Developing Human Brain
Floyd H Gilles and Marvin D. Nelson Jr

Clinics in Developmental Medicine No. 193
2012 ▪ 424pp ▪ hardback ▪ 978-1-908316-41-7
£110.00 / €132.00 / $170.00

This book treats the embryonic and fetal brain as an exciting way to explore growth and aberrations of the most complicated structure in the human body, focusing on the second half of gestation and the neonatal period. It is a unique resource, with its emphasis on quantitative methods and more than 200 pathologic and radiologic images.

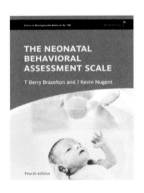

The Neonatal Behavioral Assessment Scale, 4th edition
T. Berry Brazelton and J. Kevin Nugent

Clinics in Developmental Medicine No. 190
2011▪ 184pp ▪ hardback ▪ 978-1-907655-03-6
£50.00 / €60.00 / $63.95

The Neonatal Behavioral Assessment Scale (NBAS) is the most comprehensive examination of newborn behaviour available today and has been used in clinical and research settings around the world for more than 35 years. The scale assesses the newborn's behavioral repertoire with 28 behavioral items and also includes an assessment of the infant's neurological status on 20 items.

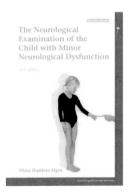

The Neurological Examination of the Child with Minor Neurological Dysfunction, 3rd edition
Mijna Hadders-Algra

A practical guide from Mac Keith Press
2010▪ 148pp ▪ softback ▪ 978-1-898683-98-8
£49.95/ €60.00 / $72.00

Bert Touwen's classic handbook has been updated to reflect contemporary clinical practice. This refined, sensitive and age-appropriate technique is designed to take into account the developmental aspects of the child's rapidly changing nervous system. The accompanying DVD contains videos illustrating typical and atypical performance and also provides an electronic assessment form.

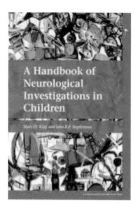

A Handbook of Neurological Investigations in Children
Mary D. King and John B. P. Stephenson

A practical guide from Mac Keith Press
2009 ▪ 400pp ▪ softback ▪ 978-1-898683-69-8
£41.95 / €50.40 / $73.95

This book sets out the investigations that are really needed to establish
the cause of neurological disorders. Its problem-oriented approach starts
with the patient's presentation, not the diagnosis, with more than 60
case vignettes to illustrate clinical scenarios.

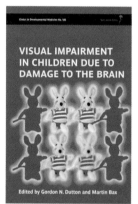

Visual Impairment in Children due to Damage to the Brain
Gordon N Dutton and Martin Bax (Eds)

Clinics in Developmental Medicine No. 186
2010 ▪ 352pp ▪ hardback ▪ 978-1-898683-86-5
£83.95 / €100.00 / $142.00

This book sets out novel concepts which will be of great practical value
to those who care for children with visual impairment due to brain
injury. Summaries of the more specialist chapters as well as clear
diagrams and a glossary enhance the book's accessibility to a broader
readership.

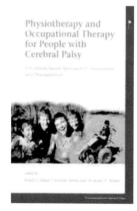

Physiotherapy and Occupational Therapy for People with Cerebral Palsy
Karen J. Dodd, Christine Imms, Nicholas F. Taylor (Eds)

A practical guide from Mac Keith Press
2010 ▪ 320pp ▪ softback ▪ 978-1-898683-68-1
£29.95/ €36.00 / $41.99

This clinically relevant resource has been written by therapists for
therapists. It takes an innovative problem-based approach to assessment
and management, using real-life situations to demonstrate the practical
use of the approaches described.

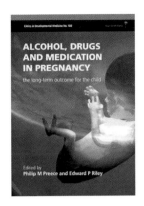

Alcohol, Drugs and Medication in Pregnancy: The Long-Term Outcome for the Child
Philip M. Preece and Edward P. Riley (Eds)

Clinics in Developmental Medicine No. 188
2011 ▪ 290pp ▪ hardback ▪ 978-1-898683-88-9
£68.50 / €82.20 /$99.95

This book documents the consequences of the exposure of infants to the influence of intrauterine chemicals. In setting out the evidence for these outcomes, the authors demonstrate that decisions about care and management can and should be made as early as possible. This should allow professionals to provide protective management and prevent the delays that are so often seen in this area of medical and social care.

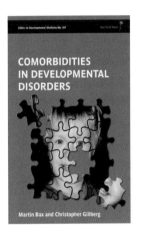

Comorbidities in Developmental Disorders
Martin Bax and Christopher Gillberg (Eds)

Clinics in Developmental Medicine No. 187
2010 ▪ 156pp ▪ softback ▪ 978-1-907655-00-5
£63.50 / €76.20 /$100.95

In the last decade the term 'comorbidity' has gained popularity in the field of paediatric neurodisability, with the increasing recognition that many conditions are rarely present in isolation. Within this field, the term is often used to refer to the co-occurrence of conditions more frequently than would be expected by chance. Whether it is valid to use the term 'comorbidity' in all these situations, and how precisely it should be used, is something that the contributors to this book grapple with in their own fields of interest.

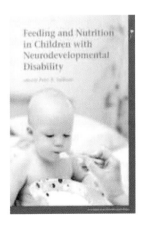

Feeding and Nutrition in Children with Neurodevelopmental Disability
Peter B. Sullivan (Ed)

A practical guide from Mac Keith Press
2009 ▪ 196pp ▪ softback ▪ 978-1-898683-60-5
£20.00 / €25.20/ $43.00

This highly practical guide is for all those who have responsibility for the nutritional and gastrointestinal care of children with neurodisability, providing an up-to-date account of the practicalities of assessment and management of feeding problems in these children.

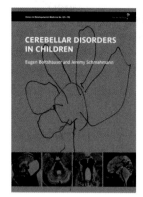

Cerebellar Disorders in Children
Eugen Boltshauser and Jeremy Schmahmann (Eds)

Clinics in Developmental Medicine No. 191-192
2012 ▪ 456pp ▪ hardback ▪ 978-1-907655-01-2
£125.00 / €147.00 / $200.00

This clinically orientated text by an international group of experts is the first definitive reference book on disorders of the cerebellum in children. It presents a wealth of practical clinical experience backed up by a strong scientific basis for the information and guidance given. This is followed by sections on clinical conditions grouped according to common characteristics such as aetiology and symptomatology.

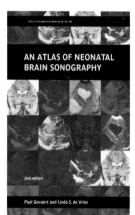

An Atlas of Neonatal Brain Sonography, 2nd edition
Paul Govaert and Linda S de Vries

Clinics in Developmental Medicine No. 182-183
2010 ▪ 400pp ▪ hardback ▪ 978-1-898683-56-8
£158.00/ €189.60 / $253.00

This Atlas covers the entire spectrum of brain disease as studied with ultrasound, illustrated throughout with superb-quality images. It is aimed at neonatologists and radiologists confronted with everyday clinical questions on the neonatal ward. This second edition of the Atlas has been brought up to date to include the many advances in technique and interpretation that have been made in the past decade. The images have been replaced with new ones of higher quality, and all the line artwork has been standardised and improved.

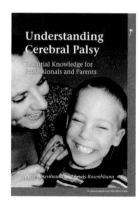

Understanding Cerebral Palsy: Essential Knowledge for Professionals and Parents
Peter Rosenbaum and Lewis Rosenbloom

A practical guide from Mac Keith Press
July 2012 ▪ 176pp ▪ softback ▪ 978-1-908316-50-9
£29.95 / €36.10 / $41.99

The book has been designed to provide readers with an understanding of cerebral palsy (CP) as a developmental as well as a neurological condition. It details the nature of CP, its causes and its clinical manifestations. Using clear, accessible language (supported by an extensive glossary) the authors have blended current science with metaphor both to explain the biomedical underpinnings of CP.

International Review Series of Child Neurology

Published for the International Child Neurology Association by Mac Keith Press www.mackeith.co.uk

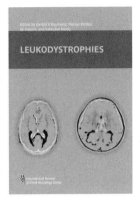

Leukodystrophies

Gerald Raymond, Florian Eichler, Ali Fatemi, and Sakkubai Naidu (Eds)

2011 ▪ 240pp ▪ hardback ▪ 978-1-907655-09-8
£80.00 / €96.00 / $125.50

This book is the only up-to-date, comprehensive text on leukodystrophies. Its purpose is to summarize for the reader all aspects of the inherited disorders of myelin in children and adults. After a wide-ranging overview of myelin and the role of oligodendrocytes, astrocytes and microglia in white matter disease, chapters are then devoted to individual disorders, covering their biochemical and molecular basis, genetics, pathophysiology, clinical features, diagnosis, treatment and screening.

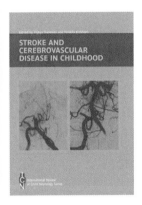

Stroke and Cerebrovascular Disease in Childhood

Vijeya Ganesan and Fenella Kirkham (Eds)

2011 ▪ 412pp ▪ hardback ▪ 978-1-898683-34-6
£145.00 / €174.00 / $199.95

This book for the first time summarizes the state of the art in this field. A team of eminent clinicians, neurologists and researchers provide an up-to-the-minute account of all aspects of stroke and cerebrovascular disease in children, ranging from a historical perspective to future directions, through epidemiology, the latest neuroimaging techniques, neurodevelopment, comorbidities, diagnosis and treatment. The authors' practical approach to the clinical problems makes this essential reading for practising clinicians and researchers in the field.

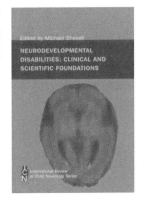

Neurodevelopmental Disabilities: Clinical and Scientific Foundations

Michael Shevell (Ed)

2009 ▪ 492pp ▪ softback ▪ 978-1-898683-67-4
£80.00 / €96.00 / $125.50

This book takes a comprehensive approach to addressing the challenges of neurodevelopmental disabilities in child health, with a special focus on global developmental delay and developmental language impairment. It presents the scientific basis of these disorders and their underlying causes. Issues related to medical management, rehabilitation, and eventual outcomes are also addressed in detail.

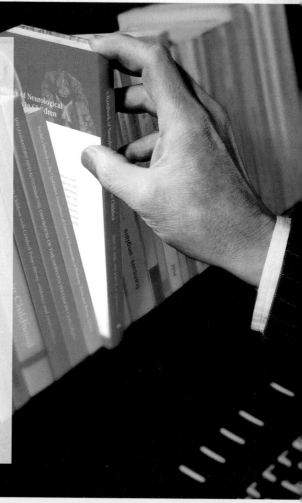
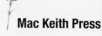

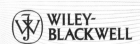